STEM CELLS - LABORATORY AND CLINICAL RESEARCH

PLURIPOTENT STEM CELLS

STEM CELLS - LABORATORY AND CLINICAL RESEARCH

Focus on Stem Cell Research
Erik V. Greer (Editor)
2004. ISBN: 1-59454-043-8

Trends in Stem Cell Research
Erik V. Greer (Editor)
2005. ISBN: 1-59454-315-1

New Developments in Stem Cell Research
Erik V. Greer (Editor)
2006. ISBN: 1-59454-847-1

Neural Stem Cell Research
Erik V. Greer (Editor)
2006. ISBN: 1-59454-846-3

Stem Cell Therapy
Erik V. Greer (Editor)
2006. ISBN: 1-59454-848-X

Embryonic Stem Cell Research
Erik V. Greer (Editor)
2006. ISBN: 1-59454-849-8

Frontiers in Stem Cell Research
Julia M. Spanning (Editor)
2006. ISBN: 1-60021-294-8

Stem Cells and Cancer
Devon W. Parsons (Editor)
2007. ISBN: 1-60021-517-3

Hematopoietic Stem Cell Transplantation Research Advances
Karl B. Neumann (Editor)
2008. ISBN: 978-1-60456-042-8

Stem Cell Applications in Diseases
Mikkel L. Sorensen (Editor)
2008. ISBN: 978-1-60456-241-5
2008. ISBN: 978-1-60876-925-4 (E-book)

Leading-Edge Stem Cell Research
Prasad S. Koka (Editor)
2008. ISBN: 978-1-60456-268-2

Stem Cell Research Progress
Prasad S. Koka (Editor)
2008. ISBN: 978-1-60456-308-5
2008. ISBN: 978-1-60876-924-7 (E-book)

Progress in Stem Cell Applications
Allen V. Faraday and Jonathon T. Dyer (Editors)
2008. ISBN: 978-1-60456-316-0

Developments in Stem Cell Research
Prasad S. Koka (Editor)
2008. ISBN: 978-1-60456-341-2
2008. ISBN: 978-1-60741-213-7 (E-book)

Gut Stem Cells: Multipotent, Clonogenic and the Origin of Gastrointestinal Cancer
Shigeki Bamba and William R. Otto
2008. ISBN: 978-1-60456-968-1

Stem Cell Transplantation, Tissue Engineering and Cancer Applications
Bernard N. Kennedy (Editor)
2008. ISBN: 978-1-60692-107-4

Stem Cells
Philippe Taupin
2009. ISBN: 978-1-60692-214-9
2009. ISBN: ISBN: 978-1-61668-577-5 (E-book)

Stem Cell Plasticity
Suraksha Agrawal, Piyush Tripathi and Sita Naik
2009. ISBN: 978-1-60741-473-5

Neural Stem Cells and Cellular Therapy
Philippe Taupin
2009. ISBN: 978-1-60876-017-6
2009. ISBN: 978-1-61668-660-4 (E-book)

Adult Stem Cells Survival
Anatoly Konoplyannikov, Sergey Proskuryakov, and Mikhail Konoplyannikov
2010. ISBN: 978-1-61668-035-0

Pluripotent Stem Cells
Derek W. Rosales and Quentin N. Mullen
2010. ISBN: 978-1-60876-738-0

STEM CELLS - LABORATORY AND CLINICAL RESEARCH

PLURIPOTENT STEM CELLS

DEREK W. ROSALES
AND
QUENTIN N. MULLEN
EDITORS

Nova Science Publishers, Inc.
New York

For permission to use material from this book please contact us:
Telephone 631-231-7269; Fax 631-231-8175
Web Site: http://www.novapublishers.com

LIBRARY OF CONGRESS CATALOGING-IN-PUBLICATION DATA

Pluripotent stem cells / editors, Derek W. Rosales and Quentin N. Mullen.
p. ; cm.
Includes bibliographical references and index.
ISBN 978-1-60876-738-0 (hardcover)
1. Stem cells. 2. Cell differentiation. I. Rosales, Derek W. II. Mullen, Quentin N.
[DNLM: 1. Pluripotent Stem Cells. QU 325 P737 2009]
QH588.S83P58 2009
616'.02774--dc22

2009048917

Published by Nova Science Publishers, Inc. ✢ New York

CONTENTS

PREFACE

Pluripotent cells of the early embryo originate all types of somatic cells and germ cells of adult organism. Pluripotent stems cell lines were derived from mammalian embryos and adult tissues using different techniques and from different sources. Despite different origin, all pluripotent stem cell lines demonstrate considerable similarity of the major biological properties. This book examines the fundamental mechanisms which regulate normal development of pluripotent cells into different lineages and are disrupted in cancer initiating cells. Analysis gene expression profiles, differentiation potentials and cell cycle of normal and mutant pluripotent stem cells provide new data to search molecular targets to eliminate malignant cells in tumors. In this book, the authors also aim to present a global picture of how extracellular signals, intracellular signal transduction pathways and transcriptional networks cooperate together to determine the cell fate of pluripotent stem cells. Practical, ethical and legal considerations that must be addressed before induced pluripotent stem (iPS) cells can realize their potential in the treatment of degenerative disease is discussed as well. Recent advancements in the cancer stem cell hypothesis are also summarized and the challenges associated with targeting resistant cancers in the context of stem cell microenvironments are presented.

Pluripotent cells of the early embryo originate all types of somatic cells and germ cells of adult organism. Pluripotent stem cell lines were derived from mammalian embryos and adult tissues using different techniques and from different sources—inner cell mass of the blastocyst, primordial germ cells, parthenogenetic oocytes, and mature spermatogonia — as well as by transgenic modification of various adult somatic cells. Despite different origin, all pluripotent stem cell lines demonstrate considerable similarity of the major biological properties: unlimited self-renewal and differentiation into various somatic and germ cells in vitro and in vivo, similar gene expression profiles, and similar cell cycle structure. Their malignant counterpart embryonal teratocarcinoma stem cell lines have restricted developmental potentials caused by genetic disturbances that result in deregulation of proliferation and differentiation balance. Numerous studies on the stability of different pluripotent stem cell lines demonstrated that, irrespective of their origin, long-term in vitro cultivation leads to the accumulation of chromosomal and gene mutations as well as epigenetic changes that can cause oncogenic transformation of cells. In Chapter 1, the authors' research of signaling pathways and pattern of specific gene expression in pluripotent stem cells and teratocarcinoma cells is focused on discovery of fundamental mechanisms that regulate normal development of pluripotent cells into different lineages and are disrupted in cancer initiating cells. Analysis gene expression profiles, differentiation potentials and cell cycle of normal and mutant pluripotent stem cells provide new data to search molecular targets to eliminate malignant cells in tumors.

The idea of growing human cells *in vitro* to yield a renewable s'ce of cells for transplantation has captured the imagination of scientists for many years. The derivation of human embryonic stem cells (hESC) represented a major milestone in achieving this goal. hESC are pluripotent and can proliferate *in vitro* indefinitely, rendering them an ideal source for cell replacement therapy. Moreover, recent advances in reprogramming somatic cells into induced pluripotent stem cells (iPS cells) have enabled us to unravel some of the key master regulators of stem cell pluripotency. By integrating recent findings of molecular mechanism involved in maintenance of these different pluripotent stem cell types, Chapter 2 aims to present a global picture of how extracellular signals, intracellular signal transduction pathways and transcriptional networks cooperate together to determine the cell fate of pluripotent stem cells. Unraveling the signaling networks that control stem cell pluripotency will be helpful in deriving novel methods to maintain these pluripotent stem cells *in vitro*.

Proviral expression of early development genes Oct4 and Sox2, in concert with cMyc and Klf4 or Nanog and Lin28, can induce differentiated cells to adopt morphological and functional characteristics of pluripotency indistinguishable from embryonic stem cells. Termed induced pluripotent stem (iPS) cells, in mice the pluripotency of these cells was confirmed by altered gene/surface antigen expression, remodeling of the epigenome, ability to contribute to embryonic lineages following blastocyst injection and commitment to all three germ layers in teratomas and liveborn chimeras. Importantly, i*n vitro* directed differentiation of iPS cells yield cells capable of treating mouse models of humanized disease. Despite these impressive results, iPS cell conversion is frustratingly inefficient.

Also, the unpredictable and random mutagenesis imposed on the host cell genome, inherent with integrative viral methodologies, continues to hamper use of these cells in a therapeutic setting. This has initiated exploration of non-integrating strategies for generating iPS cells. In Chapter 3, the authors review mechanisms that drive conversion of somatic cells to iPS cells and the strategies adopted to circumvent integrative viral strategies. Finally, the authors discuss practical, ethical and legal considerations that require addressing before iPS cells can realize their potential as patient-specific cells for treatment of degenerative disease.

Human amniotic fluid has been used in prenatal diagnosis for more than 70 years. It has proven to be a safe, reliable, and simple screening tool for a wide variety of developmental and genetic diseases. However, there is now evidence that amniotic fluid may be used as more than simply a diagnostic tool. It may be the source of a powerful therapy for a multitude of congenital and adult disorders. A subset of cells found in amniotic fluid and placenta has been isolated and found to be capable of maintaining prolonged undifferentiated proliferation as well as able to differentiate into multiple tissue types encompassing the three germ layers. It is possible that in the near future, we will see the development of therapies using progenitor cells isolated from amniotic fland and placenta for the treatment of newborns with congenital malformations, as well as adults with various disorders, using cryopreserved amniotic fluid and placental stem cells. In Chapter 4, the authors describe a number of experiments that have isolated and characterized pluripotent progenitor cells from amniotic fland and placenta. The authors also discuss various cell lines derived from amniotic fluid and placenta and future directions for this area of research.

Research investigations on various sources of stem cells have been conducted for potential to exert tissue regeneration, reverse immune-enhancement, and protect against tissue insult. At a more distant goal, it is likely that stem cells could be applied to medicine via organogenesis. However, the field of stem cells is not new since immune replacement via bone marrow transplantation is considered a successful form of cell therapy. There is evidence that stem cell therapies are close for several disorders such as neurodegeneration, immune hyperactivity, and functional insufficiencies such as Type I diabetes mellitus. The field of stem cell biology is gaining a strong foothold in science and medicine as the molecular mechanisms underlying stem cell behavior are gradually being unraveled. Although stem cells have tremendous therapeutic applicability in the aforementioned conditions, their uniqueness may also confer adverse properties, rendering them a double-edged sword. The discovery that stem cells have immortal and resilient characteristics has shed insight into the link between stem cells and tumorigenesis. Specifically, recent advancements in cancer research have implicated that a stem cell may be responsible for the refractoriness of cancers to conventional treatment such as chemotherapy and radiation. Chapter 5 summarizes the recent advancements in the cancer stem cell hypothesis and presents the challenges associated with targeting resistant cancers in the context of stem cell microenvironments.

Terminal somatic cell differentiation is not irreversible. The same route that transforms embryonic stem cells (ESCs) into specific lineages can be walked backwards, e.g. by means of the "induced pluripotent stem (iPS) cell" technology discovered by Shinya Yamanaka in 2006. The implications of iPS are out of proportion and its ease and reproducibility has made it a favorite option compared to other existing approaches including cell fusion or somatic cell nuclear transfer (SCNT). iPS allows the generation of patient specific embryonic-like stem cells that are devoid of ethical concerns and may be used for transplantation. iPS has also proven useful to create *in vitro* models that mimic human diseases and this could be used for high throughput drug screening. Besides, thanks to iPS we are now compelled to think of differentiation processes in a bidirectional way, which may be as well cell type and transcription factor specific. Therefore, knowledge is flourishing that will benefit Stem Cell Biology as much as unrelated disciplines. But the pace of discovery has been so quick that every technical advance has raised new issues, creating confusion. In Chapter 6 the authors will briefly define and try to answer some key questions that in the authors' opinion will shape iPS research and application in following years.

Holometabolous insects recruit a wide array of stem cell types to fulfil the growth of larval organs at moulting and their remodelling at metamorphosis, thus achieving the final body organization of the adult.

Over the years a large number of different stem cells, with specific roles in growth and renewal of insect tissues, have been identified in Lepidoptera and Diptera. A particular interest for the stem cells residing within the insect gut is now emerging and the early morphological studies that analyzed the behaviour of these cells are progressively supported by new cellular and molecular data.

After a brief summary of the current knowledge on insect intestinal stem cells, Chapter 7 will focus on some characteristics of the stem cells in culture of the larval midgut of *Bombyx mori*. These cells can be released from the midgut just before the fourth moult and, once placed in an appropriate medium, they multiply and differentiate in mature cells that are able to perform normal absorptive and digestive functions *in vitro*.

Thereafter the authors will discuss the use of this reliable *in vitro* system as a tool to study intestinal morphogenesis and differentiation, to investigate the specific roles and reciprocal relationships of autophagy and apoptosis during midgut remodelling, and to analyze physiological functions of midgut cells, such as their ability to internalize different substrates and the mechanisms involved. Studies on midgut stem cells appear of key importance in consideration of the extensive similarities evidenced among mammalian and insect intestinal epithelia in their development, organization and molecular regulatory mechanisms.

As discussed in Chapter 8, it is estimated that as many as 1 in 3 individuals in the United States might benefit from regenerative medicine therapy. Most regenerative medicine therapies have been postulated to require the use of embryonic stem (ES) cells for optimal effect. Unfortunately, ES cell therapies are currently limited by ethical, political, regulatory, and most importantly biological hurdles. These limitations include the inherent allogenicity of this stem cell source and the accompanying threat of immune rejection. Even with use of the rapidly developing iPS technology, the issues of low efficiency of ES/iPS derivation and the threat of teratoma formation limit ES applications directly in patients. The time and cost of deriving and validating mature, differentiated tissues for clinical use further restricts its use to a small number of well-to-do patients with a limited number of afflictions. Thus, for the foreseeable future, the march of regenerative medicine to the clinic for widespread use will depend upon the development of non-ES cell therapies. Current sources of non-ES cells easily available in large numbers can be found in the bone marrow, adipose tissue and umbilical cord blood. Each of these types of stem cells has already begun to be utilized to treat a variety of diseases.

In Chapter 9, using mouse pluripotent teratocarcinoma PCC4aza1 cells and proliferating spleen lymphocytes the authors obtained a new type of hybrids, in which marker lymphocyte genes were suppressed, but expression the *Oct-4* gene was not effected; the hybrid cells were able to differentiate to cardiomyocytes. In order to specify the environmental factors which may affect the genetic stability and other hybrid properties, the authors analyzed the total chromosome number and differentiation potencies of hybrids respectively to conditions of their cultivation. Particular attention was paid to the number and transcription activity of chromosomal nucleolus organizing regions (NORs), which harbor the most actively transcribed– ribosomal – genes. The results showed that the hybrids obtained are characterized by a relatively stable chromosome number which diminished less than in 5% during 27 passages. However, a long-term cultivation of hybrid cells in non-selective conditions resulted in preferential elimination of some NO-chromosomes, whereas the number of active NORs per cell was increased due to activation of latent NORs. On the contrary, in selective conditions, i.e. in the presence of hypoxantine, aminopterin and thymidine, the total number of NOR-bearing chromosomes was not changed, but a partial inactivation of remaining NORs was observed. The higher number of active NORs directly correlated with the capability of hybrid cells for differentiation to cardiomyocytes.

The derivation of human embryonic stem cell lines from blastocyst stage embryos, first achieved almost a decade ago, demonstrated the potential to prepare virtually unlimited numbers of therapeutically beneficial cells *in vitro*. Assuming that large-scale production of differentiated cells is attainable, it is imperative to develop strategies to prevent immune responses towards the grafted cells following transplantation. Chapter 10 presents recent advances in the production of pluripotent cell lines using three emerging techniques: somatic cell nuclear transfer into enucleated oocytes and zygotes, parthenogenetic activation of unfertilized oocytes and induction of pluripotency in somatic cells. These techniques have a remarkable potential for generation of patient-specific pluripotent cells that would be tolerated by the immune system.

As explained in Chapter 11, pluripotent cells of the early preimplantation embryo originate all types of somatic cell and germ cells of the adult organism. Permanent pluripotent cell lines (ES and EG cells) that were derived from an inner cell mass of blastocysts and primordial germ cells have a high proliferative potential and ability to differentiate in vitro into a wide variety of somatic and extraembryonic tissues as well as germ cells and to contribute to different organs of chimeric animals. In some cases pluripotent cells and primordial germ cells can generate teratomas, teratocarsinomas and some kinds of seminomas as the results of damages of differentiation programme of these cells. Experimental teratomas which formed after transplantation of undifferentiated ES and EG cells into immunocompromiced mice may provide a unique opportunity to study pluripotent cell specification and to develop novel approaches in carcinogenesis investigations. Research of signaling and metabolic pathways regulating the pluripotent cell maintenance and their multilineage differentiation are essential to search molecular targets to eliminate undifferentiated cells in tumors. Analysis of interactions between pluripotent cells and differentiated cells of the recipient animals, identification of the factors that may drive differentiation ES and EG cells in vivo contribute in understanding the mechanisms involved in the determination of cell fate during normal development and tumorigenesis. These data are important for development of effective and safe stem cell based technologies for prospective clinical treatment.

In: Pluripotent Stem Cells
Editors: D.W. Rosales et al, pp. 1-45

ISBN: 978-1-60876-738-0

Chapter 1

NORMAL AND PATHOLOGICAL DEVELOPMENT OF PLURIPOTENT STEM CELLS

Olga F. Gordeeva
Institute of Developmental Biology of Russian Academy of Sciences, Moscow, 119334, Russia

Abstract

Pluripotent cells of the early embryo originate all types of somatic cells and germ cells of adult organism. Pluripotent stem cell lines were derived from mammalian embryos and adult tissues using different techniques and from different sources—inner cell mass of the blastocyst, primordial germ cells, parthenogenetic oocytes, and mature spermatogonia — as well as by transgenic modification of various adult somatic cells. Despite different origin, all pluripotent stem cell lines demonstrate considerable similarity of the major biological properties: unlimited self-renewal and differentiation into various somatic and germ cells in vitro and in vivo, similar gene expression profiles, and similar cell cycle structure. Their malignant counterpart embryonal teratocarcinoma stem cell lines have restricted developmental potentials caused by genetic disturbances that result in deregulation of proliferation and differentiation balance. Numerous studies on the stability of different pluripotent stem cell lines demonstrated that, irrespective of their origin, long-term in vitro cultivation leads to the accumulation of chromosomal and gene mutations as well as epigenetic changes that can cause oncogenic transformation of cells. Our research of signaling pathways and pattern of specific gene expression in pluripotent stem cells and teratocarcinoma cells is focused on discovery of fundamental mechanisms that regulate normal development of pluripotent cells into different lineages and are disrupted in cancer initiating cells. Analysis gene expression profiles, differentiation potentials and cell cycle of normal and mutant pluripotent stem cells provide new data to search molecular targets to eliminate malignant cells in tumors.

Introduction

The development of higher multicellular animals starts from a totipotent zygote. The developmental potential of blastomeres of mammalian embryos changes during the period of cleavage and pluripotent cells appear in the inner cell mass of the blastocyst, they continue to proliferate in epiblast and then differentiate into multipotent precursor cells of different somatic lineages which will give rise to terminally differentiated specialized cells. Pluripotent cells appear for a short period of mammalian embryonic development—from cleavage to pre-gastrulation stages. This cell type underlies the development of all somatic cell types including extraembryonic structures and germline cells. Pluripotent embryonic cells transferred to in vitro conditions maintain their features and self-renew as undifferentiated cells during long-term culture. Pluripotent stem cell lines were derived from early embryos and they were experimentally converted from adult somatic cells. Today there exist different approaches and methods of pluripotent stem cell line derivation. The traditional ways are isolation of pluripotent cells from preimplantation embryos and conversion of embryonic and adult germ line cells (embryonic germ cells, EGCs, spermatogonial stem cells and partenogenetic and androgenetic embryonic stem cells, PG and AG ESC) into pluripotent cells. Another approach is an experimental alteration of differentiated cell potential using different reprogramming procedures, that is: somatic nuclear transfer to enucleated oocyte, fusion of pluripotent and somatic cells and pluripotency induction by retroviral transduction of pluripotency-related genes into somatic cells or without transgen integration using piggyBack transposon and episomal delivery (Figure 1).

Despite different origin, all pluripotent stem cell lines demonstrate considerable similarity of the major biological properties: high self-renewal rate and differentiation into various somatic and germ cells in vitro and in vivo, and therefore the nature of pluripotent stem cells make them an ideal source of cell-based products for regenerative medicine. Each pluripotent stem cell line can give rise to multiple somatic cell types that can be used for cell therapy for different diseases treatment and injured tissue recovery. Development of technologies that create an individual patient –specific pluripotent stem cell lines (cloning ES cells and iPS cells) can resolve the histocompatibility problem for transplanted cell derivatives. Establishment of standard model system for research of pluripotent stem cell lines of different origin maintained in strictly defined conditions is very important for development of effective and safe cell-based technologies as well as for drug discoveries.

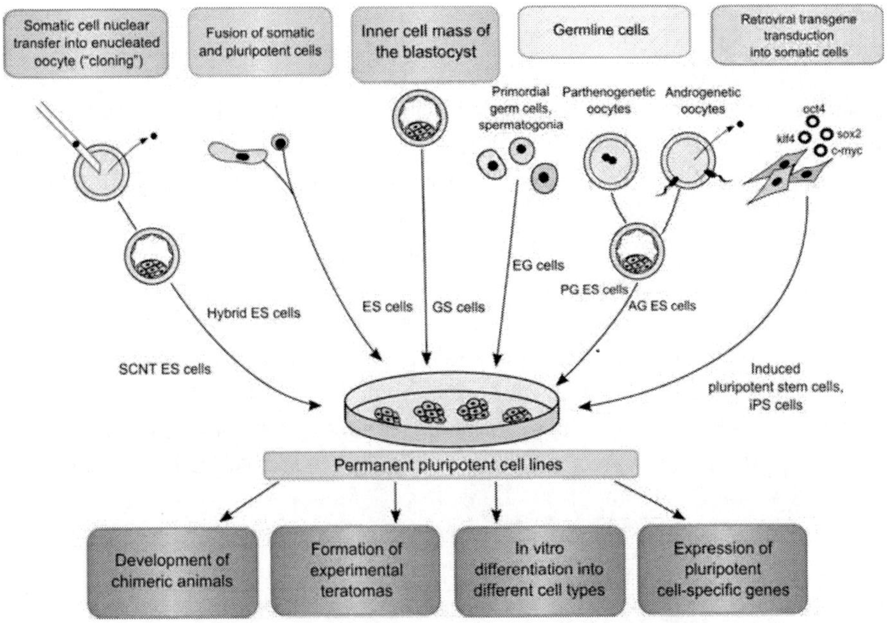

Figure 1. Pluripotent stem cells generated by different technologies.

Pluripotent stem cells can be derived from embryonic and adult somatic cells with diverse epigenetic state and transcriptional and metabolic activity. This initial background may have an influence on proliferation rate maintenance and subsequent differentiation pattern of different pluripotent stem cell lines. Therefore, role of intrinsic cell factors governing pluripotent cell differentiation programme and influence of micro environmental extrinsic factors that present in artificial niche of pluripotent stem cells – culture media - must be determined and clarified.

Utilizing the whole range of pluripotent cell lines of different origin as experimental models can entirely expose the mechanisms of normal and pathological development of various cell types in human and mammalian ontogeny. The models of permanent pluripotent cell lines derived from preimplantation embryos as well as from committed and differentiated cells by experimental manipulations are widely exploited in the research of fundamental problems of developmental biology related to the mechanisms of cell potential realization during embryogenesis and carcinogenesis.

Pluripotent Stem Cell Lines of Different Origin

Pluripotent cells are present only transiently in embryos at early stages of embryogenesis, as they quickly differentiate into various somatic cells through development. During this short period pluripotent cells fall within diverse cell environment and are affected by different extracellular signals that promote subsequent developmental events. To improve the research of early mammalian development there were established permanent embryo-derived cell lines – embryonic stem cells (ES cells), trophoblast stem (TS cells) cells, extraembryonic endoderm cells(XEN) and epiblast stem cells (EpiS cells) [1-6].

First mouse pluripotent ES cell lines were derived from the inner cell mass of blastocyst in 1981 [1, 2]. Isolated inner cell mass of mouse blastocyst was placed onto mitotically inactivated mouse primary embryonic fibroblasts and was grown in media conditioned by teratocarcinoma cells supplemented by fetal bovine serum [2]. At present, these conditions with mouse fibroblast feeder cells are most effective for derivation of ES cell lines of different species including human ES cells and most suitable for the propagation and expansion ES cells in vitro and preservation their stability [4, 7]. Monkey ES cell lines were isolated by Thomson et al. in 1995, and three years later the first human ES cell lines were derived in this laboratory [4, 8]. Initially, human ES cell lines were derived from the blastocysts discarded after in vitro fertilization procedures; later, from the morulae and individual blastomeres in the early embryos [4, 9, 10]. The efficiency of monkey and human ES cell line generation varies (10-25%) largely depending on the blastocysts quality. To date, numerous animal ES cell lines and more than 400 different lines and sublines of human and monkey ES have been derived. These lines are widely used in fundamental and applied research, and the techniques for the production, maintenance, and differentiation of pluripotent cells are still improved [1, 4, 8-13]. More recently, epiblast stem cell lines (EpiS cells) have been established from epiblasts isolated from E5.5 to E6.5 post-implantation mouse and rat embryos that differ significantly from mouse ES cells but share key features with human ES cells [5,6]. For example, EpiSCs derivation failed in the presence of LIF and/or BMP4, the two factors required for the derivation and self-renewal of mouse ES cells. In contrast, similar to human ES and iPS cells, FGF and TGFβ1/Activin/Nodal signaling appear critical for EpiSC derivation. Gene expression profile of EpiS cells closely reflects their post-implantation epiblast origin and is distinct from mouse ES cells. Nevertheless, EpiSCs do share the two key features characteristic of ES cells: prolonged proliferation in vitro and multilineage differentiation. On the other side, EpiSC lines from post-implantation epithelialised epiblast are unable to colonise the embryo even though they express the core pluripotency genes Oct4, Sox2 and Nanog [4, 5, 14]. ES cells can readily become EpiSCs in response to growth factor cues but EpiSCs do not change into ES cells without reprogramming.

The ability to derive pluripotent stem cells from early post-implantation embryos is consistent with early extrauterine embryo transplantation experiments where transplanted mouse embryos at stages ranging from one cell to egg cylinders (E8) are able to form teratocarcinomas, but this ability is quickly lost with further development [15,16].

Mouse embryonic germ cell lines were derived from primordial germ cells of different developmental stages and their pluripotency were confirmed using in vitro and in vivo tests [17-20]. In 1998, the first five human EG cell lines were derived from primordial germ cells of the rudimentary gonads in 5-9-week-old human fetuses and characterized [21]. Human EG cell lines closely resemble human ES cell lines and demonstrate the ability to differentiate into different somatic cells in vitro and in teratomas formed after transplantation into immune-deficient mice.

Pluripotent stem cell lines can be generated from germ line cells of the later stages of development – from spermatogonial cells of newborn and adult mice. Mouse spermatogonial stem cells (GS cells) derived from neonatal and adult mouse testis display ES-like morphology, express pluripotent cell marker, form teratomas after transplantation into immunocompromised mice and give rise to chimerical animals with germ line transmission [22, 23]. Thus, primordial germ cells and spermatogonial cells that are committed unipotent cells can be reprogrammed in vitro without experimental manipulation in cell population which has similar features with ES cells.

Another method to produce pluripotent cells from germline cells is the generation of parthenogenetic and androgenetic ES cell lines. Such lines of mammalian pluripotent stem cells were successfully produced and characterized in several laboratories [24-31]. Although the parthenogenetic and androgenetic embryos die during early postimplantation stages, the parthenogenetic (PG) and androgenetic (AG) ES cell lines can grow in culture and differentiate. Murine PG ES cells and AG ES cells retain the pluripotency in vitro and in vivo conditions and contribute to somatic tissues and germ cells of chimeric embryos as well as in tetraploid embryos but different cell lines show variable developmental potential

[31,34]. At the same time, their clinical applicability is limited since the resulting zygote develops from the activated oocytes with uniparental genome and it does not express a number of imprinted genes correctly. Nevertheless, these ES cell lines are interesting models to study the role of genome imprinting in histogenesis of different tissues.

The fundamental research made it possible to develop several major strategies to produce pluripotent cell lines histocompatible with each patient as a biological material for cell therapy. The first approach includes the generation of ES cell lines using somatic cell nuclear transfer into enucleated oocytes (NTES cells). A blastocyst develops from the reconstructed zygote and to give rise to an ES cell line with the genotype of the somatic nuclear donor (therapeutic cloning strategy). In this case, active molecules in the oocyte required for the normal development are the reprogramming factors.

The first successes in generating reconstructed ES-like cell lines from somatic cells via nuclear transfer reported have been performed in the cow, and then the mouse [34-36]. These ES -like cell -lines are believed to possess the same capacities for unlimited self-renewal and pluripotency as conventional ES cell lines derived from normal embryos produced by fertilization. Interestingly, NTES cell lines can be established with success rates 10 times higher than reproductive cloning [37-40].

The technique for reconstructed NTES cell line production is laborious and has limitations. First, limited human oocytes number are available for reprogramming manipulations; second, the rate of embryos developed to the blastocyst stage is low due to mechanical and chemical damage of different kinds. These technical problems are supplemented with biological limitations resulting from abnormal reactivation of the genetic and epigenetic programs of development in somatic cell nuclei. The top efficiency of producing reconstructed mouse ES cell lines is 20% for this technique [37, 40]; and if a similar efficiency is reached for human ES cell lines, it will become very promising for cell therapy. The attempts to produce human and monkey reconstructed blastocysts, which are required for ES cell line isolation, failed for a long period. The first progress in the technique development was made in 2007 when two rhesus monkey ES cell lines, CRES1 and CRES2, were obtained [41]. In this case, the technique of pronuclear removal has been improved using the new Oosight Spindle Imaging System, and the rate of viable reconstructed blastocysts increased from 1 to 16%. Attempts to produce human reconstructed cell lines are currently underway [42]. Generation of interspecific cell hybrids using the donor oocytes from monkey (as the closest species to human) and human somatic cell nuclei is also a promising approach to derivation of reconstructed human ES cell lines.

Reprogrammed ES cell lines were derived by the fusion of different somatic cells from the adult tissues and ES cells, which yielded stable human tetraploid ES cell lines with the properties and characteristics of pluripotent cells [43-45]. Nevertheless, despite the relative simplicity of production technique, these lines have not the clinical value, since hybrid cells contain a foreign genome, and differentiated somatic cells are recognized by the recipient immune system. In addition, the instability of the tetraploid genome in hybrid cells can lead to malignant transformation. On the other hand, the reactivation mechanisms of genes controlling the pluripotent status as well as the mechanisms of gene expression inactivation in specialized cells during reprogramming can be successfully studied using this experimental system.

A new revolutionary method to produce pluripotent stem cell lines (iPS cells) by reprogramming somatic cells was proposed by Shinya Yamanaka et al, and it was tested first on mouse cells and then on human cells [46-48]. This technique involves the production of ES cell-like lines from different somatic cells (embryonic and adult fibroblasts, keratinocytes, neural, blood, stomach cells, and other) using transgenic modification of their genome with viral vectors carrying pluripotency-related genes [46-52]. In this case, the integration (or not) of viral vectors into the somatic cell genome and subsequent transient expression of the regulatory genes Oct4, Sox2, C-myc, and Klf4 reprograms the somatic cell genome and reverts terminally differentiated cells to the pluripotent state. After several weeks of culture, about 0.1% of transduced cells demonstrate a dramatic change in their morphology and potential. The experiments with mouse induced pluripotent stem cells showed that they can provide for the development of chimeric animals, which completely confirms their pluripotent state. At the same time, some of these mice had laryngeal cancer, which points to the altered developmental program in pluripotent cells with such transgenic modification [53, 54]. These experiments shed new light on the changes in cell potential and on the mechanisms controlling the cell pluripotent state; however, further studies on induced pluripotent stem cells are needed. Despite a very low rate of reprogramming cells, their number suffices for a relatively rapid production of cell lines with a particular genotype. The safety of such pluripotent cell lines for clinical use remains questionable, since the degree of reprogramming correctness in somatic cells remains unclear. The generation of induced pluripotent cells involves viral vectors, which may cause genetic instability and tumorigenicity; especially if they include the C-myc oncogene that is overexpressed in the most of studied human cancers. The use of such cell lines in cell therapy requires the exclusion of this oncogene from the technique. The experiments in this direction demonstrated that lines of induced pluripotent cells can still be generated after such modification but the method efficiency considerably decreases [48, 55].

Malignant teratocarcinoma cell lines were established in the 70s of 20th century. That was significantly earlier than ES cells were derived [56-61]. These cell lines were the first model system for study mechanisms of early development. Embryonal teratocarcinoma lines (EC cells) were isolated from mouse and human ovarian and testicular tumors and they displayed variable developmental potential therefore they can be considered as malignant pluripotent stem cells. The most of teratocarcinoma cell lines demonstrate restricted differentiation potential and cannot contribute to germ line of chimeric embryos, some of these lines, nullipotent cell lines, completely lost the ability to differentiate into somatic or germ cells with the exception of extraembryonic endoderm cells [60]. Current studies of EC cells provide unique opportunities to dissect mechanisms of cancer initiation at the earliest stages of development and its progression with different spectrum of developmental disturbances.

Pluripotent Stem Cell Characteristics

Irrespective of the cell sources and production techniques, all pluripotent cell lines share the same biological properties but demonstrate individual variation in some culture properties, the capacity to differentiate into different somatic cell types, and maintenance of genetic and epigenetic stability. The revealed differences can be due to genetic background of cell sources that initiate pluripotent stem cell lines, to individual sensitivity to different adaptive effects of in vitro cultivation, and to methodical variations of culture maintenance in different laboratories.

Similar in vitro culture systems are used to generate and maintain ES cells as well as induced pluripotent stem cells. These systems include various feeder cell types or extracellular matrix protein components and fetal serum or serum replacement, various growth factors such as leukemia inhibitory factor basic fibroblast growth factor (bFGF), Activin, and Nodal [62-69]. Routine ES cell cultivation includes enzymatic treatment for passaging. The characteristic feature of monkey and human ES cells is low survival rate of individual cells and accordingly low clonogenic capacity, and therefore, in this case, cultures are separated into cell clusters rather than into individual cells to increase the survival rate and to support the cell growth. Monkey and human ES cells are more prone to in vitro differentiation compared to mouse ones; accordingly, differentiated cells should be removed from the population to maintain the major line properties. To allow in vitro differentiation pluripotent cells are placed in media containing differentiation promoting growth factors or small molecules. In course of spontaneous in vitro differentiation, pluripotent stem cells as well as malignant teratocarcinoma cells form three-dimensional cell aggregates that recapitulate the early pregastrulation stages of mammalian embryo development (Figure 2, 4B).

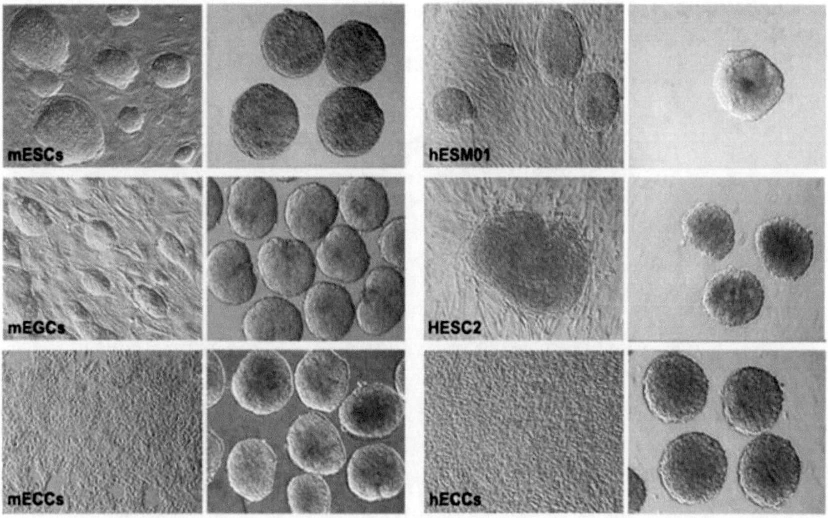

Figure 2. The initial stages of in vitro differentiation of pluripotent mES, mEG, hES cells and their malignant counterparts mEC, hEC cells. These cell lines can form embryoid bodies of similar morphology despite their different origins.

Several tests were developed to characterized pluripotent cell lines. The "gold standard" of mouse ES cell pluripotency is their capacity to contribute into development of different tissues and organs of chimeric animals developed from the blastocyst injected with ES cells. However, ethical restrictions does not allow this test for human ES cells, and the described and novel ES cell lines of human and primates are assigned to pluripotent cell lines based on other properties that are largely the same for mice, primates, and human.

The pluripotency is primarily evaluated using the teratoma test, i.e., the capacity of ES, EG, and iPS cells to form teratomas in immune-deficient animal models (Nude or SCID mice). The classical teratomas formed from pluripotent cells contain rudiments of different tissues and structures derived from the three germ layers [70, 71]. On the contrary, EC cells being malignant counterparts of pluripotent stem cells demonstrate restricted differentiation potential or undifferentiated tumor cell growth only after transplantation into different tissue sites of immune-deficient mice (Figure 3).

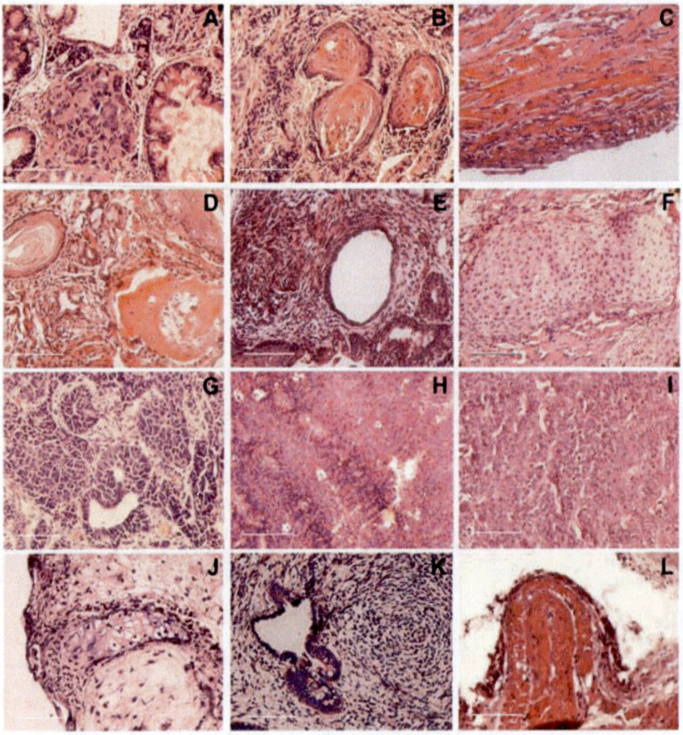

Figure 3. Differentiation of mouse and human pluripotent and teratocarcinoma cells in experimental teratomas formed after transplantation into of immunedeficient mice. Histological sections of teratomas, formed by mESCs (A-C), mEGCs (D-G), hESCs (J-L) and teratocarcinomas, developed by nullipotent mECCs (H) and hECCs (I). Teratomas contained various types of differentiated somatic cells, including ectodermal, mesodermal and endodermal lineages: neural rosettes (G), ciliated epithelium of intestinal type (A,K), striated muscles (C, L), keratinized epithelium (B, D), hyaline cartilage (F, J), and intestinal cysts (D, F). Teratocarcinomas included undifferentiated cells solely (H, I). Bar, 100μm.

All undifferentiated pluripotent cell lines are morphologically identical; they grow in vitro as colonies of small densely packed cells with a high nuclear—cytoplasmic ratio (Fig. 2). All cells in a colony express specific transcription factors (Oct4 and Nanog) and membrane proteins (stage-specific embryonic antigens SSEA3, SSEA4, as well as CD9 and keratin sulfate antigens TRA-160 and TRA-1-81) and demonstrate high telomerase and alkaline phosphatase activities (Figure 4A).

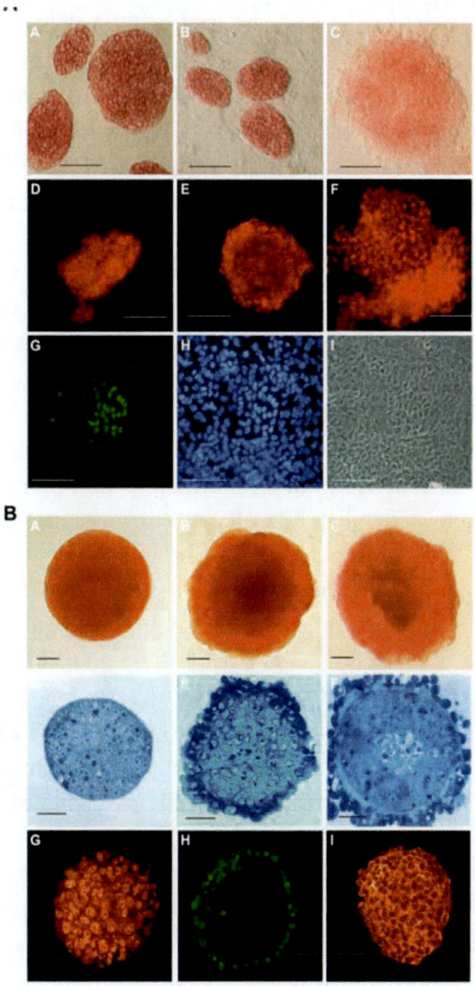

Figure 4. Activity of alkaline phosphatase and expression of Oct4 and GATA4 in mouse ES, EG and EC cells and in embryoid bodies. **(A)** Alkaline phosphatase (A-C) and Oct4 (D-F) are highly expressed in all undifferentiated ES (A,D), EG (B, E) and EC (C, F) cells. Minor fraction of EC cells expressed marker of extraembryonic endoderm Gata4 (G-I). Bar, 100μm. **(B)** Embryoid bodies developed after in vitro differentiation of ES cells on day 1(A, D), 3(B, E, G-I), 5(C, F). Activity of alkaline phosphatase were retained in undifferentiated cells (A-C) but marker of extraembryonic endoderm Gata4 were already expressed in the outer cells of embryoid bodies. Morphological reorganization in embryoid bodies reproduce the early stages of embryogenesis (D-F) and epiblast-like inner cells of embryoid bodies are in contact using adherent cell junction (E-cadherin, I). Bar, 100μm (A-C), 50 μm (D-I).

The transcription profiles of pluripotent cell lines and their differentiated derivatives have been studied in detail using the Microarray technology. The results of these studies demonstrate that the expression level of many genes can vary in different pluripotent stem cell lines; however, all studied mouse, monkey and human stem cell lines showed high expression level of stem cell-specific factors, Pou5f1(Oct4), Sox2, Nanog, Tdgf/Cripto, Lefty2, Dnmt3b, GDF3, and Gabrb3 [41, 47, 72-78]. Comparative analysis of transcriptional profiles of mouse ES and EG cell lines with diverse genetic backgrounds showed that ES cells and EG cells are indistinguishable based on global gene expression patterns alone. All pluripotent cell lines showed similar gene expression patterns, which separated them clearly from other tissue stem cells with lower developmental potency. Differences between pluripotent lines derived from different sources were smaller than differences between lines derived from different mouse strains (129 vs. C57BL/6). Even in the differentiation-promoting conditions, these pluripotent cells showed the same general trends of gene expression changes regardless of their origin and genetic background [77] . Similarly, the study of 59 human ES cell lines obtained and maintained in 17 laboratories worldwide demonstrated expression variations of components of signaling pathways and regulators of proliferation, FGF4, LEFTYB, EBAF(LEFTYA), NODAL, TDGF1, IFITM1, FOXD3, GAL, LIN28, TERT, UTF1, etc. [76]. The causes of the expression variation in different human ES cell lines are unclear. Probably, like in mouse pluripotent stem cells, the revealed heterogeneity of the expression profiles may be attributed to different genotypes of embryonic cell sources. This variation can also be due to the initial events during ES cell line isolation, since cells in the inner cell mass of the blastocyst are to a certain extent a heterogeneous population and adapt differently to the artificial environment. One cannot exclude that the observed variations result from different processing algorithms of experimental data obtained using the microarray technology.

Recently, it was shown that somatic/ES cell hybrid cell lines resemble their pre-fusion ES cell partners in terms of behavior in culture and pluripotency. However, they contain unique expression profiles that are similar but not identical to normal ES cells [45]. A study of gene expression profiles of mouse and human ES cells and iPS cells suggests that, while iPS cells are quite similar to their embryonic counterparts, a recurrent gene expression signature appears in iPS cells regardless of their origin or the method by which they were generated. Upon extended culture, human iPS cells adopt a gene expression profile more similar to human ES cells; however, they still retain a gene expression signature unique from ES cells that extends to miRNA expression. Genome-wide data suggested that the iPS cell signature gene expression differences are due to differential promoter binding by the reprogramming factors. High-resolution array profiling demonstrated that there is no common specific subkaryotypic alteration that is required for reprogramming and that reprogramming does not lead to genomic instability. Based on these data iPS cells can be considered as unique subtype of pluripotent cell [78].

The capacity of ES cell lines of different origin, EG cell lines, and iPS cell lines to in vitro multilineage differentiation is also a pluripotency test for each line. Numerous studies of in vitro differentiation of various mammalian pluripotent cell lines have developed protocols to produce different types of differentiation cells in culture: neurons and glial cells, cardiomyocytes, hematopoietic, endothelial, osteogenic, insulin-producing, and hepatocyte-like cells, adipocytes, melanocytes, keratinocytes, trophoblast and prostate cells [31, 79-85]. The fundamental studies of the mechanisms underlying the regulation of different histogeneses using the pluripotent cell lines of different origins gave an impetus to the development of techniques to produce particular cell types for clinical use.

Self-Renewal and Maintenance of Genomic Integrity in Pluripotent Stem Cells

Pluripotent cells actively self-renew during prolonged cultivation in vitro, and their proliferation rate is comparable to that in immortalized or transformed cells. Studies on the mechanisms of self-renewal of pluripotent cells in different animals demonstrated that the cell cycle regulation in ES, EG and other types of pluripotent cells indeed has some specific properties and considerably differs from that in normal somatic cells. First, mouse, monkey, and human pluripotent stem cells remain in S-phase more than a half of the cell cycle, while the G1 and G2 periods are substantially reduced [86-90]. Analysis of cell cycle stage distribution in ES, EG as well as EC cells demonstrate that the most of undifferentiated cells, 60-70% are in S-phase and only 15-25% cells in G1. This indicates that their cell cycle is specifically regulated so that newly formed cells start new DNA replication nearly immediately after the previous mitosis. However, in contrast to cancer cells, ES cells have mechanisms providing for their high sensitivity to differentiation promoting factors and not preventing death of abnormal cells [86-90]. Characteristics of mouse ES cell cycle regulation are the lack of dependence on serum stimulation and mitogen-activated protein kinase kinase (MEK)–associated signaling [91, 92]. Mouse ES cells rely on phosphatidyl inositol-3 kinase (PI3K) dependent signaling for progression through the G1 phase as well as for inhibition of differentiation [92, 93]. However, PI3K activity is not dependent on persistent serum stimulation but rather largely relies on both on stimulation of the leukemia inhibitory factor (LIF) receptor and on expression of the ESC-specific Eras factor [92, 94].

Studies of mechanisms underlying cell cycle control in ES cells from different mammals demonstrate kind-specific differences in the regulation of pluripotent stem cell self-renewal despite high similarity of cell cycle structure. For instance, hyperphosphorylated Rb and cyclin E (proteins specific for the S and G2/M phases) proved to be present in mouse, monkey and human ES cells throughout their cell cycle; however, in contrast to mouse ES cells, cyclin A is not continuously expressed in monkey ES cells, and Rb protein dynamic is similar in mouse and human ES cells. In mouse ES cells, there is compelling evidence that the G1/S transition is not dependent on a functional cyclin D-Cdk4/6 and RB-E2F pathway [87, 88, 95-97] and that rapid progression through the cell cycle relies largely on constitutively active cyclin E-Cdk2 and cyclin A-Cdk2 complexes [98]. Monkey ES cells also express cyclin E during all phases of the cell cycle, suggesting that ectopic cyclin E-Cdk2 kinase activity may also be a characteristic feature of primate ESCs. However, monkey ES cell line ORMES-1 cells did not express cyclin A in all phases of their cell cycle, in contrast to mouse ESCs [89]. Thus, heterogeneous cell cycle duration that characterizes rhesus ESCs could result from discontinuous expression of cyclin A.

Analysis of the expression profiles of human ES cells demonstrated the absent or low-level expression of the p53 gene as well as of p16, p19 *and* p21 involved in the cell cycle regulation. Conversely, mouse ES cells demonstrated high expression level of these genes and their negative regulators MDM genes [99, 100]. It is assumed that the inactivation of the p53- and Rb-dependent pathways is nevertheless an essential component of the cell cycle regulation in pluripotent cells of different mammals [101]. In addition, the mitotic cycle regulation in ES cells features the independence of the stimulation by serum factors as well as of the mitogen-activated protein kinase kinase pathway [87].

Recently, there was shown that human ES cells express all G1-specific CYCLINs (D1, D2, D3 and E) and cyclin-dependent kinases CDK2, CDK4 and CDK6 at variable levels. In contrast to murine ES cells, most of the cell cycle regulators in hES cells show cell cycle-dependent expression, thus revealing important differences in the expression of cell cycle regulatory components between these two embryonic cell types. Knockdown of CDK2 using RNA interference resulted in hES cells arrest at G1 phase of the cell cycle and differentiation to extraembryonic lineages [102]. Moreover, it was shown that NANOG, a master transcription factor, regulates S-phase entry in human embryonic stem cells via transcriptional regulation of cell cycle regulatory components. Chromatin immunoprecipitation combined with reporter-based transfection assays reveal that the C-terminal region of NANOG binds to the regulatory regions of CDK6 and CDC25A genes under normal physiological conditions. Decreased CDK6 and CDC25A expression in human ES cells suggest that both CDK6 and CDC25A are involved in S-phase regulation. The effects of NANOG overexpression on S-phase regulation are mitigated by the down-regulation of CDK6 or CDC25A alone. Overexpression of CDK6 or CDC25A alone can rescue the impact of NANOG down-regulation on S-phase entry, suggesting that CDK6 and CDC25A are downstream cell cycle effectors of NANOG during the G1 to S transition [103].

The experiments on monkey ES cells demonstrated that gamma-irradiation does not arrest their cell cycle in G1, which points to the absence of the G1/S checkpoint typical of untransformed cells and required for DNA damage repair. On the other side, irradiated human ES cells were accumulated in G1 stage. The apoptotic factors are activated and aberrant cells with damaged DNA are rapidly eliminated in mouse, primate, and human ES cells [88, 89]. Genetically damaged human ES cells demonstrated changed biosynthesis of histone proteins: mRNA transcription and processing are affected and H4 mRNA is destabilized, which disrupts the normal mitotic process [90]. An alternative pathway for damaged cells has been demonstrated: p53 can repress the promoter of the pluripotent cell-specific Nanog gene in mouse ES cells, which induces irreversible differentiation of these cells and, thus, eliminates them from the pool of undifferentiated cells but not from the total cell population [104].

On the other hand, efficient mechanisms of protection from oxidative stress-induced damage and DNA repair are active in undifferentiated mouse and human ES cells. The resistance of ES cells to damage can be due to high activity of multiple drug resistance transporter of verapamil, heat shock proteins, and double-stranded DNA damage repair systems. Interestingly, that high ES cell resistance to active oxygen species mediated by the glutathione/thioredoxin system is observed only in undifferentiated cells, and its efficiency substantially reduces during early differentiation [105, 106]. Analysis of the transcription profiles of human ES cell lines demonstrates high expression levels of various genes including APEX, RAD, MSH, and genes involved in DNA repair, which provides for secure protection of the genetic material. Nevertheless, the data on the control mechanisms of cell cycle and resistance to various stress factors in different pluripotent cell types or their differentiated derivatives are limited, and these problems require further investigation.

Despite the cell cycle similarity in ES cells of different mammals, the mechanisms providing for the unique proliferative potential of pluripotent cells in different species and types of cell lines derived from different sources remain unclear, since almost no published data are available on this problem. In summary, one can propose that the mechanisms controlling the active proliferation of pluripotent cell lines in culture slightly differ from those in the embryo. A high rate of cell division to yield the required cell mass is the priority task during early embryogenesis; however, the extraembryonic structures, trophoectoderm and extraembryonic endoderm, differentiate during this short period, i.e., the mechanisms inhibiting differentiation are not active in them. Self-renewal of pluripotent cell lines in artificial in vitro culture continues over long periods, and the maintenance of this cell status requires external stimuli maintaining high rate of cell divisions and preventing differentiation events at the same time. Under such suboptimal conditions, appearance of genetically transformed cells in population is inevitable within long-term cultivation. Apparently, pluripotent line founder cells that can faster adapt to in vitro conditions, faster proliferate, and don't respond to differentiation signals during their short G1 period are selected during the establishment of pluripotent cell line. Thus, in terms of pluripotent cell adaptation to artificial in vitro conditions as a process of minimum transformation, one can propose that the variants with a shorter cycle and low sensitivity to differentiation and damaging factors have a selective advantage. In other words, artificial conditions of in vitro culture maintaining high growth rate of pluripotent cells are the proper factors initiating the genetic and epigenetic alterations in these cells.

Genetic Mutation and Epigenetic Modification in Pluripotent Stem Cells and Problem of Cancer Transformation.

The maintenance of genome stability in pluripotent cells is the crucial factor of their structural and functional integrity, which is manifested as the normal balance between proliferation and differentiation in different cell types in vitro and in vivo. Long-term ES cell cultures can accumulate cells with different genetic aberrations and epigenetic changes. Analysis of the karyotype in long-term cultures of different human ES cell lines (passages 34-140) demonstrated aneuploidy of chromosomes X, 12, and 17 [107-113]. Preferred trisomy of chromosomes 12 and 17 has been revealed in lines HUES, H1, H14, BG01, and BG02 [107, 108, 113-115]. Trisomy of chromosomes 13 and 3 has been revealed in lines SA002 and Miz-hES13, respectively [116-118]. Cytogenetic analysis of

18 ORMES lines of rhesus monkey ES cells using G-banding demonstrated a diploid set of 42 chromosomes in 15 lines; various chromosomal abnormalities including balanced translocations t(11;16), t(5;19), and t(1;18) in three lines (ORMES-1, -2, and -5); and a pericentric inversion in chromosome 1 in one line. However, these aberrations were observed in ES cells at early passages (9) that suggest that these abnormalities could be initially present in the source embryos [81]. Aneuploidy have also been found in one out of seven parthenogenetic lines of human ES cells (karyotype phESC-7, 47,XXX, and 48,XXX+6) at early passages, which also suggests that this mutation was inherited from germ cells [30].

One of two monkey ES cell lines (CRES-1) generated by somatic cell nuclear transfer had normal karyotype 42,XY; while the other line (CRES-2) demonstrated chromosomal aberrations at early passages. The Y chromosomes was missing in 12% of cells, while other cells contained the Y isochromosome with two extra copies of the long arm (karyotype 41,X[3]/42,Xi(Y)q10[17]) [41].

Note that the trend to accumulate chromosomal abnormalities is not observed in all human and primate ES cell lines. Sporadic aneuploidy that can have no selective advantage is sometimes observed. For instance, SA002c cells with trisomy of chromosome 13 had no advantage in clonal growth and disappeared from the population in subsequent passages [118]. Another study demonstrated that seven novel isolated lines of human ES cells from blastocyst-stage embryos diagnosed as aneuploid in preimplantation genetic screening exhibited morphology and markers typical of human ES cells and the capacity for long-term proliferation. The derived hES cell lines manifested pluripotent differentiation potential both in vivo and in vitro. Surprisingly, karyotype analysis of these lines that were derived from aneuploid embryos showed that the cell lines carry a normal euploid karyotype. Because authors showed that the euploidy was not achieved through chromosome duplication, they suggest that the euploid human ES cell lines originated from mosaic embryos consisting of aneuploid and euploid cells, and in vitro selection occurred to favor euploid cells [119].

It remains unclear what gives rise to aberrant cells -- different susceptibility of particular genotypes to mutations or specific ES cell culture conditions. For instance, Mitalipova et al. analyzed the karyotype of two human ES cell lines, BG01 and BG02, at early and late passages using different culture techniques: mechanical and enzymatic (using trypsin or collagenase) dissociation of colonies into clusters [113]. In the case of enzymatic treatment, both ES cell lines contained cells with trisomy of chromosomes 12 and 17 and sometimes extra copies of chromosomes 14, 20, and X; while no abnormalities were observed after mechanical dissociation up to passage 105. In other cases, chromosomal aberrations have been revealed after mechanical passage but not after enzymatic passaging [118, 120, 121]. One can propose that the genetic damage of ES cells can also be promoted by extra cycles of cell cryopreservation and thawing.

Studies of various mutant human ES cell sublines demonstrated no significant changes in the transcriptional profiles in most cases; however, the expression level can vary for some genes [113,115]. Many authors reported that human ES cells carrying extra copies of chromosomes 12 and 17 rapidly become dominant in the population and demonstrate advantages growth and higher clonal activity [108, 115, 122, 123]. The isochromosome 12p has been found previously in some germ cell tumors of the gonads including human teratocarcinomas [109,124,125], while the amplification 17q is associated with some neuroblastomas [126]. These chromosomes contain the genes controlling self-renewal and differentiation, NANOG, STELLAR, GDF3, GRB2, and STAT3, whose altered expression in the case of the corresponding extra copies of chromosomes can modulate the cell potential in ES cell lines [88,125]. A comparative study of human ES cell lines BG01 and BG01V and human hyperpolyploid teratocarcinoma NTERA demonstrated that the properties of the abnormal line BG01V are more similar to the original line BG01 rather than to the teratocarcinoma NTERA. BG01V cells differentiated in experimental teratomas with the formation of various ectodermal, entodermal, and mesodermal structures; however, a higher number of undifferentiated cells was observed compared to the BG01 teratomas [115].

A detailed study of the genetic changes in 10 human ES cell lines in long-term culture demonstrated (passages 22--105) one (or more) genetic damages that are commonly observed in various cancer cells in eight out of nine studied lines [112]. According to these data, the aberrations in ES cells included different changes in the number of gene copies (45%), sequence changes in mitochondrial DNA (22%), and changes in the methylation level in some gene promoters (90%). In particular, some ES cell lines at late passages studied in this work demonstrated the amplification of gene loci containing the C-MYC oncogene that are present in nearly all cancer types including that after spontaneous transformation of mesenchymal stem cells of the bone marrow during in vitro culture (127, 128]. All data available to date indicate that long-term culture of all ES cell lines leads to their genetic damage that can considerably change the cell phenotype and introduce oncogenic properties to mutant cells.

Different epigenetic modifications of chromatin take place together with the structural changes of the genome in long-term in vitro cultures of pluripotent stem cell lines. The epigenetic changes in chromatin structure are the key factors in the regulation of gene imprinting, expression of non-imprinted genes, X chromosome inactivation, and genome stability [129,130]. A set of different epigenetic modifications in DNA and associated histone proteins is known to determine the timing of gene activation in the cell. The epigenetic modifications of chromatin include cytosine methylation in gene promoter regions, repetitive sequences, and imprinted genes as well as histone methylation and acetylation. In most cases, DNA methylation in the promoter or differentially methylated region inactivates the corresponding gene expression. Abnormal DNA methylation pattern in the cells results developmental defects and various pathologies including carcinogenesis [131- 139]. For instance, the inactivation of oncogenesis suppressor genes in some tumors results from the hypermethylation of their promoters, and conversely, the hypomethylation of the regulatory regions of oncogenes can induce their ectopic transcription.

Genomic imprinting is a form of the epigenetic program including the modification of different gene loci, whose expression during development and cell differentiation is monoallelic according to the parental origin of a particular allele. Imprinted genes have a trend to cluster in "imprinting centers" in the genome. One of such centers is located on chromosome 15 (15q11-q13) and is associated with the Prader-Willi and Angelman syndromes; and another one on chromosome 11 (11p15.5), with the Beckwith-Wiedemann syndrome [140-142]. Imprinting in these regions is controlled in *cis* by so-called imprinting centers (ICs) that regulate parent-specific expression of target genes bidirectionally over long distances. ICs are subject to parent-specific epigenetic modifications including DNA methylation and histone changes recognized by specific factors such as DNA-binding proteins that in turn, activate downstream effects leading to appropriate mono-allelic gene expression. These epigenetic modifications must be reprogrammed during development, involving first erasure of old epigenetic marks during germ cell development and establishment of new marks in a gender-specific manner. Methylation of CpG dinucleotides within ICs is proposed to be one of the initial mechanisms differentially marking parental chromosomes in gametes. Once established, locus-specific DNA methylation profiles must be stably maintained in future generations of cells.

During development, DNA methylation is provided by coordinated activity of DNA methyltransferases including Dnmtl and de novo DNA methyltransferases Dnmt3a and Dnmt3b. DNMT3 deficiency in humans causes substantial demethylation of the centromeric minor satellite repeats, and such individuals demonstrate rare genetic disease, ICF syndrome (or Immunodeficiency, Centromere instability and Facial anomalies syndrome) [143, 144].

The methylation profile alterations in the promoter regions of some genes in pluripotent cell lines of different origin demonstrated that specific in vitro culture conditions can modulate the methylation of imprinted genes, although, not in all human and monkey ES cell lines and largely at late passages [145-147]. Monoallelic expression of imprinted genes H19, KCNQ1, PEG10, and NDNL1 was observed in human ES cell lines SHhES1 and HUES-7 at both early and late passages, and the corresponding methylation status of imprinted genes KCNQ1, IGF2, SCL22A18, NESP55, and SNRPN has also been revealed at early and late passages in lines H9, H7, HUES-3, and HSF6. After a long-term culture of the H9 line, the changes in the methylated region of the H19 gene were recorded without the gametic imprinting loss [146, 147]. It is of interest that the normal methylation profile of the imprinted genes H19, SNRPN, and DLK1/MEG3 was conserved in the genetically abnormal human ES cell line BG01V [115]. A study of expression of 10 imprinted genes SNRPN, IPW, KCNQ10T1, PEG3, IGF2, MEST, H19, NESP55, MEG3, and SCL22A18 in 59 human ES cell lines demonstrated monoallelic expression in 80% of cases and expression from the other parental allele or biallelic expression in the other 20% of samples [76]. Overall, these data indicate high stability of the methylation status in imprinted genes in human ES cell lines.

On the other hand, a study of the methylation status and expression pattern of imprinted genes in primate ES cell lines demonstrated biallelic expression of the IGF2 and H19 genes in all studied lines, while the SNRPN and NDN genes demonstrated normal expression of the parental allele only. Conversely, the normal expression of the parental IGF2 allele and maternal H19 allele was detected in the rhesus monkey blastocysts that were the sources of ES cell lines. These data suggest that the changes in the IGF2 and H19 methylation status in monkey ES cells took place at the initial stages of line isolation [81,148].

As mentioned above, the changes in the DNA methylation of non-imprinted gene loci is associated in many cases with the development of various malignant tumors; that is why analysis of the methylation status stability in oncogenes and tumor suppressor genes in different ES cell lines is important to understand the evolution of these lines in long-term in vitro cultures [149]. DNA hypermethylation in the promoter regions of oncosuppressor genes RASSF1 and PTPN6 has been found in long-term cultures of human ES cell lines BG01, BG02, BG03, HUES-2, HUES-3, H7, H9, SA001, and SA002; while the methylation of the TNFRSF10C promoter was observed only in two of these lines, HUES-2 and SA002 [112].

Significant variation in the expression level of DNA methyltransferase DNMT3B in different human ES cell lines was reported in numerous studies [8, 150-152]. Different levels of this enzyme expression and activity can be the main variation factor of the methylation status and epigenetic stability in different pluripotent cell lines. The ES cell genome is largely hypomethylated (in a 'transcription-ready' state), and the expression of many genes specific for different cell types is basically regulated at the post-transcriptional level [153].

The overexpression of genes located on the X chromosome during cell differentiation is known to be compensated by the inactivation of one of X chromosomes in the cells with the female genotype as a result of DNA methylation, histone modification, and expression of the noncoding XIST mRNA. Several publications demonstrated considerable variation in XIST expression indicative of the X chromosomes inactivation in both undifferentiated and differentiated cells of different ES cell lines with the female genotype [8, 76, 154]. Noteworthily, XIST mRNA was detected at early passages of undifferentiated cells of euploid human ES cell line H7, and it was undetectable at the late passages; while XIST expression was not detected even in differentiated cells of the aneuploid subline of H7 [122]. What underlies such heterogeneity in different ES cell lines remains unclear. Presumably, it can be due to the X chromosome inactivation status in cells of the inner cell mass of the embryo that served as line sources, or it was affected by in vitro culture conditions. Thus, the epigenetic modifications revealed in different human and primate ES cell lines take place during the adaptation to culture conditions at different passages in individual cells of the same line. These changes as well as the genetic aberrations can contribute to genome instability and cell transformation.

Regulation of Pluripotent State Maintenance and the Initial Stage of Differentiation of Pluripotent Stem Cells

Pluripotent stem cells retain their features to differentiate into all cell types of organism including germ line and extraembryonic tissue even after prolonged cultivation in artificial microenvironment which significantly differs from embryonic niche. However, pluripotent stem cell can realize their potential completely only if they are returned to blastocysts which are their natural niche. After injection of pluripotent stem cells into ectopic adult tissue sites they develop teratomas which represent chaotic development of different tissue structure of different degree of maturation. Pluripotent stem cells can recapitulate several elements of developmental program of mammalian embryo during in vitro differentiation but they can reproduce the histogenesis of some somatic tissues only after experimental modulation of signaling and growth factors' gradients. Though, pluripotent stem cells of different origin differentiate asynchronously and incompletely even after step-by-step treatment by different differentiation inductors. One of the challenges of pluripotent stem cell-based technology for regenerative medicine is uncompleted differentiation and as the result - variable percentage of residual undifferentiated cells that can form teratomas. Therefore, role of intrinsic cell factors governing pluripotent cell differentiation programme and influence of extrinsic factors that drive the in vitro differentiation of pluripotent stem cells must be determined and clarified.

The pluripotency is maintained by a complex of extracellular and intracellular factors that set up a specific pattern of the gene expression. Molecular signaling network working in pluripotent cells controls self-renewal and maintenance of the pluripotent cell identity. When the external signals from the environment niche (it is culture media for pluripotent cell lines) do change and the balance of proliferation and differentiation promoting factors alters then the pluripotent cells are involved in the lineages' determination.

One of the core regulator of pluripotent state is octamer-binding homeobox transcriptional factor POU family Oct4 which was the first identified factor that sustained pluripotent phenotype in cells of pre-implantation embryo and in germ cells as well as in ES, EG, iPS cells and expressed in different EC cell lines [46, 75, 155, 156,]. Two other transcriptional factors Sox2 and FoxD3 can interact with Oct4, in particular, Sox2 and Oct4 bind to adjacent cites within the enhancer of several target genes and act cooperatively to stimulate the transcription [157]. The second identified pluripotency-related homeodomain transcription factor Nanog was identified in mouse and human pluripotent and teratocarcinoma cells. Pattern of Nanog expression is differed from Oct4 and detected firstly in late morula stage and then it decreases in epiblast cells. Nanog is detectable in migrating primordial germ cells and in residing early gonocytes but it is not expressed in adult gonads [158-161].

Obviously, Oct4, Nanog and Sox2 function as suppressors of differentiation of inner cell mass into extraembryonic lineages – trophoblast and extraembryonic endoderm but they act cooperatively with many other genes that are elements of developmental programme of pluripotent cells. These core genes control expression of numerous target genes that are involved in cell cycle progression and lineages determination [103, 162]. Expression of Oct4, Nanog and Sox2 was detected in various mouse and human teratocarcinoma cells with different differentiation potential and mRNA Oct4 has been found in some other tumors too (breast, pancreas and colon cancer) [8, 163, 164].

Yamanaka et al, have demonstrated that ectopic expression of four transcription factors Oct4, Sox2, Klf4, and c-Myc can reprogram mouse and human somatic cells to induced pluripotent stem (iPS) cells. As it was mentioned above, Oct4, Sox2 together with Nanog are key genes underlying pluripotency. The fourth gene Kruppel-like factor 4 (Klf4) cooperates with Oct4 and Sox2 to activate Lefty1expression, and that Klf4 acts as a mediating factor that specifically binds to the proximal element of the Lefty1promoter [165]. Recently it was shown, after using PiggyBac transposition to introduce a single reprogramming factor, Klf4, into EpiS cells a fraction of cells formed undifferentiated ES-like colonies. These EpiSC-derived induced pluripotent stem (Epi-iPS) cells activated expression of ES cell-specific transcripts including endogenous Klf4, and down regulated markers of lineage specification. They produced high-contribution chimaeras that yielded germline transmission. These properties were maintained after Cre-mediated deletion of the Klf4 transgene, formally demonstrating complete and stable reprogramming of developmental phenotype. Thus, re-expression of Klf4 in an appropriate environment can regenerate the ground state from EpiSCs [14].

In mouse ES cells, Klf4 is mainly activated by the Jak-Stat3 pathway and preferentially activates Sox2, whereas Tbx3 is preferentially regulated by the phosphatidylinositol-3-OH kinase-Akt and mitogen-activated protein kinase pathways and predominantly stimulates Nanog. In the absence of LIF, artificial expression of Klf4 or Tbx3 is sufficient to maintain pluripotency while maintaining Oct4 expression. Notably, overexpression of Nanog supports LIF-independent self-renewal of mouse ES cells in the absence of Klf4 and Tbx3 activity. Therefore, Klf4 and Tbx3 are involved in mediating LIF signaling to the core circuitry but are not directly associated with the maintenance of pluripotency, because ES cells keep pluripotency without their expression in the particular context [162].

Another component of the regulation of gene expression pattern in mouse and human ES cells is polycomb group (PcG) proteins which directly repress a large cohort of differentiation regulators. Using genome-wide location analysis in murine ES cells, there was found that the Polycomb repressive complexes PRC1 and PRC2 co-occupied 512 genes, many of which encode transcription factors with important roles in development [166, 167]. The polycomb repressor complex PRC2 is involved in the initiation of silencing and contains histone methyltransferases that can methylate histone H3 lysine 9 and 27, which are marks of silenced chromatin. The PRC2 is involved in the initiation of silencing and contains EZH2, the histone methyltransferase that places the histone methylation modification HeK27me. On the other side, the PRC1 complexes contain chromo domain proteins such as the CBX family that recognize the HeK27me mark, and the key stem cell protein Bmi1, which can silence the p16 gene (a key gene epigenetically silenced early in cancers). Enrichment of EZH2 and the H3K27me mark is a property of the promoters of DNA hypermethylated and silenced genes as is the sirtuin deactylase SIRT1, which has been associated with PRC2 complexes found in stem and cancer cells. Steady-state levels of EZH2, Bmi1, and other PcG complex members are increased in cancer too. Thus, dysregulation of the PcG system potentially links cancer formation to stem cell biology [168].

The investigation of signaling pathways that underlay pluripotent state maintenance demonstrated that there exist several differences between mouse and human ES cells. It was shown that leukemia inhibitory factor (LIF) is essential for self-renewal mouse ES and EG cells but doesn't require for pre-gastrulation mouse development and for derivation and maintenance of EpiS cells [169-172, 5, 6]. LIF is binding to the LIF receptor and activates the signal transducer and activator of transcription 3 (Stat-3). Phosphorilated Stat-3 translocates into nucleus and regulates target genes transcription. Mouse ES cells growing without feeder cells begin to differentiate after several days of LIF withdrawal. On the other hand, human ES cells are not sensitive to LIF absence and the supplement to this factor to culture media does not prevent the differentiation [173]. With the presence of LIF, bone morphogenetic protein 4 (BMP4) enhance the self-renewal of ES cells and activate Id (inhibitor of differentiation) genes. Opposite, without LIF, BMP4 activates other signaling cascades that promote the differentiation of mouse ES cells. BMP4 also stimulates human ES cells to differentiate into trophoblast cells or mesodermal precursors [79, 161, 174, 175].

Nanog and Stat3 were found to bind to and synergistically activate Stat3-dependent promoters, moreover, Nanog binds to NFkappa B proteins and inhibits transcriptional activity of NFkappa B proteins. Endogenous NFkappa B activity and target-gene expression increased during differentiation of ES cells. Overexpression of NFkappa B proteins promoted differentiation, whereas inhibition of NF kappa B signalling, either by genetic ablation of the Ikbkg gene or overexpression of the Ikappa B alpha super-repressor, increased expression of pluripotency markers. Thus, Nanog can repress the pro-differentiation activities of NFkappaB and can cooperate with Stat3 to maintain pluripotency [176].

Although Stat-3 signaling is involved in mouse ES cell self-renewal, stimulation of this pathway does not support self-renewal of human ES cells. However, activation of the canonical Wnt pathway is sufficient to maintain self-renewal of both human and mouse ES cells. Wnt pathway activation by 6-bromoindirubin-3'-oxime (BIO), a specific pharmacological inhibitor of glycogen synthase kinase-3 (GSK-3), maintains the undifferentiated phenotype in both types of ES cells and sustains expression of the specific pluripotentcy-related transcription factors Oct4, Rex-1 and Nanog. Wnt signaling is endogenously activated in undifferentiated mouse ES cells and is downregulated upon differentiation. In addition, BIO-mediated Wnt activation is functionally reversible, as withdrawal of the compound leads to normal multilineage differentiation in human and mouse ES cells [177]. Functional screening identifies Wnt5A and Wnt6 as feeder cell-produced factors that potently inhibit ES cell differentiation in a serum-dependent manner. Furthermore, direct activation of beta-catenin without disturbing the upstream components of the Wnt/β-catenin pathway fully recapitulates the effect of Wnts on ES cells. In addition, the WNT/β-catenin pathway up-regulates the mRNA for Stat3, that suggests that LIF is able to mimic the serum effect to act synergistically with Wnt proteins to inhibit ES cell differentiation [178].

Specific signals that determine the cell fate in early embryogenesis are modulated via interactions of several signaling pathways to form a unique regulatory cell network, essential for differentiation of a certain cell type. Factors of TGFβ family (Activin, Nodal, Lefty, BMP, GDF and TGFβ) are involved in the regulation of specialization of the precursors of ecto-, endo-, and mesoderm, as well as of germline cells [179-182]. These factors are implicated in the regulation of morphogenesis, formation of polarity axes of vertebrate embryos. Factors of the TGFβ family control proliferation, differentiation, migration, adhesion and apoptosis of different cell types in adult tissues and alterations in their activity are often found in various tumors [182,183].

Previously, genetic studies demonstrated that TGFβ family signaling regulates the maintenance of pluripotent cell identity because it was shown that mouse embryos deficient in Smad4 (signal transducer in TGFβ signaling) display defective epiblast proliferation and delayed outgrowth of the inner cell mass and that Nodal-deficient mouse embryos had reduced epiblast cell population which expressed very low level of Oct4 [184-186]. Large-scale gene profiling of ES cells has revealed that TGFβ family signaling has important role in the maintance pluripotency and in cell lineages commitment [99]. Several groups demonstrated that the preserving of undifferentiated state of human ES cells requires Activin and Nodal signaling interaction with FGF2 cascade [68,187]. Inhibition of Activin and Nodal signaling by pharmacological inhibitor of receptor kinases SB-431542 resulted in a decreased expression of pluripotent cell specific genes [188]. On the contrary, hES cell treatment by BMP, TGFβ and Cripto led to the stimulation of their differentiation and the number of Oct4-positive cells was significantly decreased [68, 189]. Inhibition of signals from Activin/Nodal receptors also led to the initiation of differentiation of human ES cells even in the presence of FGF [68; 188].

The developmental fate of differentiating ES cells depends on the complex combination of growth factors and extracellular matrix proteins constituting the developmental niche in which these stem cells exist. The numerous findings suggest important parallels of TGFβ family signaling in germ layer specification between embryogenesis and ES cells in vitro differentiation systems. For instance, embryoid bodies derived from either Lefty or Cerb-S (Nodal antagonists) overexpressing human ES cells showed increased expression of neuroectoderm markers Sox1, Sox3, and Nestin. Conversely, they were negative for a definitive endoderm marker Sox17 and did not generate beating cardiomyocyte structures in conditions that allowed mesendoderm differentiation from WT hESCs. Embryoid bodies derived from either Lefty or Cerb-S expressing hES cells also contained a greater abundance of neural rosette structures as compared to controls and generated a dense network of beta-tubulin III positive neuritis. SB431542 treatments reproduced the neuralising effects of Lefty overexpression in human ES cells. These results show that inhibition of Nodal signaling promotes neuronal specification, indicating a role for this pathway in controlling early neural development of pluripotent cells [190].

On the other side, several lines of evidence have demonstrated the role of TGFβ family signaling in the development of the cardiac lineage from ES cells. BMP2 and Cripto have been shown to promote or improve cardiomiocytes differentiation but they act as stimulators of mesoderm precursor differentiation. Interestingly, transient inhibition of BMP signaling in undifferentiated ES cells by noggin dramatically induces cardiomycyte differentiation of mouse ES cells [191-193].

The embryonic stem cell differentiation system was used to define the roles of the Activin/Nodal, BMP, and canonical Wnt signaling pathways at three distinct developmental stages during hematopoietic ontogeny: induction of a primitive streak-like population, formation of Flk1(+) mesoderm, and induction of hematopoietic progenitors. It was shown that Activin/Nodal and Wnt, but not BMP, signaling is required for the induction of the primitive streak. Although BMP is not required for primitive streak induction, it displays a strong posteriorizing effect on this population. All three signaling pathways regulate induction of Flk1(+) mesoderm. The specification of Flk1(+) mesoderm to the hematopoietic lineages requires VEGF and Wnt, but not BMP or Activin/Nodal signaling. Specifically, Wnt signaling is essential for commitment of the primitive erythroid, but not the definitive lineages. These findings highlight dynamic changes in signaling requirements during different lineages' development from pluripotent stem cells [194].

Our research of the earliest stages of human and mouse ES, EG and EC differentiation is focused on the study of the interaction between different branches of TGFβ family signaling that regulate the pluripotency and specification of different embryonic cell populations and on determining which of them are impaired in malignant teratocarcinoma cells.

Comparative analysis of cell growth dynamic of mouse pluripotent ES, EG and nullipotent EC cells demonstrates that ES and EG cells and EC cells respond to serum factors and LIF in different ways [75, 195]. ES and EG cell growth was insensitive to serum factors but depended on LIF presence. After LIF withdrawal ES and EG cells initiated differentiation and their growth rate was diminished in serum containing and serum-free conditions. Cell cycle distribution test revealed that spontaneous differentiation of ES and EC cells but not EC cells was accompanied by cell accumulation in G1 phase of the cell cycle. Proportion of ES and EG cells l in G1 phase of the cell cycle went up to 11-17% after 5day LIF withdrawal and no changes were found in cell cycle distribution of EC cell population (Figure 5).

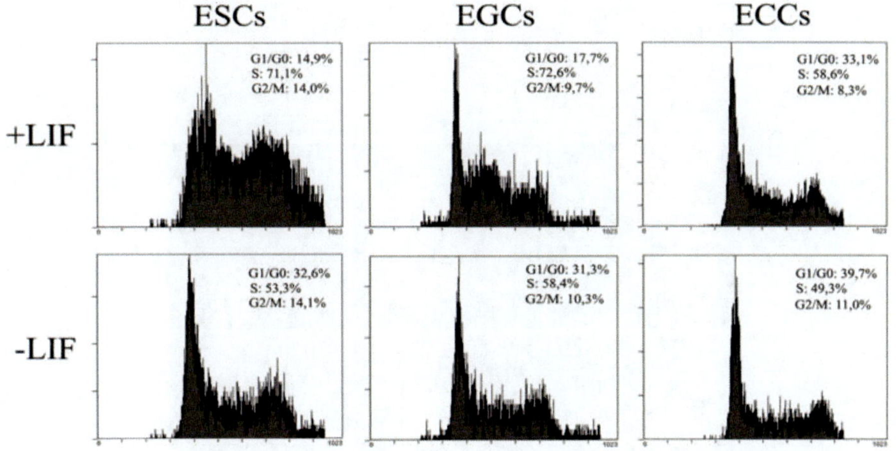

Figure 5. Cell cycle distribution in undifferentiated (+LIF) and differentiating (-LIF) ES, EG, EC cell populations. EC cells don't initiate differentiation after LIF withdrawal within 5 days.

Therewith, in spontaneously differentiating ES and EG cells the expression of Oct4, Nanog and alkaline phosphatase activity were down-regulated but the expression of markers of all three germ layers and extraembryonic endoderm GATA4, 6, AFP, Nestin, Pax6, Bry was up-regulated. On the contrary, LIF-independent EC cells reduced their proliferation rate in serum-free conditions more than twice but expression of Oct4 and alkaline phosphatase was invariable in serum and serum-free culture systems (Figure 6). We have found that in course of spontaneous differentiation of ES and EG cells expression level of ActivinA, Nodal, Lefty1, 2 and GDF3 was down regulated together with Oct4 and Nanog expression while expression of other member of TGFβ family, BMP4 and TGFβ1, was at the steady level. Interestingly, that expression of genes that are the components of TGFβ family signaling (receptors Teri, ActrI,ActrII, BmprI and signal transducers Smad2,4,5) was sensibly constant.

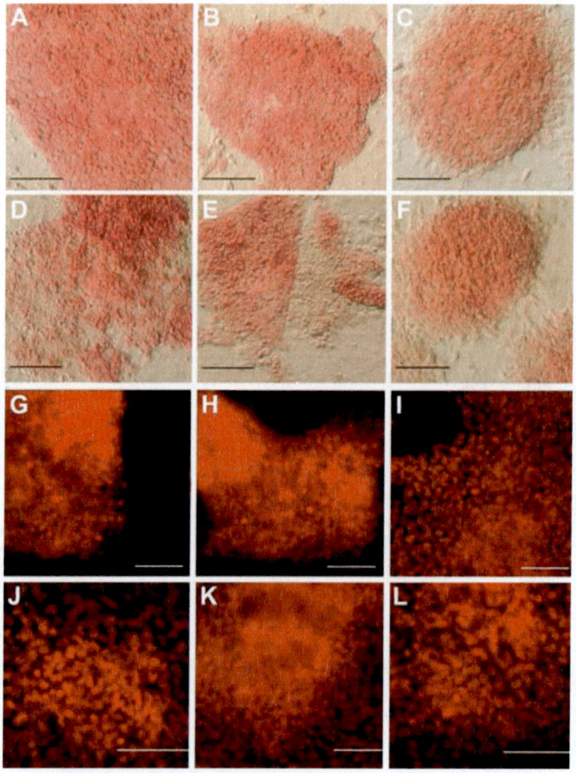

Figure 6. Activity of alkaline phosphatase (A-F) and expression of Oct4 (G-L) in mouse ES (A,D,G,F), EG (B,E,H,K) and EC(C,F,I,L) cells growing in LIF-supplemented media (A-C, G-I) and after LIF withdrawal (D-F, J-L) within 5 days. Bar, 100μm.

On the other side, in teratocarcinoma cells expression of pluripotency-related genes and GATA4, 6, Pax6 as well as signal ligands, receptors and signal transducers has not changed. We have revealed that nullipotent EC cells don't express ActivinA as apposed to pluripoten stem cells. These data indicate that malignant transformation of pluripotent stem cells to teratocarcinoma cells may be conducted with the initiation of new mechanisms regulating self-renew and differentiation which are LIF and ActivinA independent. Disturbed signaling network in EC cells results in deregulation of proliferation and differentiation balance. Note that we have revealed similar trends in transcriptional profiles of human ES and EC cells that argue for the conservative mechanism of malignant teratocarcinoma transformation [196]. However, the origin of these disturbances remains unclear and our study of these defective mechanisms will be continued in future.

Conclusion

Numerous pluripotent stem cell lines derived from different sources using different techniques demonstrate their considerable similarity in the basic biological properties as well as individual variations. More than twenty years of intense studies of the stability of different pluripotent stem cell lines demonstrated the accumulation of chromosomal and gene mutations and epigenetic alterations during their long term in vitro culture, which can lead to malignant transformation. It is generally accepted that the line stability maintenance requires continuous monitoring of the line karyotype, epigenetic profile, and carcinogenesis-associated gene mutations. One of the most important lessons that came from the recent studies of stem cells biology postulates that the deregulation of signaling pathways involved in control of self-renewal and differentiation stem cells and progenitors leads to carcinogenesis in embryonic and adult tissues. In the context of clinical use of pluripotent stem cell lines, the maintenance of the genetic and epigenetic stability is crucial for the development of safe and efficient cell technologies. Considering the high risk of carcinogenesis, the outlooks of clinical application of induced pluripotent stem cell lines still remain questionable despite relative simplicity of producing patient-specific lines. Nevertheless, the available data clearly indicate that the elucidation of the evolutionary patterns of cell lines with different genotypes and the development of techniques providing their stability in long-term in vitro cultures are the main goals in the production and application of permanent pluripotent stem cell lines. Correct studies of the basic mechanisms regulating pluripotent cell self-renewal and specialization into different cell types clearly require the validation of the main cell parameters in the model lines. This also applies to the utilization of ES cells as test systems to study the efficiency and toxicity of new drugs.

Acknowledgments

This work was supported by the Russian Foundation for Basic Research (project no. 08-04-09307).

References

[1] Evans, M. J. and Kaufman, M. H. (1981). Establishment in culture of pluripotential cells from mouse embryos. *Nature*, **292**, 154-156.

[2] Martin, G. R. (1981). Isolation of pluripotent cell line from early mouse embryo cultured in medium conditioned by teratocarcinoma stem cells. *Proc. Natl. Acad. Sci. USA*., **78**, 7634-7638.

[3] Rossant, J. (2001). Stem cells from mammalian blastocyst. *Stem Cells*, **19**, 477-482.

[4] Thomson, J. A., Itskovitz-Eldor, J., Shapiro, S. S., Waknitz, M. A., Swiergiel, J. J, Marshall, V. S. and Jones J. M. (1998). Embryonic stem cell lines derived from human blastocysts. *Science*, **282**(5391), 1145-1147.

[5] Brons, I. G., Smithers, L. E., Trotter, M. W., Rugg-Gunn, P., Sun, B., Chuva de Sousa Lopes, S. M., Howlett, S. K., Clarkson, A., Ahrlund-Richter, L., Pedersen, R, A. and Vallier, L. (2007). Derivation of pluripotent epiblast stem cells from mammalian embryos. *Nature*, **448**(7150), 191-195.

[6] Tesar, P. J,, Chenoweth, J. G,, Brook, F. A, Davies, T, J., Evans, E. P., Mack, D. L., Gardner, R. L. and McKay, R. D. (2007). New cell lines from mouse epiblast share defining features with human embryonic stem cells. *Nature*, **448**(7150), 196-199.

[7] Mitalipova, M. M., Rao, R. R. and Hoyer, D. M., et al. (2005). Preserving the genetic integrity of human embryonic stem cells. *Nat. Biotechnol*, **23**, 19-20.

[8] Thomson, J. A., Kalishman, J. and Golos, T. G. et al. (1995). Isolation of a primate embryonic stem cell line. *Proc. Natl. Acad. Sci. U S A*, **92**(17), 7844-7848.

[9] Strelchenko, N., Verlinsky, O., Kukharenko, V., Verlinsky, Y. (2004). Morula-derived human embryonic stem cells. *Reprod. Biomed. Online*, **9**(6), 623-629.

[10] Klimanskaya, I., Chung, Y. and Becker, S. et al. (2006). Human embryonic stem cell lines derived from single blastomeres. *Nature*, **444**(7118), 481-485.

[11] Nagy, A., Rossant, J. and Nagy, R. et al. (1993). Embryonic stem cells alone are able to support fetal development in the mouse. *Proc. Natl. Acad. Sci. U S A*, **90**, 8424-8428.

[12] Suemor, i. H., Tada, T. and Torii, R. et al. (2001). Establishment of embryonic stem cell lines from cynomolgus monkey blastocysts produced by IVF or ICSI. *Devel. Dyn.*, **222**, 273-279.

[13] Mitalipov, S., Kuo, H.C., Byrn, e. J. et al. (2006). Isolation and characterization of novel rhesus monkey embryonic stem cell lines. *Stem Cells*, **24**, 2177-2186.

[14] Guo, G., Yang, J., Nichols, J,, Hall, J. S., Eyres, I., Mansfield, W. and Smith, A. (2009). Klf4 reverts developmentally programmed restriction of ground state pluripotency. *Development*, **136**(7), 1063-9.

[15] Stevens, L.C. (1970). The development of transplantable teratocarcinomas from intratesticular grafts of pre- and postimplantation mouse embryos. *Dev. Biol.,* **21**, 364-382.

[16] Solter, D., Skreb, N. andmjanov, I. (1970). Extrauterine growth of mouse egg-cylinders results in malignant teratoma. *Nature*, **227**, 503-504.

[17] Matsui, Y., Zsebo, K. and Hogan, B. L. (1992). Derivation of pluripotential embryonic stem cells from murine primordial germ cells in culture. *Cell*, **70**, 841-847.

[18] Resnick, J. L., Bixler, L. S., Cheng, L. and Donovan, P. J. (1992). Long-term proliferation of mouse primordial germ cells in culture. *Nature*, **359**, 550-551.

[19] Stewart, C. L., Gadi, I. and Bhatt, H. (1994). Stem cells from primordial germ cells can reenter the germ line. *Dev. Biol.*, **161**, 626–628.

[20] Labosky, P. A., Barlow, D. P. and Hogan, B.L. (1994). Mouse embryonic germ (EG) cell lines: transmission through the germline and differences in the methylation imprint of insulin-like growth factor 2 receptor (Igf2r) gene compared with embryonic stem (ES) cell lines. *Development*, **120**, 3197–3204.

[21] Shamblott, M. J., Axelman, J., Wang. S. et al. (1998). Derivation of pluripotent stem cells from cultured human primordial germ cells. *Proc. Natl. Acad. Sci. U S A*, **95**, 13726-13731.

[22] Kanatsu-Shinohara, M., Inoue, K., Lee, J., Yoshimoto, M., Ogonuki, N., et al. (2004). Generation of pluripotent stem cells from neonatal mouse testis. *Cell*, **119**, 1001-1012.

[23] Guan, K., Nayernia, K., Maier, L. S., Wagner, S., Dressel, R., Lee, J. H., Nolte, J., Wolf, F., Li, M., Engel, W. and Hasenfuss, G. (2006). Pluripotency of spermatogonial stem cells from adult mouse testis. *Nature*, **440**, 1199-1203.

[24] Robertson, E. J., Evans, M. J. and Kaufman, M. H. (1983). X-chromosome instability in pluripotential stem cell lines derived from parthenogenetic embryos. *J. Embryol. exp. Morph.*, **74**, 297-309.

[25] Mann, J. R., Gadi, I., Harbison, M. L., Abbondanzo, S. J. and Stewart, C. L. (1990). androgenetic mouse embryonic stem cells are pluripotent and cause skeletal defects in chimeras: Implications for genetic imprinting. *Cell,* **62**, 251-260.

[26] Mann, J. R. and Stewart, C. L. (1991). Development to term of mouse androgenetic aggregation chimeras. *Development*, **113**, 1325-1333.

[27] Cibelli, J. B., Grant, K. A., Chapman, K. B. et al. (2002). Parthenogenetic stem cells in nonhuman primates. *Science*, **295**, 819.

[28] Vrana, K. E., Hipp, J. D., Goss, A.M. et al. (2003). Nonhuman primate parthenogenetic stem cells. *Proc. Natl. Acad. Sci. U S A,* **100**, 11911-11916.

[29] Lin, G., OuYang, Q., Zhou, X. et al. (2007). A highly homozygous and parthenogenetic human embryonic stem cell line derived from a one-pronuclear oocyte following in vitro fertilization procedure. *Cell Res.*, **17**(12), 999-1007.

[30] Revazova, E. S., Turovets, N. A., Kochetkova, O. D. et al. (2007). Patient-specific stem cell lines derived from human parthenogenetic blastocysts. *Cloning Stem Cells*, **9**(3), 432-449.

[31] Eckardt, S., Dinger, T. C., Kurosaka, S., Leu, N. A., Müller, A. M. and McLaughlin, K. J. (2008). In vivo and in vitro differentiation of uniparental embryonic stem cells into hematopoietic and neural cell types. *Organogenesis*, **4**(1), 33-41.

[32] Dighe, V., Clepper, L., Pedersen, D. et al. (2008). Heterozygous embryonic stem cell lines derived from nonhuman primate parthenotes. *Stem Cells*, **26**(3), 756-766.

[33] Allen, N. D., Barton, S. C., Hilton, K., Norris, M. L. and Surani, M. A. (1994). A functional analysis of imprinting in parthenogenetic embryonic stem cells. *Development,* **120**(6), 1473-82

[34] Cibelli, J. B., Stice, S. L., Golueke, P. J., et al. (1998). Transgenic bovine chimeric offspring produced from somatic cell-derived stem-like cells. *Nat. Biotechnol.*, **16**, 642-646.

[35] Kawase, E., Yamazaki, Y., Yagi, T., et al. (2000). Mouse embryonic stem (ES) cell lines established from neuronal cell-derived cloned blastocysts. *Genesis*, **28**, 156-163.

[36] Munsie, M. J., Michalska, A. E., O'Brien, C. M., et al. (2000). Isolation of pluripotent embryonic stem cells from reprogrammed adult mouse somatic cell nuclei. *Curr. Biol.*, **10**, 989-992.

[37] Wakayama, T., Tabar, V., Rodriguez, I., et al. (2001). Differentiation of embryonic stem cell lines generated from adult somatic cells by nuclear transfer. *Science*, **292**, 740-743.

[38] Wakayama, S., Jakt, M. L., Suzuki, M., et al. (2006). Equivalency of nuclear transfer-derived embryonic stem cells to those derived from fertilized mouse blastocysts. *Stem Cells*, **24**, 2023-2033.

[39] Wakayama, S., Mizutani, E. and Kishigami, S., et al. (2005). Mice cloned by nuclear transfer from somatic and ntES cells derived from the same individuals. *J. Reprod. Dev.*, **51**, 765-772.

[40] Wakayama, S., Ohta, H., Kishigami, S., et al. (2005). Establishment of male and female nuclear transfer embryonic stem cell lines from different mouse strains and tissues. *Biol. Reprod.*, **72**, 932-936.

[41] Byrne, J. A., Pedersen, D. A., Clepper, L. L., et al. (2007). Producing Primate Embryonic Stem Cells by Somatic Cell Nuclear Transfer. *Nature*, **450**, 497-505.

[42] French, A. J., Adams, C. A., anderson, L. S. et al. (2008). Development of human cloned blastocysts following somatic nuclear transfer (SCNT) with adult fibroblast. *Stem Cells*, **26**, 485-493.

[43] Cowan, C. A., Atienza, J., Melton, D. A. and Eggan, K. (2005). Nuclear reprogramming of somatic cells after fusion with human embryonic stem cells. *Science*, **309**, 1369-1373.

[44] Yu, J., Vodyanik, M. A., He, P., Slukvin, I. I., and Thomson, J. A. (2006). Human embryonic stem cells reprogram myeloid precursors following cell–cell fusion. *Stem Cells*, **24**, 168–176.

[45] Ambrosi, D. J., Tanasijevic, B., Kaur, A., Obergfell, C., O'Neill, R. J., Krueger, W., Rasmussen, T. P. (2007). Genome-wide reprogramming in hybrids of somatic cells and embryonic stem cells. *Stem Cells*, **25**(5), 1104-13.

[46] Takahashi, K., Yamanaka, S. (2006). Induction of pluripotent stem cells from mouse embryonic and adult fibroblast cultures by defined factors. *Cell*, **126**. P. 663–676.

[47] Takahashi, K., Tanabe, K., Ohnuki, V. et al. (2007). Induction of pluripotent stem cells from adult human fibroblasts by defined factors. *Cell*, **131**, 861-872.

[48] Yu, J., Vodyanik, M., Smuga-Otoo, K. et al. (2007). Induced pluripotent stem cell lines derived from human somatic cells. *Science*, **318**, 1917-1920.

[49] Lowry, W. E., Richter, L., Yachechko, R., et al. (2008). Generation of human induced pluripotent stem cells from dermal fibroblasts. *Proc. Natl. Acad. Sci.,* **105**, 2883–2888.

[50] Park, I. H., Zhao, R., West, J. A., et al. (2008). Reprogramming of human somatic cells to pluripotency with defined factors. *Nature*, **451**,141–146.

[51] Aoi, T., Yae, K., Nakagawa, M., et al. (2008). Generation of pluripotent stem cells from adult mouse liver and stomach cells. *Science*, **321**(5889), 699-702.

[52] Hanna, J., Markoulaki, S., Schorderet, P., et al. (2008). Direct reprogramming of terminally differentiated mature B lymphocytes to pluripotency. *Cell*, **133**(2), 250-64.

[53] Maherali, N., Sridharan, R., Xie, W. et al.(2007). Directly reprogrammed fibroblasts show global epigenetic remodeling and widespread tissue contribution. *Cell Stem Cell*, **1**, 55–70.

[54] Okita, K., Ichisaka, T. and Yamanaka, S. (2007). Generation of germ-line competent induced pluripotent stem cells. *Nature*, **448**, 13–317.

[55] Nakagawa, M., Koyanagi1, M., Tanabe, K. et al. (2008). Generation of induced pluripotent stem cells without Myc from mouse and human fibroblasts. *Nat. Biotech.*, **26**, 101-106.

[56] Kleinsmith, L. J. and Pierce, G. B. (1964). Multipotentiality of single embryonal carcinoma cells. *Cancer Res.*, **24**, 1544–1552.

[57] Hogan, B., Fellows, M., Avner, P. and Jacob, F. (1977) Isolation of a human teratoma cell line which expresses F9 antigen. *Nature*, **270**, 515–518.

[58] Lee, V. M.-Y. and andrews, P. W. (1986). Differentiation of NTERA-2 clonal human embryonal carcinoma cells into neurons involves the induction of all three neuro. Lament proteins. *J. Neurosci.,* **6**, 514–521.

[59] Rossant, J. and McBurney, M.W (1982). The developmental potential of a euploid male teratocarcinoma cell line after blastocyst injection. *J Embryol Exp Morphol*, **70**, 99-112.

[60] andrews, P. W. (2002). From teratocarcinomas to embryonic stem cells. *Philos Trans R Soc Lond B Biol Sci.*, **357**, 405-417.

[61] Blelloch, R. H., Hochedlinger, K., Yamada, Y., Brennan, C., Kim, M., Mintz, B., Chin, L. and Jaenisch, R. (2004). Nuclear cloning of embryonal carcinoma cells. *Proc Natl Acad Sci U S A,* **101**, 13985-13990.

[62] Xu, C., Inokuma M. S., Denham J. et al. (2001). Feeder-free growth of undifferentiated human embryonic stem cells. *Nat Biotechnol.*, **19**(10), 971-974.

[63] Xu, C., Jiang, J., Sottile V. et al. (2004). Immortalized fibroblast-like cells derived from human embryonic stem cells support undifferentiated cell growth. *Stem Cells*, **22**(6), 972-980.

[64] Xu, C., Rosler E., Jiang J. et al. (2005). Basic fibroblast growth factor supports undifferentiated human embryonic stem cell growth without conditioned medium. *Stem Cells*, **23**(3), 315-323.

[65] Hovatta, O., Mikkola, M., Gertow, K. et al. (2003). A culture system using human foreskin fibroblasts as feeder cells allows production of human embryonic stem cells. *Hum. Reprod.*, **18**, 1404-1409.

[66] Rosler, E. S., Fisk, G. J., Ares, X. et al. (2004). Long-term culture of human embryonic stem cells in feeder-free conditions. *Dev. Dyn.*, **229**, 259-274.

[67] Beattie, G. M., Lopez, A. D., Bucay, N. et al. (2005) Activin A maintains pluripotency of human embryonic stem cells in the absence of feeder layers. *Stem Cells*, **23**, 489-495.

[68] Vallier, L., Alexander, M. and Pedersen, R. A. (2005). Activin/Nodal and FGF pathways cooperate to maintain pluripotency of human embryonic stem cells. *J. Cell Sci.,* **118**, 4495-4509.

[69] Bigdeli, N., andersson, M. and Strehl, R. et al. (2008). Adaptation of human embryonic stem cells to feeder-free and matrix-free culture conditions directly on plastic surfaces. *J. Biotechnol.,* **133**(1), 146-153.

[70] Przyborski, S. A. (2005). Differentiation of Human Embryonic Stem Cells After Transplantation in Immune-Deficient Mice. *Stem Cells*, **23**, 1242-1250.

[71] Gordeeva, O.F. Pluripotent cells in embryogenesis and in teratoma formation. In: Parsons D.W, editor. *Stem cells and cancer*. N.Y.: Nova Sci. Publ. Ink.; 2007; 62-85.

[72] Ramalho-Santos, M., Yoon, S., Matsuzaki, Y., Mulligan, R. C. andFigureMelton, D. A. (2002). «Stemness»: transcriptional profiling of embrionic and adult stem cells. *Science*, **298**, 597-600.

[73] Sato, N., Sanjuan, I. M., Heke, M., et al. (2003). Molecular signature of human embryonic stem cells and its comparison with the mouse. *Dev. Biol.,* **260**, 404-413.

[74] Gordeeva, O. F., Krasnikova, N. Yu., Larionova, A. V., et al. (2006). Analysis of Expression of Genes Specific for Pluripotent and Primordial Germ Cells in Human and Mouse Embryonic Stem Cell Lines. *Dokl. Akad. Nauk*, **406**(6), 835-839.

[75] Gordeeva, O. F., Lifantzeva, N. V. and Nikonova, T. M. (2009). Regulation of in vitro and in vivo differentiation of embryonic stem, embryonic germ and teratocarcinomal cell by factors of TGFβ family. *Ontogenez*, **40**(6), 403-418.

[76] Adewumi, O., Aflatoonian, B., Ahrlund-Richter, L. et al. (2007). Characterization of human embryonic stem cell lines by the International Stem Cell Initiative. *Nat. Biotech.*, **25**, 803-816.

[77] Sharova, L. V., Sharov, A. A., Piao, Y., et al. (2007). Global gene expression profiling reveals similarities and differences among mouse pluripotent stem cells of different origins and strains. *Dev Biol.* **307**(2), 446-59.

[78] Chin, M. H., Mason, M. J., Xie, W., et al. (2009). Induced pluripotent stem cells and embryonic stem cells are distinguished by gene expression signatures. *Cell Stem Cells*, **5**(1), 111-23.

[79] Gerami-Naini, B., Dovzhenk, O. V., Durning, M. et al. (2004). Trophoblast differentiation in embryoid bodies derived from human embryonic stem cells. *Endocrinology*, **145**, 1517-1524.

[80] Fang, D., Leishear, K., Nguyen,T. K. et al. (2006). Defining the conditions for the generation of melocytes from human embryonic stem cells. *Stem Cells*, **24**, 1668-1677.

[81] Mitalipov, S., Kuo, H.C., Byrne, J. et al. (2006). Isolation and characterization of novel rhesus monkey embryonic stem cell lines. *Stem Cells*, **24**, 2177-2186.

[82] Schwanke, K., Wunderlich, S., Reppel, M. et al. (2006). Generation and characterization of functional cardiomyocytes from rhesus monkey embryonic stem cells. *Stem Cells*, **24**, 1423-1432.

[83] Shin, S., Mitalipova, M., Noggle, S., et al. (2006). Long-term proliferation of human embryonic stem cell–derived neuroepithelial cells using defined adherent culture conditions. *Stem Cells*, **24**, 125-138.

[84] Taylor, R. A., Cowin, P. A. and Cunha, G. R. et al. (2006). Formation of human prostate tissue from embryomic stem cells. *Nat. Methods.*, **3**, 179-181.

[85] Rajesh, D., Chinnasamy, N., M. Mitalipov, S. M. et al. (2007). Differential Requirements for Hematopoietic Commitment Between Human andRhesus Embryonic Stem Cells. *Stem Cells*, **25**, 490-499.

[86] Savatier, P., Huang, S., Szekely, L., et al. (1994). Contrasting patterns of retinoblastoma protein expression in mouse embryonic stem cells and embryonic fibroblasts. *Oncogene*, **9**, 809-818.

[87] Savatier, P., Lapillonne, H., Grunsven van, L.A., et al. (1996). Withdrawal of differentiation inhibitory activity/leukemia inhibitory factor up-regulates D type cyclins and cyclin-dependent kinase inhibitors in mouse embryonic stem cells. *Oncogene*, **12**, 309-322.

[88] Burdon, T., Smith, A. and Savatier, P. (2002). Signaling, cell cycle and pluripotency in embryonic stem cells. *Trends Cell Biol.*, **12**, 432-438.

[89] Fluckiger, A. C., Marcy, G., Marchand, M., et al. (2006). Cell cycle features of primate embryonic stem cells. *Stem Cells*, **24**, 547-556.

[90] Becker, K. A., Stein, J. L., Lian, J. B., et al. (2007). Establishment of histone gene regulation and cell cycle checkpoint control in human embryonic stem cells. *J. Cell Physiol.*, **210**, 517-526.

[91] Burdon, T., Stracey, C., Chambers, I., et al. (1999). Suppression of SHP-2 and ERK signaling promotes self-renewal of mouse embryonic stem cells. *Dev. Biol.,* **210**, 30–43.

[92] Jirmanova, L., Afanassieff, M., Gobert-Gosse, S., et al. (2002). Differential contributions of ERK and PI3-kinase to the regulation of cyclin D1 expression and to the control of the G1/S transition in mouse embryonic stem cells. *Oncogene*, **21**, 515–5528.

[93] Paling, N. R., Wheadon, H., Bone, H. K., et al. (2004). Regulation of embryonic stem cell self-renewal by phosphoinositide 3-kinase-dependent signaling. *J. Biol. Chem.,* **279**, 48063– 48070.

[94] Takahashi, K., Mitsui, K. and Yamanaka, S. (2003). Role of ERas in promoting tumourlike properties in mouse embryonic stem cells. *Nature*, **423**, 541–545.

[95] Dannenberg, J. H., van Rossum, A., Schuijff, L., et al. (2000). Ablation of the retinoblastoma gene family deregulates G(1) control causing immortalization and increased cell turnover under growth-restricting conditions. *Genes Dev.*, **14**, 3051–3064.

[96] Sage, J., Mulligan, G. J., Attardi, L. D., et al. (2000). Targeted disruption of the three Rb-related genes leads to loss of G(1) control and immortalization. *Genes Dev.*, **14**, 3037–3050.

[97] White, J., Stead, E. and Faast, R., et al. (2005). Developmental activation of the Rb-E2F pathway and establishment of cell cycle regulated Cdk activity during embryonic stem cell differentiation. *Mol. Biol. Cell*, **16**, 2018 –2027.

[98] Stead, E., White, J., Faast, R., et al. (2002). Pluripotent cell division cycles are driven by ectopic Cdk2, cyclin A/E and E2F activities. *Oncogene*, **21**, 8320–8333.

[99] Brandenberger, R., Wei, H., Zhang, S. et al. (2004). Transcriptome characterization elucidates signaling networks that control human ES cell growth and differentiation. *Nat. Biotechnol.*, **22**(6), 707-716.

[100] Miura, T., Luo, Y., Khrebtukova, I. et al. (2004). Monitoring early differentiation events in human embryonic stem cells by massively parallel signature sequencing and expressed sequence tag scan. *Stem Cells Devel.*, **13**, 694–715.

[101] Zeng X. (2007). Human embryonic stem cells: mechanisms to escape replicative senescence? *Stem Cell Rev.,* **3**, 270-279.

[102] Neganova, I., Zhang, X., Atkinson, S.and Lako, M. (2009). Expression and functional analysis of G1 to S regulatory components reveals an important role for CDK2 in cell cycle regulation in human embryonic stem cells. *Oncogene*, **28**(1), 20-30.

[103] Zhang, X., Neganova, I., Przyborski, S., et al. (2009). A role for NANOG in G1 to S transition in human embryonic stem cells through direct binding of CDK6 and CDC25A. *J. Cell Biol.,* **184**(1), 67-82.

[104] Lin, T., Chao, C., Saito, S., et al. (2005). p53 induces differentiation of mouse embryonic stem cells by suppressing Nanog expression. *Nat. Cell Biol.*, **7**, 165–171.

[105] Saretzki, G., Armstrong, L., Leake, A., et al. (2004). Stress defense in murine embryonic stem cells is superior to that of various differentiated murine cells. *Stem Cells*, **22**(6), 962-971.

[106] Saretzki, G., Walter, T., Atkinson, S., et al. (2008). Downregulation of multiple stress defense mechanisms during differentiation of human embryonic stem cells. *Stem Cells*, **26**(2), 455-464.

[107] Brimble, S. N., Zeng, X., Weiler, D. A., et al. (2004). Karyotypic stability, genotyping, differentiation, feeder-free maintenance, and gene expression sampling in three human embryonic stem cell lines derived prior to August 9, 2001. *Stem Cells Dev.*, **13**, 585-597.

[108] Cowan, C. A., Klimanskaya, I., McMahon, J. et al. (2004). Derivation of embryonic stem-cell lines from human blastocysts. *N. Engl. J. Med.,* **50**, 1353-1356.

[109] Draper, J. S., Smith, K., Gokhale, P., et al. (2004). Recurrent gain of chromosomes 17q and 12 in cultured human embryonic stem cells. *Nat. Biotechnol.*, **22**, 53-54.

[110] Inzunza, J., Sahlen, S., Holmberg, K., et al. (2004). Comparative genomic hybridization and karyotyping of human embryonic stem cells reveals the occurence of an isodicentric X chromosome after long-term cultivation. *Mol. Hum. Reprod.*, **10**, 461-466.

[111] Hanson, C. and Caisander, G.. (2005). Human embryonic stem cells and chromosome stability. *Apmis*, **113**, 751-755.

[112] Maitra, A., Arking, D. E. and Shivapurkar, N., et al. (2005). Genomic alterations in cultured human embryonic stem cells. *Nat. Genet.,* **37**, 1099-1103.

[113] Mitalipova, M. M., Rao, R. R., Hoyer, D. M., et al. (2005). Preserving the genetic integrity of human embryonic stem cells. *Nat. Biotechnol.,* **23**, 19-20.

[114] Lakshmipathy, U., Pelacho, B., Sudo, K., et al. (2004). Efficient transfection of embronic and adult stem cells. *Stem Cells*, **22**, 531-543.

[115] Plaia, T. W., Josephson, R., Liu, Y., et al. (2005). Characterization of a new NIH registers variant human embryonic stem cell line BG01V: a tool for human embryonic stem cell research. *Stem Cells*, **24**, 531-546.

[116] Heins, N., Englund, M. C., Sjoblom, C., et al. (2004). Derivation, characterization, and differentiation of human embryonic stem cells. *Stem Cells*, **22**, 367-376.

[117] Kim, S. J., Lee, J. E., Park, J. H. et al. (2005). Efficient derivation of new human embryonic stem cell lines. *Mol. Cells*, **19**, 46-53.

[118] Caisander, G., Park, H., Frej, K. et al. (2006). Chromosomal integrity maintained in five human embryonic stem cell lines after prolonged in vitro culture. *Chromosome Res*, **14**, 131-137.

[119] Lavon, N., Narwani, K., Golan-Lev, et al. (2008). Derivation of euploid human embryonic stem cells from aneuploid embryos. *Stem Cells*, **7**, 1874-82.

[120] Thomson, A., Wojtacha, D., Hewitt, Z., et al. Human embryonic stem Buzzard, J. J., Gough, N. M., Crook, J. M. and Colman A. (2004). Karyotype of human ES cells during extended culture. *Nat. Biotechnol.*, **22**, 381-382.

[121] cells passaged using enzymatic methods retain a normal karyotype and express CD30. *Cloning Stem Cells*, **10**(1), 89-106.

[122] Enver, T., Soneji, S., Joshi, C., et al. (2005). Cellular differentiation hierarchics in normal and culture-adapted human embryonic stem cells. *Hum. Mol. Genet.,* **14**, 3129-3140.

[123] Herszfeld, D., Wolvetang, E., Langton-Bunker, E., et al. (2006). CD30 is a survival factor and a biomarker for tranformed human pluripotent stem cells. *Nat. Biotechnol.*, **24**, 351-357.

[124] Skotheim, R. I., Monni, O. and Mousses, S., et al. (2002). New insights into testicular germ cell tumorigenesis from gene expression profiling. *Cancer Res.*, **62**, 2359-2364.

[125] Clark, A. T., Rodrigues, R. T. and Bodnar, M. S., et al. (2004). Human STELLAR, NANOG, and GDF3 genes are expressed in pluripotent cellsand map to chromosome 12p13, a hotspot for teratocarcinoma. *Stem Cells*, **22**, 169-179.
[126] Westermann, F. and Schwab, M. (2002). Genetic parameters of neuroblastomas. *Cancer Lett.*, **184**, 127-147.
[127] Secombe, J., Pierce, S. B. and Eisenman, R. N. (2004). Myc: a weapon of mass destruction. *Cell*, **117**, 153-156.
[128] Miura, M., Miura, Y. and Padilla-Nash, H. M. et al. (2005). Accumulated chromosomal instability in murin bone marrow mesenchymal stem cells leads to malignant transformation. *Stem Cells,* **24**, 1095-1103.
[129] Onyango, P., Jiang S. and Uejima, H. et al. (2002). Monoallelic expression and methylation of imprinted genes in human and mouse embryonic germ cell lineages. *Proc. Natl. Acad. Sci.* U S A, **99**, 10599-10604.
[130] Jaenisch, R., and Bird, A. (2003). Epigenetic regulation of gene expression: how the genome integrates intrinsic and environmental signals. *Nat. Genet.*, **33**, 245-254.
[131] van Gurp, R. J., Oosterhuis, J. W. and Kalscheuer, V., et al. (1994). Biallelic expression of the H19 and IGF2 genes in human testicular germ cell tumors. *J. Natl. Cancer Inst.*, **86**, 1070-1075.
[132] Szabo, P. E. and Mann, J. R. (1995). Biallelic expression of imprinted genes in the mouse germ line: implications for erasure, establishment, and mechanisms of genomic imprinting. *Genes Devel.*, **9**, 1857-1868.
[133] Nonomura, N., Miki, T. and Nishimura, K., et al. (1997). Altered imprinting of the H19 and insulin-like growth factor II genes in testicular tumors. *J. Urol.,* **157**, 1977-1979.
[134] Nakagawa, H., Chadwick, R. B., Peltomaki, P., et al. (2001). Loss of imprinting of the insulin-like growth factor II gene occurs by biallelic methylation in a core region of H19-associated CTCF-binding sites in colorectal cancer. *Proc. Natl. Acad. Sci. U S A*, **98**, 591-596.
[135] Takai, D., Gonzales, F.A., Tsai, Y.C., et al. (2001). Large scale mapping of methylcytosines in CTCF-binding sites in the human H19 promoter and aberrant hypomethylation in human bladder cancer. *Hum. Mol. Genet.*, **10**, 2619-2626.
[136] Cui, H., Onyango, P., Brandenburg, S., et al. (2002). Loss of imprinting in colorectal cancer linked to hypomethylation of H19 and IGF2. *Cancer Res.,* **62**, 6442-6446.
[137] Hernandez, L., Kozlov, S., Piras, G. and Stewar, C. L. (2003). Paternal and maternal genomes confer opposite effects on proliferation, cell-cycle length,

senescence, and tumor formation. *Proc. Natl. Acad. Sci. U S A,* **100**, 13344-13349.

[138] Ulaner, G. A., Vu, T. H., Li, T., et al. (2003). Loss of imprinting of IGF2 and H19 in osteosarcoma is accompanied by reciprocal methylation changes of a CTCF-binding site. *Hum. Mol. Genet.*, **12**, 535-549.

[139] Feinberg, A. P. and Tycko, B. (2004). The history of cancer epigenetics. *Nat. Rev. Cancer*, **4**, 143-153.

[140] Nicholls, R. D. and Knepper, J. L. (2001). Genome organization, function, and imprinting in Prader-Willi and Angelman syndromes. *Annu. Rev. Genomics Hum. Genet*, **2**, 153-175.

[141] Weksberg, R., Smith, A. C., Squire, J. and Sadowski, P. (2003). Beckwith-Wiedemann syndrome demonstrates a role for epigenetic control of normal development. *Hum. Mol. Genet.*, **12**, 61-68.

[142] Soejima, H. and Wagstaff, J. (2005). Imprinting centers, chromatin structure, and disease. *J. Cell Biochem.*, **95**, 226-233.

[143] Okano, M., Bell, D. W., Haber and D. A., Li, E. (1999). DNA methyltransferases Dnmt3a and Dnmt3b are essential for de novo methylation and mammalian development. *Cell*, **99(**3), 247-257.

[144] Xu, G. L., Bestor, T. H., Bourc'his, D., et al. (1999). Chromosome instability and immunodeficiency syndrome caused by mutations in a DNA methyltransferase gene. *Nature*, **402** (6758), 187-191.

[145] Fujimoto, A., Mitalipov, S. M., Clepper, L. L. and Wolf, D. P. (2005). Development of a monkey model for the study of primate genomic imprinting. *Mol. Hum. Reprod.* , **11**, 413-422.

[146] Rugg-Gunn, P. J., Ferguson-Smith, A. C. and Pedersen, R. A. (2005). Epigenetic status of human embryonic stem cells. *Nat. Genet*, **37**, 585-587.

[147] Sun, B. W., Yang, A. C., Feng, Y., et al. (2006). Temporal and parental-specific expression of imprinted genes in a newly derived Chinese human embrionic stem cell line and embryoid bodies. *Hum. Mol. Genet.*, **15**, 65-75.

[148] Mitalipov, S., Clepper, L., Sritanaudomchai, H., et al. (2007). Methylation status of imprinting centers for H19/IGF2 and SNURF/SNRPN in primate embryonic stem cells. *Stem Cells*, **25**, 581-588.

[149] Burbee, D. G., Forgacs, E., Zochbauer-Muller, S., et al. (2001). Epigenetic inactivation of RASSF1A in lung and breast cancers and malignant phenotype suppression. *J. Natl. Cancer Inst.,* **93**, 691-699.

[150] Bhattacharia, B., Miura, T., Brandenberger, R., et al. (2004). Gene expression in human embryonic stem cell lines: unique molecular signature. *Blood*, **103**(8), 2956-2961.

[151] Rao, R. R., Calhoun, J. D., Qin, X., et al. (2004). Comparative transcriptional profiling of two human embryonic stem cell lines. *Biotech. Bioengin.*, **88**(3), 273-286.

[152] Skottman, H., Mikkola, M., Lundin, K., et al. (2005). Gene expression signatures of seven individual human embryonic stem cell lines. *Stem Cells,* **23**, 343-1356.

[153] Ohm, J. E., McGarvey, K. M., Yu, X., et al. (2007). A stem cell–like chromatin pattern may predispose tumor suppressor genes to DNA hypermethylation and heritable silencing. *Nat. Genet.*, **39**, 237-242.

[154] Hoffman, L. M., Hall, L., Batten, J. L., et al. (2005). X-inactivation status varies in human embryonic stem cell lines. *Stem Cells*, **23**, 1468-1478.

[155] Palmieri, S. L., Peter, W., Hess, H. and Scholer, H.R. (1994). Oct-4 transcription factor is differentially expressed in the mouse embryo during establishment of the first two extraembryonic cell lineages involved in implantation. *Dev. Biol.,* **166**, 259-267.

[156] Niwa, H., Miyazaki. J. and Smith, A.G. (2000). Quantitative expression of Oct-3/4 defines differentiation, dedifferentiation or self-renewal of ES cells. *Nat. Genet.*, **24**, 372-376.

[157] Boiani, M. and Schöler, H. R. (2005). Regulatory networks in embryo-derived pluripotent stem cells. *Nat. Rev. Mol. Cell Biol.*, **6,** 872-884.

[158] Chambers, I., Colby, D., Robertson, M., Nichols, J., Lee, S., Tweedie, S. and Smith, A. (2003). Functional expression cloning of Nanog, a pluripotency sustaining factor in embryonic stem cells. *Cell*, **113**, 643-655.

[159] Mitsui, K., Tokuzawa, Y., Itoh, H., Segawa, K., Murakami, M., Takahashi, K., Maruyama, M., Maeda, M. and Yamanaka, S. (2003). The homeoprotein Nanog is required for maintenance of pluripotency in mouse epiblast and ES cells. *Cell*, **113**, 631-642.

[160] Hart, A. H., Hartley, L., Ibrahim, M. and Robb, L. (2004). Identification, cloning and expression analysis of the pluripotency promoting Nanog genes in mouse and human. *Dev Dyn.*, **230**, 187-198.

[161] Chambers, I. and Smith, A. (2004). Self-renewal of teratocarcinoma and embryonic stem cells. *Oncogene*, **23**, 7150-7160.

[162] Niwa, H., Ogawa, K., Shimosato, D. and Adachi, K. (2009). A parallel circuit of LIF signalling pathways maintains pluripotency of mouse ES cells. *Nature*, **460**(7251), 118-22.

[163] Josefson, R., Ording, J. C., Liu, Y., et al. (2007). Qualification of Embryonal Carcinoma 2102Ep As a Reference for Human Embryonic Stem Cell Research. *Stem Cells*, **25**, 437–446.

[164] Monk, M. and Holding, C. (2001). Human embryonic genes re-expressed in cancer cells. *Oncogene,* **20**, 8085-8091

[165] Nakatake, Y., Fukui, N., Iwamatsu, Y., et al. (2006). Klf4 cooperates with Oct3/4 and Sox2 to activate the Lefty1 core promoter in embryonic stem cells. *Mol. Cell Biol.*, **20**, 7772-82.

[166] Boyer, L. A., Plath, K. and Zeitlinger, J., et al. (2006). Polycomb complexes repress developmental regulators in murine embryonic stem cells. *Nature*, **441**, 349-353.

[167] Lee, T. I., Jenner, R. G., Boyer, L. A., et al. (2006). Control of developmental regulators by Polycomb in human embryonic stem cells. *Cell*, **125**, 301-313.

[168] Jones, P. A., Stephen B. and Baylin, S. B. (2007). The Epigenomics of Cancer. *Cell*, **128**, 683–692.

[169] Smith, A. G., Heath, J. K., Donaldson, D. D., Wong, G. G., Moreau, J., Stahl, M. and Rogers, D. (1988). Myeloid leukaemia inhibitory factor maintains the developmental potential of embryonic stem cells. *Nature*, **336**, 684-687.

[170] Boeuf, H., Hauss, C., Graeve, F. D., Baran, N. and Kedinger, C. (1997). Leukemia inhibitory factor-dependent transcriptional activation in embryonic stem cells. *J Cell Biol.,* **138**, 1207-1217.

[171] . Niwa, H., Burdon, T., Chambers, I. and Smith, A. (1998). Self-renewal of pluripotent embryonic stem cells is mediated via activation of STAT3. *Genes Dev.*, **12**, 2048-2060.

[172] Nichols, J., Davidson, D., Taga, T., Yoshida, K., Chambers, I. and Smith, A. (1996). Complementary tissue-specific expression of LIF and LIF-receptor mRNAs in early mouse embryogenesis. *Mech Dev.*, **57**, 123-131.

[173] Daheron, L., Opitz, S. L., Zaehres, H., Lensch, W. M., andrews, P. W., Itskovitz-Eldor, J. and Daley, G. Q. (2004). LIF/STAT3 signaling fails to maintain self-renewal of human embryonic stem cells. *Stem Cells*, **22**, 770-778.

[174] Ying, Q. L., Nichols, J., Chambers, I. and Smith, A. (2003). BMP induction of Id proteins suppresses differentiation and sustains embryonic stem cell self-renewal in collaboration with STAT3. *Cell*, **115**, 281-292.

[175] Schuldiner, M., Yanuka, O., Itskovitz-Eldor, J., Melton, D. A. and Benvenisty, N. (2000). Effects of eight growth factors on the differentiation of cells derived from human embryonic stem cells. *Proc Natl Acad Sci* U S *A,* **97**, 11307-11312.

[176] Torres, J. and Watt, F. M. (2008). Nanog maintains pluripotency of mouse embryonic stem cells by inhibiting NFkappaB and cooperating with Stat3. *Nat Cell Biol.*, **10**(2), 194-201.

[177] Sato, N., Meijer, L., Skaltsounis, L., Greengard, P. and Brivanlou, A. H. (2004). Maintenance of pluripotency in human and mouse embryonic stem cells through activation of Wnt signaling by a pharmacological GSK-3-specific inhibitor. *Nat Med.*, **10**, 55-63.

[178] Hao, J., Li, T. G., Qi, X., Zhao, D. F. and Zhao, G. Q. (2006). WNT/beta-catenin pathway up-regulates Stat3 and converges on LIF to prevent differentiation of mouse embryonic stem cells. *Dev Biol.*, **290**, 81-91.

[179] Saijoh, Y., Adachi, H., Mochida, K., Ohishi, S., Hirao, A. and Hamada, H. (1999). Distinct transcriptional regulatory mechanisms underlie left-right asymmetric expression of lefty-1 and lefty-2. *Genes Dev.*, **13**, 259-269.

[180] Tremblay, K. D., Dunn, N. R. and Robertson, E. J. (2001). *Mouse embryos lacking Smad1* signals display defects in extra-embryonic tissues and germ cell formation. *Development*, **128**, 3609-3621.

[181] Panchision, D. M., Pickel, J. M., Studer, L., Lee, S. H., Turner, P. A., Hazel, T. G. and McKay, R. D. (2001). Sequential actions of BMP receptors control neural precursor cell production and fate. *Genes Dev.*, **15**(16), 2094-2110.

[182] Vincent, S. D., Dunn, N. R., Hayashi, S., Norris, D. P., Robertson, E. J. (2003). Cell fate decisions within the mouse organizer are governed by graded Nodal signals. *Genes Dev.,* **17**, 1646-1662.

[183] Derynck, R., Akhurst, R. J. and Balmain, A. (2001). TGF-β signaling in tumor suppression anf cancer progression. *Nat. Genet.,* **29**, 117-129.

[184] Sirard, C., de la Pompa, J. L., Elia, A., et al. (1998). The tumor suppressor gene Smad4/Dpc4 is required for gastrulation and later for anterior development of the mouse embryo. *Genes Dev.*, **12**, 107-119.

[185] Conlon, F. L., Lyons, K .M., Takaesu, N., et al. (1994). A primary requirement for nodal in the formation and maintenance of the primitive streak in the mouse. *Development*, **120**, 1919-1928.

[186] Robertson, E. J., Norris, D. P., Brennan, J. and Bikoff, E. K. (2003). Control of early anterior-posterior patterning in the mouse embryo by TGF-β signaling. *Philos. Trans. R. Soc. Lond. B Biol. Sci.*, **358**, 1351-1357.

[187] Beattie, G. M., Lopez, A. D., Bucay, et al. (2005). Activin A maintains pluripotency of human embryonic stem cells in the absence of feeder layers. *Stem Cells*, **23**, 489-495,

[188] James D, Levine A, J., Besser, D. and Hemmati-Brivanlou, A. (2005). TGFbeta/activin/nodal signaling is necessary for the maintenance of

pluripotency in human embryonic stem cells. *Development*, **132**, 1273-1282.

[189] Xu, R. H., Peck, R. M., Li, D. S., et al. (2005). Basic FGF and suppression of BMP signaling sustain undifferentiated proliferation of human ES cells. *Nat. Methods.*, **2**, 185-190.

[190] Smith, J. R., Vallier, L., Lupo, G., Alexander, M., Harris, W. A. and Pedersen, R. A. (2008). Inhibition of Activin/Nodal signaling promotes specification of human embryonic stem cells into neuroectoderm. *Dev Biol.*, **313**(1), 107-17.

[191] Parisi, S., D'andrea, D., Lago, C. T., Adamson, E. D., Persico, M. G. and Minchiotti, G. (2003). Nodal-depend Cripto signaling promotes cardiomyogenesis and redirects the neural fate of embryonic stem cells. *J. Cell Biol.*, **163**, 303-314.

[192] Kawai, T., Takahashi, T., Esaki, M., Ushikoshi, H., Nagano, S., Fujiwara, H. and Kosai, K. (2004). Efficient cardiomyogenic differentiation of embryonic stem cells by fibroblast growth factor 2 and bone morphogenetic proteins 2. *Circ. J.*, **68**, 691-702.

[193] Yuasa, S., Itabashi, Y., Coshimizu, U., Tanaka, T., Sugimura, K., Kinoshita, M., Hattori, F., Fukami, S., Shimazaki, T., Okano, H., et al. (2005). Transient inhibition of BMP signaling by Noggin induces cardiomyocyte differentiation of mouse embryonic stem cells. *Nat. Biotechnol.*, **23**, 607-611.

[194] Nostro, M. C., Cheng, X., Keller, G. M. and Gadue, P. (2008). Wnt, activin and BMP signaling regulate distinct stages in the developmental pathway from embryonic stem cells to blood. *Cell Stem Cell.*, **2**(1), 60-71.

[195] Krasnikova. N. Iu. and Gordeeva, O. F. (2007). Comparative analysis of expression of TGFbeta family factors and their receptors in mouse embryonic stem and embryonic teratocarcinoma cells. *Ontogenez*, **38**(2), 126-135.

[196] Krasnikova, N. Y. and Gordeeva, O. F. (2006). Nodal signaling in the regulation of pluripotent state ofhuman and mouse ES and EC cells. *FEBS*, **273**(suppl 1), 126.

In: Pluripotent Stem Cells
Editors: D.W. Rosales et al, pp. 47-79
ISBN: 978-1-60876-738-0

Chapter 2

MOLECULAR MECHANISM INVOLVED IN THE MAINTENANCE OF PLURIPOTENT STEM CELLS

Raymond Ching-Bong Wong[1], Peter J. Donovan[1,2] and Alice Pébay[3]

[1]Department of Biological Chemistry,
[2]Department of Developmental and Cell biology, University of California Irvine, Irvine, CA 92697, USA
[3]Centre for Neuroscience, Department of Pharmacology The University of Melbourne, Parkville, Vic 3010, Australia and Bernard O'Brien Institute, Fitzroy, VIC 3065, Australia.

Abstract

The idea of growing human cells *in vitro* to yield a renewable source of cells for transplantation has captured the imagination of scientists for many years. The derivation of human embryonic stem cells (hESC) represented a major milestone in achieving this goal. hESC are pluripotent and can proliferate *in vitro* indefinitely, rendering them an ideal source for cell replacement therapy. Moreover, recent advances in reprogramming somatic cells into induced pluripotent stem cells (iPS cells) have enabled us to unravel some of the key master regulators of stem cell pluripotency. By integrating recent findings of molecular mechanism involved in maintenance of these different pluripotent stem cell types, we aim to present a global picture of how extracellular signals, intracellular signal transduction pathways and transcriptional networks cooperate together to determine the cell fate of pluripotent stem cells. Unraveling the signaling networks that control stem cell pluripotency will be helpful in deriving novel methods to maintain these pluripotent stem cells *in vitro*.

Introduction

Human embryonic stem cells (hESC) were originally derived from the inner cell mass of human blastocysts (Thomson, Itskovitz-Eldor et al. 1998; Reubinoff, Pera et al. 2000). They possess the remarkable ability to self-renew indefinitely *in vitro* while maintaining the potential to differentiate into cells representative of the three primary germ layers (Pera, Reubinoff et al. 2000). hESC have great potential for regenerative medicine, and serve as a great model to study the underlying mechanisms of self-renewal and differentiation during human embryo development. Recently, several signaling pathways have emerged to be important players in the maintenance of hESC pluripotency. Moreover, the development of induced pluripotent stem cells˙(iPS cells) has demonstrated that several key 'stemness' transcription factor can be used to reprogram somatic cells to a pluripotent state (Takahashi, Tanabe et al. 2007; Yu, Vodyanik et al. 2007). In this chapter we review current knowledge of the molecular mechanism that defines cell pluripotency, focusing mainly on human pluripotent stem cells. Learning how to control stem cell pluripotency may point to new methods of up-scaling the production of undifferentiated hESC as well as deriving efficient methods to generate patient-specific iPS cells.

Signal Transduction Pathways that Maintain Pluripotency

Differences in Signal Transduction Pathways that Maintain Pluripotency in mESC and hESC

Emerging evidence has suggested that growth factor requirements for maintaining mouse embryonic stem cells (mESC) and hESC are rather different. In mESC, a combination of Leukemia inhibitory factor (LIF) and bone morphogenetic factor 4 (BMP4) can alleviate the need for serum and feeder cells to maintain undifferentiated mESC (Ying, Nichols et al. 2003). However, LIF signaling fails to maintain self-renewal in hESC (Daheron, Opitz et al. 2004; Humphrey, Beattie et al. 2004), and BMP signaling promotes differentiation of hESC (Xu, Chen et al.

2002; Pera, Andrade et al. 2004). Wnt signaling has also emerged as a key player in maintaining mESC pluripotency (Sato, Meijer et al. 2004), but many studies have failed to maintain hESC by activating this signaling pathway (Cheon, Kim et al. 2005; Dravid, Ye et al. 2005). Moreover, Fibroblast growth factor (FGF)-4 stimulation of Erk1/2 signaling caused differentiation in mESC (Kunath, Saba-El-Leil et al. 2007), whereas in hESC the same signaling cascades promote self-renewal (Mayshar, Rom et al. 2008). These results highlight the differences in signaling requirement for pluripotency in hESC and mESC. Instead, recent evidence suggested that the signaling requirement for determining cell fate in hESC is more similar to pluripotent cells derived from the mouse epiblast, termed mouse epiblast stem cells (Brons, Smithers et al. 2007; Vallier, Touboul et al. 2009). Since research in mouse epiblast stem cells is still in its early stage, in this section we will focus on reviewing our current knowledge of the role of various signaling pathways in regulating cell pluripotency in hESC.

The STAT3 Pathway and LIF in hESC

LIF belongs to the Interleukin 6 class cytokine and exert its biological effects by binding to its receptor complex constituted of the transmembrane proteins gp130 and LIFRβ. In turn, receptor activation induces the recruitment of the Janus Kinases (JAK), activation of the Signal Transducer and Activator of Transcription 3 (STAT3) pathway, and transcription of self-renewal genes in mESC (Burdon, Chambers et al. 1999; Burdon, Smith et al. 2002). LIF also activates the Mitogen-Activated Protein Kinases (MAPK)-Extracellular Signal-Regulated Kinase (ERK) 1 and 2 pathway which is involved in mESC differentiation but also proliferation (Burdon, Chambers et al. 1999; Burdon, Stracey et al. 1999; Burdon, Smith et al. 2002). In hESC, LIF activates the STAT3 and the ERK pathways but it is not sufficient to maintain hESC (Thomson, Itskovitz-Eldor et al. 1998; Reubinoff, Pera et al. 2000; Daheron, Opitz et al. 2004; Humphrey, Beattie et al. 2004; Sato, Meijer et al. 2004). Similarly, constitutive activation of STAT3 also fails to maintain hESC (Daheron, Opitz et al. 2004; Humphrey, Beattie et al. 2004), indicating a major difference in signaling requirements between mESC and hESC. It has been hypothesized that the fate of hESC is dependent on the phosphorylation site of the transcription factor STAT3 (Androutsellis-Theotokis, Leker et al. 2006), with the JAK-dependent phosphorylation of Tyr705 leading to hESC differentiation and the JAK-independent Ser727 phosphorylation promoting hESC survival (Androutsellis-Theotokis, Leker et al. 2006). However, as LIF promotes hESC differentiation and induces the phosphorylation of both sites (Daheron, Opitz et al. 2004), further study is needed to confirm this hypothesis.

The Smad Pathways and the TGFβ Superfamily

A number of studies converge to suggest that the Transforming Growth Factor (TGF) β superfamily control essential aspects of hESC pluripotency. The TGFβ superfamily consists of two subfamilies: the TGFβ/Activin/Nodal subfamily which activates the downstream Smad 2/3 proteins; and the BMP/GDF/MIS subfamily which activates Smad 1/5/8 proteins (Figure 1; Miyazawa, Shinozaki et al. 2002; Shi and Massague 2003). TGFβ ligands bind to serine/threonine kinase type II receptors which induce the recruitment of the serine/threonine kinase type I receptors, leading to the activation of either Smad2/3 or Smad 1/5/8 signaling pathways. Subsequently, this induces binding with Smad4 and translocation into the nucleus and regulation of gene expression (Letamendia, Labbe et al. 2001). Activin and nodal bind to type I (Alk4/ActR-IB) and type II (ActR-IIB) receptors, and nodal also binds to another type I (Alk7) receptor (Reissmann, Jornvall et al. 2001; Shi and Massague 2003). This signaling pathway can be regulated by Cripto, an extracellular GPI-linked protein which acts as an accessory receptor (Shi and Massague 2003). On the other hand, BMP act through the receptors BMPIα (Alk2, Alk3) BMPI β (Alk6) and BMPII.

Previous studies demonstrated that the feeder layer of MEF express multiple ligands in the TGFβ superfamily, including TGFβ 1, 2, 3, BMP-2, 4 and Activin A (Beattie, Lopez et al. 2005; Wang, Zhang et al. 2005) as well as the BMP antagonists gremlin and noggin (Pera, Andrade et al. 2004; Xu, Peck et al. 2005). On the other hand, hESC express TGFβ 1, 2, 3, activin, nodal, cripto, BMP-2, BMP-4, BMP-7 and the receptors TGFβR1, 2, 3, BMPIα, BMPIβ and BMPII (Besser 2004; Vallier, Reynolds et al. 2004; Vallier, Alexander et al. 2005; Wang, Zhang et al. 2005; Rho, Yu et al. 2006). Therefore, a paracrine signaling circuit between MEF and hESC as well as an autocrine signaling between hESC is likely to occur to maintain hESC undifferentiated. In undifferentiated hESC, the Smad2/3 pathway is active with Smad 2/3 proteins found to be present within the hESC nucleus (James, Levine et al. 2005; Vallier, Alexander et al. 2005), while the Smad 1/5/8 signaling pathway is repressed. Upon hESC differentiation, Smad2/3 signaling is decreased while Smad1/5/8 is activated (James, Levine et al. 2005; Xu, Peck et al. 2005). It was recently described that the transcriptional regulator TAZ is required for the nuclear accumulation of Smad2/3 and thus regulate the maintenance of hESC by TGFβ (Varelas, Sakuma et al. 2008). In this regard, Activin can induces the phosphorylation of Smad2/3 in hESC (Vallier, Alexander et al. 2005; Wong, Tellis et al. 2007), whereas BMP-4 stimulates the Smad1/5/8 pathway and their subsequent nuclear translocation, an effect independent of the ERK1/2 pathway (Vallier, Alexander et al. 2005). Hence, these results suggested that stimulating Smad 2/3 or repressing Smad1/5/8 would be expected to maintain hESC while the opposite would be hypothesized to induce hESC differentiation.

However, although activin is used to promote hESC self-renewal at lower concentration (5-50 ng/ml), it can promotes definite endoderm differentiation of hESC at a high concentration of 100 ng/ml (D'Amour, Agulnick et al. 2005). Whether its sole incubation is sufficient to maintain hESC in culture on the long-term is somewhat controversial. For instance Vallier et al. (2005) reported that activin delays the short term differentiation of hESC and needs to be co-incubated with bFGF to maintain the long-term hESC pluripotency (Vallier, Alexander et al. 2005). Contrary to this result, Xiao et al. (2006) showed that activin A on its own is able to maintain self-renewal and pluripotency of hESC (Xiao, Yuan et al. 2006). Microarray analysis of gene expression showed that the up-regulation of activin A in hESC is correlated with an increase in the expression of Oct4 and Nanog, and of genes involved in the FGF, Nodal/Activin, Wnt and Hedgehog signaling pathways (Xiao, Yuan et al. 2006). Furthermore, activin A stimulation of Smad2/3 nuclear translocation could also cross-talks with the Wnt signaling (Beattie, Lopez et al. 2005; James, Levine et al. 2005). Clearly, further analysis of the role of activin signaling in hESC is required.

Another member of the TGFβ superfamily, Nodal has also been shown to be involved in maintenance of hESC pluripotency. Indeed, its over-expression in hESC is correlated with a prolonged expression of pluripotent markers and an inhibition of neuroectodermal differentiation upon embryoid body formation (Vallier, Reynolds et al. 2004). Moreover, the inhibition of nodal signaling by Lefty-A down-regulates the expression of stem cell marker Oct4 (Xiao, Yuan et al. 2006), whereas inhibition of nodal by cerberus 1 is accompanied by hESC differentiation (Katoh 2006). However, similar to activin, nodal alone is not sufficient to maintain hESC undifferentiated and would require the presence of bFGF for the long-term maintenance of these cells (Vallier, Alexander et al. 2005). The effects of bFGF and nodal on hESC is dependent on the Activin/Nodal receptors as their inhibition by SB431542 reduces the expression of hESC pluripotency markers (Vallier, Alexander et al. 2005).

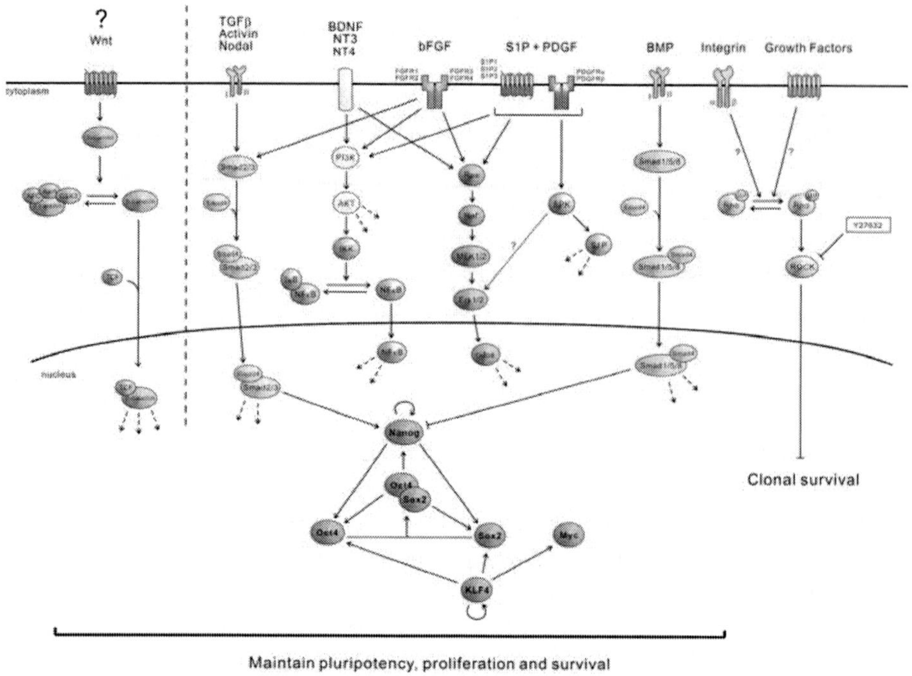

Figure 1. Proposed signaling networks in maintenance of proliferation, survival and pluripotency in hESC. Note that Wnt signaling remains controversial in its role in maintaining undifferentiated hESC. Dotted arrows indicated activation of targets yet to be identified in hESC. Abbreviations not mentioned in the text: MEK: Mitogen-activated protein kinase kinase; SPK: Sphingosine kinase; IκB: Inhibitor of kappa B; IKK: IκB kinase.

On the other hand, BMP have been shown to promote trophoblast differentiation of hESC (Xu, Chen et al. 2002), yet blockage of BMP signaling with noggin does not maintain hESC undifferentiated but promotes neural differentiation (Pera, Andrade et al. 2004; Itsykson, Ilouz et al. 2005). Instead, prolonged culture of undifferentiated hESC can be achieved by a combination of bFGF and blockage of BMP signaling by noggin (Wang, Zhang et al. 2005; Xu, Peck et al. 2005). How bFGF acts in this cooperative effect remains unclear, as it does not inhibit Smad 1/5/8 phosphorylation (Xu, Peck et al. 2005). Taken together, emerging evidence suggested an opposing role of the two Smad pathways in determining the cell fate of hESC: the activation of the Smad2/3 pathway leading to hESC maintenance, while Smad1/5/8 pathway play a pro-differentiation role in hESC (Figure 1).

The ERK, PI3K/Akt and NFκB Pathways in hESC

Various data now point to an important role of constitutively active PI3K/Akt and ERK pathways in the maintenance of hESC. Indeed, these two pathways are active in most culture media used for the maintenance of hESC (Li, Wang et al. 2007). Various pro-maintenance factors activate these signaling pathways in hESC, in particular bFGF, neurotrophins, sphingosine-1-phosphate (S1P) and platelet-derived growth factor (PDGF). The inhibition of the PI3K/Akt pathway has been shown to inhibit hESC proliferation (Li, Wang et al. 2007) and to induce hESC differentiation (Armstrong, Hughes et al. 2006; Li, Wang et al. 2007; McLean, D'Amour et al. 2007) and apoptosis (Li, Wang et al. 2007; Wong, Tellis et al. 2007). The inhibition of the ERK1/2 pathway induces differentiation and increases cell death in hESC (Armstrong, Hughes et al. 2006; Wong, Tellis et al. 2007), but the latter effect on differentiation is not observed in other study (Li, Wang et al. 2007). Similarly, inhibition of the Nuclear Factor Kappa-light-chain-enhance of activated B cells (NFκB) pathway also leads to differentiation and cell death in hESC (Armstrong, Hughes et al. 2006). How these three pathways crosstalk to each other is not well understood. Some data suggest that the PI3K/Akt pathway is upstream of the ERK1/2 and the NFκB pathways (Armstrong, Hughes et al. 2006) while others suggest that the activation of the ERK1/2 pathway in hESC is independent of the PI3K/Akt pathway (Kang, Kim et al. 2005; Li, Wang et al. 2007; Wong, Tellis et al. 2007). Hence more studies are needed to understand the interaction between these pathways that resulted in maintenance of hESC. Taken together, these results demonstrated the importance of these three pathways in hESC pluripotency, and various culture systems for hESC rely on the addition of growth factors that signal through these three pathways, including bFGF, S1P, PDGF and neurotrophins (Figure 1).

Basic Fibroblast Growth Factor and Insulin-Like Growth Factor

bFGF is a member of the FGF family that comprises of at least 22 members in human (Itoh and Ornitz 2004). Alternative splicing of the mRNA results in two different isoforms of bFGF with different cellular effects in human: a low molecular mass isoforms (LMM, 18kDa) and a higher molecular mass isoforms (HMM, 21-24 kDa) (Delrieu 2000). The HMM bFGF isoform is generally localized within the nucleus, while the LMM bFGF isoform is generally cytoplasmic and can also be secreted (Delrieu 2000; Stachowiak, Fang et al. 2003). This secreted form of bFGF can signals through binding to its receptor FGFR1b, 1c, 2c, 3c and 4 (Itoh and Ornitz 2004).. Upon ligand binding, the FGF receptors dimerize and induce phosphorylation of a set of downstream signaling molecules, capable of activating the Erk1/2 pathway, PI3K/Akt pathway and also the phospholipase C (PLC)/protein kinase C (PKC) pathway (Figure 1, Schlessinger 2004).

bFGF is a potent pro-maintenance factor of hESC. bFGF was first used at 4 ng/ml to enhance hESC clonal growth (Amit, Carpenter et al. 2000; Xu, Inokuma et al. 2001) and was subsequently used at higher concentration with unconditioned knockout serum replacement (KSR) to support hESC growth in the absence of feeder cells. Examples of higher concentrations that maintain hESC in culture include: 16 ng/ml bFGF with LIF in a feeder-free system that allowed successful derivation of hESC (Klimanskaya, Chung et al. 2005); and 20-40 ng/ml bFGF to sustain the long-term culture of hESC in some conditions (Wang, Li et al. 2005; Xu, Rosler et al. 2005; Yao, Chen et al. 2006), while 100 ng/ml bFGF is effective in propagating hESC (Levenstein, Ludwig et al. 2005; Ludwig, Levenstein et al. 2006). However, other data showed opposite results, where bFGF (up to 20 ng/ml) decreased hESC colony outgrowth (Dvorak, Dvorakova et al. 2005). The reason why bFGF needs to be added in such high concentration is not fully understood. It is hypothesized that this could be linked to a rapid degradation of bFGF in the culture medium (Levenstein, Ludwig et al. 2005), or high concentration of bFGF can suppresses the pro-differentiation effect of BMP signaling in hESC (Xu, Peck et al. 2005).

The four FGF receptors are expressed by hESC with FGFR1 being dominant, and hESC synthesize multiple members of the FGF family ligand, including FGF-4, FGF-11, FGF-13 and both LMM and HMM isoforms of bFGF (Delrieu 2000; Sato, Sanjuan et al. 2003; Sperger, Chen et al. 2003; Brandenberger, Wei et al. 2004; Ginis, Luo et al. 2004; Itoh and Ornitz 2004; Dvorak, Dvorakova et al. 2005; Kang, Kim et al. 2005; Rho, Yu et al. 2006). The secreted LMM isoform of bFGF could reach a concentration of 80-100 pg/ml in hESC-conditioned medium, suggesting an autocrine and paracrine activation of the FGF receptors within hESC (Dvorak, Dvorakova et al. 2005). It is becoming clear that there is also a paracrine signaling between the feeder layer and hESC involving bFGF. Previous study has shown that bFGF can maintain hESC in the presence of MEF conditioned medium in a feeder-free system (Xu, Inokuma et al. 2001). In a follow up study, Diecke *et al.* (2008) studied the gene expression profile of bFGF-primed MEF to assess whether MEF release pro-maintenance factors. The results showed that upon bFGF treatment MEF up-regulate such as the BMP antagonist gremlin, and molecules involved in the activation of the Smad 2/3 pathway (Diecke, Quiroga-Negreira et al. 2008). Recent study also demonstrated that hESC-derived fibroblasts respond to bFGF and secret insulin-like growth factors (IGF), which acts on hESC to maintain pluripotency by activation of the PI3K/Akt pathway (Bendall, Stewart et al. 2007; McLean, D'Amour et al. 2007). Hence, the effect of bFGF on hESC maintenance can also be indirect, by inducing IGF release from more differentiated cells that in turn signal to maintain hESC undifferentiated (Gotoh 2009).

In hESC, bFGF activates the ERK1/2 pathway with subsequent *c-fos* expression (Dvorak, Dvorakova et al. 2005; Kang, Kim et al. 2005; Li, Wang et al. 2007) but also crosstalks with members of the TGFβ superfamily (such as BMPs, TGFβ1, nodal and activin) (Amit, Shariki et al. 2004; Vallier, Alexander et al. 2005; Wang, Zhang et al. 2005; Xu, Peck et al. 2005). Indeed, addition of the BMP inhibitor noggin, together with bFGF maintain hESC undifferentiated (Wang, Zhang et al. 2005; Xu, Peck et al. 2005), yet bFGF does not inhibit BMP-4 stimulation of Smad 1/5/8 signaling in hESC (Vallier, Alexander et al. 2005), suggesting that bFGF does not act on the Smad 1/5/8 pathway *per se*. As bFGF's impact on pluripotency is dependent on the activin/nodal signaling within hESC, bFGF might be a "competence factor" for the activin/nodal signaling in hESC maintenance (Vallier, Alexander et al. 2005).

Neurotrophins

The neurotrophin family includes Nerve Growth Factor (NGF), Brain-Derived Neurotrophic Factor (BDNF) and Neurotrophins (NT) 3 and 4 which bind their specific receptors Tropomyosin Receptor Kinases (TRK) A, B and C and the p75 neurotrophin receptor (p75NGFR) (Figure 1, Lu, Pang et al. 2005). Limited research have study the role of neurotrophins in hESC. hESC express high levels of TRKB and TRKC, while MEF express NGF, BDNF, NT3 and NT4 while (Pyle, Lock et al. 2006). Importantly, neurotrophins have been shown to increase hESC clonal survival and viability, an effect that is largely attributed to activation of the PI3K/Akt pathway (Pyle, Lock et al. 2006).

Sphingosine-1-Phosphate and Platelet-Derived Growth Factor

Sphingosine-1-phosphate (S1P) is a bioactive lysophospholipid that binds its specific receptors $S1P_{1-5}$ which are coupled to at least three G protein families, G_i, G_q and G_{12} (Chun, Goetzl et al. 2002; Takuwa, Takuwa et al. 2002), while Platelet Derived Growth Factor (PDGF) binds to two specific tyrosine kinase receptors PDGFRα and PDGFRß. The two factors can cooperate to activate classical protein kinase signaling pathways, including the sphingosine kinases (SPK) which generate intracellular S1P (Figure 1). Both MEF and hESC express $S1P_{1-3}$,

PDGFRα and PDGFRß (Pebay, Wong et al. 2005; Inniss and Moore 2006). Different profiles of lipid content of sphingosine, S1P, sphingomyelin and glucosylceramide were found in hESC than in MEF (Brimble, Sherrer et al. 2007), suggesting that MEF may release bioactive sphingolipids in the culture medium which could account for some of the MEF-mediated effects on hESC. Importantly, S1P and PDGF have been demonstrated to maintain hESC pluripotency and proliferation and inhibit apoptosis (Pebay, Wong et al. 2005; Inniss and Moore 2006; Wong, Tellis et al. 2007), allowing long-term maintenance of hESC in the presence of MEF (Pebay, Wong et al. 2005). However, S1P on its own is not sufficient to maintain hESC (Pebay, Wong et al. 2005). Recently, a micro-array analysis showed that S1P up-regulates anti-apoptotic genes, cell cycle progression and cell adhesion genes and down-regulates pro-apoptotic genes (Avery, Avery et al. 2008). However, S1P also down-regulates pluripotency genes such as *nanog* and *Oct-4* (Avery, Avery et al. 2008), confirming that S1P by itself is not sufficient to maintain hESC undifferentiated. Both S1P and PDGF stimulate the ERK1/2 pathway and PDGF also stimulates the PI3K/Akt pathway, and the two pathways are necessary to the anti-apoptotic effect of S1P and PDGF in hESC (Wong, Tellis et al. 2007; Avery, Avery et al. 2008). Interestingly, neither S1P nor PDGF modifies Smad2 phosphorylation in hESC, even after two hours of incubation, thus raising the possibility that hESC maintenance can be achieved without activation of the Smad2/3 signaling pathway (Wong, Tellis et al. 2007). Moreover, S1P and PDGF also stimulate other branches of the MAPK pathways, p38 and JNK1/2 phosphorylation, with physiological consequences yet to be identified (Pitson and Pebay Submitted).

The Wnt Signaling in hESC

Wnts are lipid modified glycoproteins that bind to their membrane receptor complex constituted of Frizzled and Low-density-Lysoprotein-Related-Protein5/6 (LRP). In the absence of canonical Wnt signaling, cytoplasmic β-catenin is bound in a complex with Glycogen Synthase Kinase (GSK)-3-beta, Axin, and Adenomatosis Polyposis Coli (APC), resulting in its phosphorylation and subsequent degradation via the ubiquitin pathway. Upon Wnt binding to its receptors, the protein Dishevelled mediates the inhibition of GSK-3 phosphorylation of beta-catenin, leading to the accumulation of cytosolic β-catenin, followed by its nuclear translocation where β-catenin acts as a transcriptional cofactor of T cell factor (TCF)/ Lymphoid Enhancer Binding Factor1 (Figure 1, Cadigan and Liu 2006).

MEF express transcripts of Wnt2, Wnt4, Wnt5a, Wnt6 and the Wnt inhibitors Dkk-1 and Dkk-3 (Sato, Meijer et al. 2004; Dravid, Ye et al. 2005; Wang, Zhang et al. 2005). Although Wnt1, Wnt3, and Dkk-1 have been found to be expressed in hESC (Walsh and Andrews 2003; Rho, Yu et al. 2006), other studies found no evidence of Wnt ligands in hESC (Brandenberger, Wei et al. 2004; Davidson, Jamshidi et al. 2007). In addition, in hESC only a low level of β-catenin/TCF mediated activation were detected, suggesting that the canonical Wnt signaling pathway is inactive in undifferentiated hESC (Dravid, Ye et al. 2005). Previous report from Sato et al. (2004) claimed that the activation of the Wnt signaling pathway - by either Wnt3a or the GSK-3 inhibitor, 6-bromoindirubin-3'-oxime (BIO) maintains hESC undifferentiated and pluripotent (Sato, Meijer et al. 2004). Yet, these data were not reproduced with the use of another GSK-3 inhibitor LiCl (Sato, Meijer et al. 2004) and other studies have failed to maintain hESC using either Wnt3a, BIO, or by blocking endogenous Wnt signaling using Frizzled-Related Protein 2 (FRP2) and Dkk-1 (Cheon, Kim et al. 2005; Dravid, Ye et al. 2005). Despite its inability to maintain pluripotency, Wnt3a appears to increase single-cell survival (Hasegawa, Fujioka et al. 2006) and to stimulate proliferation in hESC, an effect that is dependent on the presence of an undefined anti-differentiation factors (Dravid, Ye et al. 2005). Candidates of such factors are hypothesized to be members of the TGFβ superfamily (James, Levine et al. 2005). More research is needed to clarify the role of Wnt signaling in the maintenance of hESC.

The Rho/ROCK Pathway in hESC

The Rho/ROCK pathway is also involved in regulating hESC clonal survival (Figure 1). Indeed, data suggest that the Rho/ROCK pathway is activated in hESC and responsible for cell-cell contacts (Harb, Archer et al. 2008), and the inhibition of ROCK significantly increases hESC single cell survival (Watanabe, Ueno et al. 2007; Damoiseaux, Sherman et al. 2008). These data have allowed the development of new techniques to improve hESC culture and cryopreservation (Li, Meng et al. 2008; Claassen, Desler et al. 2009; Heng 2009; Li, Krawetz et al. 2009). Furthermore, it is hypothesized that ROCK inhibition may not act directly by reducing apoptosis, but rather act by desensitizing cells to their environment thus limiting apoptosis (Krawetz, Li et al. 2009). Further work is now needed to confirm this hypothesis and also identify whether pro- and anti-differentiation factors modulate the Rho/ROCK signaling axis.

Transcriptional Network Governing Pluripotency in Mouse and hESC

The signaling pathways discussed previously eventually lead to activation of a transcriptional program that govern cell pluripotency, by activating genes that support self-renewal and repressing genes that promote differentiation. Several transcription factors have been identified as key regulators in this transcriptional network, including Oct4, Sox2 and Nanog. Using genome-wide mapping analysis, previous studies have demonstrated that Oct4, Sox2 and Nanog co-occupy a substantial portion of their target genes in hESC (Boyer, Lee et al. 2005) and mESC (Chen, Xu et al. 2008; Kim, Chu et al. 2008). Furthermore, they are able to regulate each other and effectively forming a core regulatory circuitry regulating stem cell pluripotency, where Oct4, Sox2 and Nanog are proposed to be the master regulators of this transcriptional network.

In addition to Oct4, Sox2 and Nanog, the recent development of iPS cells have also confirmed the important roles of other genes in regulating cell pluripotency. An elegant experiment by Takahashi et al. (2007) demonstrated that mouse somatic cells can be reprogrammed to a pluripotent state using four transcription factors Oct4, Sox2, c-Myc and Klf4 (Takahashi and Yamanaka 2006). Subsequent study by the same group has demonstrated that the same four factors used in mice can be used to generate human iPS cells (Takahashi, Tanabe et al. 2007). These suggested that although the upstream signal transduction pathways regulating pluripotency are different in mESC and hESC (see discussion in previous section), the downstream transcriptional network that defines pluripotency may be similar in mouse and human. In this aspect, studies in early mouse embryos or mESC are helpful in understanding this transcriptional network in defining hESC pluripotency. Subsequently, Nanog and Lin28 have also been used for generation of iPS cells (Yu, Vodyanik et al. 2007). In this section, we will discuss the role of these factors in regulating cell pluripotency in early mouse embryo, mESC and hESC.

Oct4

Oct4, also known as Oct3 or Pou5F1, is one of the most extensively studied transcription factors associated with pluripotent cells of the embryo (Scholer, Balling et al. 1989; Okamoto, Okazawa et al. 1990; Rosner, Vigano et al. 1990). It belongs to a family of transcription factors containing the POU DNA binding domain. In the developing mouse embryo, Oct4 is restricted to the inner cell mass, primitive ectoderm, and later in primordial germ cells (Pesce and Scholer 2001). *In vitro*, Oct4 is expressed in undifferentiated EC cells and ESC and down-regulated upon differentiation (Rosner, Vigano et al. 1990; Assou, Le Carrour et al. 2007). This restricted expression of Oct4 renders it a useful marker for stem cell pluripotency. However, this simplistic view should be treated cautiously, as Oct4 seems to regulate pluripotency in a dosage-dependent manner. Transient increase in Oct4 expression has been observed in mESC during mesodermal differentiation (Zeineddine, Papadimou et al. 2006). In support of this, previous studies have demonstrated that transgene-mediated increase of Oct4 level in mESC drives differentiation into extraembryonic endoderm, mesoderm or neuroectoderm under different conditions (Niwa, Miyazaki et al. 2000; Shimozaki, Nakashima et al. 2003; Zeineddine, Papadimou et al. 2006). Therefore, a precise level of Oct4 is required in maintaining cell pluripotency.

Pluripotency in early embryo or ESC depends on the tight control of Oct4 expression. Knockout of Oct4 in mice resulted in embryonic lethality due to failure to form the inner cell mass, and *in vitro* culture of Oct4 knockout embryos showed that the inner cell mass cells loss pluripotency and differentiate into trophectoderm cells (Nichols, Zevnik et al. 1998). Subsequent studies have shown that Oct4 can directly inhibit Cdx2, Eomes and hCG, three important regulators in trophectoderm differentiation (Liu and Roberts 1996; Liu, Leaman et al. 1997; Niwa, Toyooka et al. 2005). Therefore, Oct4 is generally viewed as a repressor for trophectoderm differentiation as well as required for maintaining pluripotency in the inner cell mass. Consistent with this idea, siRNA mediated knockdown of Oct4 resulted in trophectoderm differentiation in both hESC and mESC (Niwa, Miyazaki et al. 2000; Matin, Walsh et al. 2004; Zaehres, Lensch et al. 2005; Fong, Hohenstein et al. 2008; Hohenstein, Pyle et al. 2008).

In human, several splice variants of Oct4 are reported, including Oct4a, Oct4b and recently Oct4b1 (Takeda, Seino et al. 1992; Atlasi, Mowla et al. 2008). While Oct4a and Oct4b1 are restricted to pluripotent cells, Oct4b is expressed in many nonpluripotent cell types (Atlasi, Mowla et al. 2008). Importantly, Oct4a is expressed in the nucleus and confers stem cell pluripotency, while Oct4b is expressed in the cytoplasm and cannot sustains stem cell self-renewal (Lee, Kim et al. 2006). On the other hand, the function of Oct4b1 is not well understood. These facts point out the importance of choosing the right tools for the study of Oct4 in human, and it also suggest a more complex picture of how Oct4 act to maintain cell pluripotency.

To date, all protocols for generating iPS cells require the addition of Oct4, suggesting its importance as a master regulator in governing cell pluripotency (Feng, Ng et al. 2009). However, it is apparent that Oct4 on its own is not sufficient to induce pluripotency and the presences of binding partners determine whether the target genes are activated or repressed. For example, when Oct4 binds to FoxD3, it functions as a corepressor to inhibit FoxD3 activation of the endodermal genes FoxA1 and FoxA2, effectively preventing ESC from differentiation (Guo, Costa et al. 2002). On the other hand, Sox2 represents an important binding partner for Oct4 to activate stem cell specific genes, such as Sox2, Fbx10, FGF4 and UTF1 (Yuan, Corbi et al. 1995; Ambrosetti, Basilico et al. 1997; Okuda, Fukushima et al. 1998; Tomioka, Nishimoto et al. 2002; Tokuzawa, Kaiho et al. 2003).

Sox2

The SRY-related HMG box (Sox) gene family encodes transcription factors with a single HMG DNA-binding domain. In the developing mouse embryo, Sox2 is expressed in pluripotent cells of the inner cell mass and epiblast, primodial germ cells as well as multipotent cells of extraembryonic ectoderm (Avilion, Nicolis et al. 2003). Unlike Oct4, Sox2 expression is persistent in neural stem cells throughout development (Ellis, Fagan et al. 2004). Sox2 knockout mice die shortly after implantation due to defects in epiblast formation (Avilion, Nicolis et al. 2003). *In vitro*, Sox2 is expressed in undifferentiated ESC and can be use as a marker to select for neural progenitor cells upon embryoid bodies formation (Li, Pevny et al. 1998). Consistent with this idea, Sox2 overexpression in mESC biased the cells towards neural differentiation (Zhao, Nichols et al. 2004; Kopp, Ormsbee et al. 2008).

On the other hand, siRNA-mediated knockdown of Sox2 in hESC resulted in trophectoderm differentiation (Fong, Hohenstein et al. 2008). Similar results are seen in mESC using a dominant negative form of Sox2 (Li, Pan et al. 2007) or an inducible knockout system (Masui, Nakatake et al. 2007). However, ectopic expression of Oct4 can rescue this phenotype in mESC, suggesting that the essential function of Sox2 is to maintain Oct4 expression (Masui, Nakatake et al. 2007). Surprisingly, the expression of many Oct4/Sox2 target genes was not affected by the loss of Sox2. This suggested that the role of Sox2 may be compensated by other Sox family members, such as Sox4, Sox11 and Sox15 present in ESC.

Sox2 is involved in defining distinct cell fates that is largely dependent on its binding partner: Pax6 for lens differentiation, Brn2 for neural differentiation, and Oct4 for maintaining pluripotency in ESC (Kondoh, Uchikawa et al. 2004). In the latter case, the interaction between Sox2 and Oct4 had been implicated in stimulating expression of FGF4 (Ambrosetti, Basilico et al. 1997), UTF1 (Nishimoto, Fukushima et al. 1999; Nishimoto, Miyagi et al. 2005) and Nanog (Kuroda, Tada et al. 2005; Rodda, Chew et al. 2005), all of which are important in maintenance of ESC. Moreover, the Oct4-Sox2 complex can stimulate the expression of Oct4 and Sox2 itself, effectively forming a positive feedback loop to maintain pluripotency in ESC (Figure 1, Chew, Loh et al. 2005).

Nanog

Nanog is a homeodomain protein that was recently identified as a new master regulator for maintenance of stem cell pluripotency (Chambers, Colby et al. 2003; Mitsui, Tokuzawa et al. 2003). Similar to Oct4, Nanog is restricted to the inner cell mass, epiblast and primodial germ cells in the developing embryo. *In vitro*, Nanog is highly enriched in a number of pluripotent cells lines such as ESC, EC cells and embryonic germ (EG) cells (Chambers, Colby et al. 2003). Previous reports demonstrated an important role of Nanog in maintaining pluripotency. Overexpression of Nanog prevents mESC from differentiation (Chambers, Colby et al. 2003; Ivanova, Dobrin et al. 2006). However, in the absence of Oct4, Nanog alone is not enough to sustain self-renewal in mESC (Chambers, Colby et al. 2003). Similarly in hESC, overexpression of Nanog enables hESC to stay undifferentiated in conditions that favour differentiation (Darr, Mayshar et al. 2006).

On the other hand, Nanog-null mouse embryos fail to form inner cell mass, and *in vitro* culture has shown that the mutant inner cell mass differentiates into parietal endoderm-like cells (Mitsui, Tokuzawa et al. 2003). Moreover, reduction of Nanog drives differentiation to multi-lineage cells in mESC (Mitsui, Tokuzawa et al. 2003; Hatano, Tada et al. 2005; Ivanova, Dobrin et al. 2006) and hESC (Hyslop, Stojkovic et al. 2005; Zaehres, Lensch et al. 2005; Fong, Hohenstein et al. 2008). All of these studies point to an indispensible role of Nanog in safeguarding pluripotency. However, this view is being challenged by a recent experiment from Chambers et al. (2007), where the authors demonstrated that in the absence of Nanog undifferentiated mESC can persist with normal self-renewal and differentiation potentials (Chambers, Silva et al. 2007). Moreover, the authors show that down-regulation of Nanog expression is reversible, and transient down-regulation of Nanog does not mark commitment to differentiate unless the extrinsic conditions favour differentiation (Chambers, Silva et al. 2007). Taken together, Nanog is presented as an important regulator in pluripotency, but unlike Oct4 and Sox2, it is not essential in housekeeping stem cell pluripotency.

Nanog can physically interact with Oct4 (Wang, Rao et al. 2006) and cooperates extensively with Oct4 and Sox2 in the core-transcriptional network both in human (Boyer, Lee et al. 2005) and mESC (Chen, Xu et al. 2008; Kim, Chu et al. 2008). In this aspect, Oct4, Sox2 and Nanog can also bind to their own promoters, thus forming an autoregulation loop to maintain ESC self-renewal (Figure 1, Boyer, Lee et al. 2005). Moreover, in mESC it has been demonstrated that Nanog can also interact with Smad1 to block BMP-induced differentiation (Suzuki, Raya et al. 2006).

Klf4

The role of *Klf4* and its family members in the maintenance of pluripotency have not been realized until recently. Klf4 belongs to the Krüppel-like factor family of zinc finger transcription factors, whose members have important roles in regulating different physiological processes (McConnell, Ghaleb et al. 2007; Evans and Liu 2008). Klf4 can be an oncogene or a tumor suppressing gene depending on the cell context (Rowland and Peeper 2006). Together with Oct4, Sox2 and c-Myc, Klf4 have demonstrated its ability to reprogram somatic cells back to a pluripotent state (Takahashi and Yamanaka 2006; Takahashi, Tanabe et al. 2007). Overexpression of Klf4 also prevents differentiation into erythroid progenitors in mESC, indicating it is an important regulator of cell pluripotency (Li, McClintick et al. 2005).

Klf4 knockout mice die soon after birth due to dehydration caused by defects in the epidermal barrier of the skin (Segre, Bauer et al. 1999). However, these knockout mice are normal during early embryo development in their pluripotent stem cell populations. Similarly, although Klf4 is an abundant transcript in mESC, knocking down Klf4 does not generate an obvious phenotype (Nakatake, Fukui et al. 2006; Jiang, Chan et al. 2008). One explanation is that there may be functional redundancy among other Klf family members in ESC. Indeed, triple knockdown of the Klf2, Klf4 and Klf5 resulted in rapid differentiation in mESC (Jiang, Chan et al. 2008). Consistent with this idea, other Klf family members (Klf1, Klf2 or

Klf5) can substitute for Klf4 in the generation of iPS cells (Nakagawa, Koyanagi et al. 2008).

However, not all Klf factors have totally redundant functions. A recent study by Ema et al. (2008) demonstrated that knockout of Klf5 in mice resulted in early embryo lethality due to defects in implantation, a result in sharp contrast to Klf4 knockout mice. Furthermore, knockout of Klf5 in mESC leads to rapid differentiation whereas Klf5 overexpression confers resistance to differentiation and increase in proliferation (Ema, Mori et al. 2008). Importantly, ectopic expression of Klf4 can rescue the differentiation phenotype in Klf5-null mESC, but proliferation is markedly decreased. These results suggested that although Klf4 and Klf5 have a similar function in suppressing differentiation, they may play an opposing role in proliferation as observed in other cell types (Ghaleb, Nandan et al. 2005).

The precise mechanism of how Klf4 contributes to somatic cell reprogramming or maintaining pluripotency remains unclear. Previous studies have demonstrated that Klf4 is not essential in iPS cell generation (Yu, Vodyanik et al. 2007). But rather, Klf4 serves as a secondary factor to enhance iPS cell generation. One hypothesis is that Klf4 may act synergistically with Oct4, Sox2 and Nanog to restart the pluripotent stem cell-specific gene expression program. In mESC, Klf4 can cooperate with Oct4 and Sox2 to activate a subset of ESC specific genes (Nakatake, Fukui et al. 2006). Through global mapping of promoter analysis, in mESC Klf4 has been demonstrated to bind to the promoter of Oct4, Sox2, Nanog, Myc and Klf4 itself (Figure 1, Chen, Xu et al. 2008; Kim, Chu et al. 2008). Whether the same interaction is conversed in hESC is not confirmed yet, but in hESC Klf4 can directly bind and activate expression of Nanog (Chan, Zhang et al. 2009). Furthermore, many Klf family members share similar target genes with Nanog, suggesting Klf proteins are important components of the transcriptional network regulating cell pluripotency (Jiang, Chan et al. 2008). Another hypothesis is that Klf4 acts as an inhibitor of apoptosis which in turn help somatic cell reprogramming. Klf4 is a negative regulator of p53 (Rowland, Bernards et al. 2005), therefore this could counteract the effect of c-Myc in inducing p53-mediated apoptosis during reprogramming (Adhikary and Eilers 2005). Studies that address whether p53 depletion in somatic cells can enhance iPS cell generation will be particularly interesting in this context.

Lin28

Lin28 was first identified as a heterochronic gene that regulates the developmental timing pathway in *Caenorhabditis Elegan*s, where mutation of Lin28 leads to precocious development and gain of function allele leads to retarded development (Moss, Lee et al. 1997). Lin28 encodes for a cytoplasmic RNA binding protein that contains a cold shock domain and retroviral type zinc finger motifs and has been implicated as a translational enhancer (Polesskaya, Cuvellier et al. 2007).

Lin28 was identified as a hESC-specific gene in transcriptome study by serial analysis of gene expression (SAGE) (Richards, Tan et al. 2004). However, functional studies of Lin28 in hESC and mESC have yielded opposing results. Overexpression of Lin28 resulted in accelerated cell proliferation in mESC (Xu, Zhang et al. 2009), but seemed to slow down proliferation and cause extraembryonic endoderm differentiation in hESC (Darr and Benvenisty 2009). Conversely, knockdown of Lin28 resulted in decreased cell proliferation in mESC (Xu, Zhang et al. 2009), while in hESC there is no obvious phenotype (Darr and Benvenisty 2009). Whether Lin28 play a different role in human and mouse is unclear at the moment. However in human, Lin28 seemed to be dispensible for ESC self-renewal but is involved in differentiation commitment (Darr and Benvenisty 2009). At this point, it is worth noting that although Lin28 is used in conjunction with Nanog, Oct-4, and Sox2 to reprogram human fibroblast to pluripotency, it only has a modest effect on reprogramming (Yu, Vodyanik et al. 2007). Moreover, Lin28 can be replaced by other combinations of transcription factors (Takahashi, Tanabe et al. 2007). Together, this suggests that Lin28 may not be a core component of the transcriptional network governing ESC pluripotency, but rather an enhancer to induce pluripotency much like Klf4. Clearly, a complete understanding of the role of Lin28 in ESC self-renewal and iPS cell reprogramming awaits further study.

How Lin28 contributes to maintain ESC pluripotency is intriguing at the moment. One proposed mechanism is that Lin28 acts to block the processing of let7 microRNA family members, a group of microRNA associated with differentiation (Viswanathan, Daley et al. 2008). Moreover, let7 has been suggested to act as tumor suppressor by repressing oncogene expression such as c-Myc and Ras, therefore Lin28 may be promoting oncogenic proliferation by down-regulating let7 (Peter 2009). Another proposed mechanism of Lin28 is that it may acts to stabilize and enhance translation of certain mRNAs that are critical for pluripotency. A previous study have demonstrated that Lin28 can reside in both polysomal ribosome fractions, in which mRNA is translated, and also P-bodies, in which mRNA is degraded (Balzer and Moss 2007). Therefore, Lin28 may regulate pluripotency by selectively enhancing translation for certain mRNA while degrading other mRNA.

Myc

The Myc gene family has been intensively studied for more than two decades. c-Myc have a well documented role in cancer biology. Deregulated levels of c-Myc have been observed in human cancers and demonstrated to promote cell transformation and tumor progression (Kendall, Adam et al. 2006). c-Myc is believed to regulate the expression of 15% of all genes, including genes involved in cellular apoptosis, cell cycle control, protein biosynthesis and metabolism (Patel, Loboda et al. 2004). c-Myc has been shown to regulate its target genes through interactions with chromatin remodeling complexes, histone modifying enzymes, DNA methyltransferases and general components of the transcription machinery (Eilers and Eisenman 2008).

Research addressing the role of Myc in pluripotent cells in the pre-implantation embryo has yielded contradictory results. In mouse embryo, c-Myc expression is initiated at the four-cell stage and is highly expressed during the blastocyst stage (Paria, Dey et al. 1992). Knockdown of c-Myc using antisense DNA leads to developmental arrest before the blastocyst stage, suggesting a critical role of c-Myc in early mouse embryo (Paria, Dey et al. 1992; Naz, Kumar et al. 1994). However, knockout studies of c-Myc or another family member N-Myc in mice resulted in embryo lethality but die at a much later time at E9.5-E12.5 (Charron, Malynn et al. 1992; Stanton, Perkins et al. 1992; Davis, Wims et al. 1993). The reason for this contradiction in previous studies is unclear at this stage, and further study is needed to clarify the role of Myc in pluripotent cells in early embryo.

Previous studies have demonstrated that c-Myc play a critical role in mESC. Sustained expression of c-Myc renders mESC resistant to differentiation, whereas expression of a dominant negative form of c-Myc antagonizes self-renewal and promotes differentiation (Cartwright, McLean et al. 2005). Surprisingly, c-Myc behaves quite differently in hESC. Overexpression of c-Myc drives hESC to apoptosis and differentiation into extraembryonic endoderm and trophectoderm (Sumi, Tsuneyoshi et al. 2007). In this latter study, the authors also demonstrated that blockage of p53 and caspase signaling effectively prevent the apoptosis phenotype evoked by c-Myc, but the differentiation phenotype still occurs in c-Myc overexpressing cells. Therefore, it is unlikely that c-Myc-driven apoptotic signals are driving hESC to differentiate (Sumi, Tsuneyoshi et al. 2007).

c-Myc was identified as one of four factors able to generate both mouse and human iPS cells (Takahashi and Yamanaka 2006; Takahashi, Tanabe et al. 2007). However, subsequent studies demonstrated that somatic cell reprogramming can be achieved without addition of c-Myc, although with significantly reduced efficiency and kinetics (Nakagawa, Koyanagi et al. 2008; Wernig, Meissner et al. 2008). Moreover, Klf4 and c-Myc can be replaced by a combination of Nanog and Lin28, suggesting that c-Myc is not essential for induced pluripotency (Yu, Vodyanik et al. 2007). How c-Myc contributes to induced pluripotency is an area under intense study right now. Recent evidence suggest that c-Myc play an important part during early reprogramming by down-regulating somatic gene expressions, a process that occurs before the activation of the pluripotency gene networks (Sridharan, Tchieu et al. 2009). Genome-wide analysis of promoter binding demonstrated that c-Myc regulates a different set of target genes compared to other pluripotency factors Oct4, Sox2 and Klf4 in mESC (Chen, Xu et al. 2008; Kim, Chu et al. 2008). This suggests that the function of c-Myc in ESC maybe very different to other 'stemness' transcription factors. One proposed function of c-Myc is that it may induce a cell cycle program that is necessary for self-renewal of stem cells. Previous studies have demonstrated that c-Myc can activate proliferation-associated genes (i.e. cyclin A, cyclin E or E2F) and suppresses genes associated with growth arrest (i.e. p21, p27) (Vermeulen, Berneman et al. 2003). Moreover, Myc has a documented role in maintaining the epigenetic status of chromatin (Knoepfler, Zhang et al. 2006). Thus another proposed mechanism for c-Myc is that it can modify the chromatin structure to allow expression of genes that promote self-renewal and inhibit expression of pro-differentiation genes.

Conclusion

As summarized in Figure 1, this chapter has provided a detailed review of the signal transduction pathways and the transcriptional network regulating self-renewal in ESC. Emerging evidence suggests that no one signaling pathways is sufficient to maintain hESC undifferentiated on its own. Instead, multiple signaling pathways cooperate together to achieve self-renewal, such as activin and bFGF signaling. The interactions between these signaling pathways are still poorly understood. Similarly, in the transcriptional network not one transcription factor is sufficient to maintain ESC pluripotency, but the important genes such as Oct4, Sox2, Nanog and Klf4 often cooperate together to activate a gene expression program that governs stem cell self-renewal. As limited studies have attempted to link the upstream signaling pathways to the downstream transcriptional network that regulate cell pluripotency, this remains a major challenge for future research in hESC. For instance, in hESC activin stimulation of Smad2/3 binds and activates Nanog, whereas BMP stimulation of Smad1 binds and represses Nanog (Xu, Sampsell-Barron et al. 2008). Future research that bridges the gap between the upstream signaling pathways with the downstream transcriptional network will help to unravel this complex molecular mechanism governing stem cell pluripotency. These studies in turn will help in the goal of using human pluripotent stem cells to develop mew treatments for human disease as well as provide critical insigits into early human development.

Acknowledgments

The authors wish to thank Dr. Sandy S.C. Hung for proof reading the manuscript and helping with generating the figure. The authors are also grateful to supports from California Institute of Regenerative Medicine (Grant T1-00008 to Raymond C.B. Wong, RCI-00110 to Peter J. Donovan), National Institute of Health (Grant HD49488 and HD47675 to Peter J. Donovan), University of Melbourne, National Health and Medical Research Council of Australia (Grant 454723 to Alice Pébay) and Friedreich Ataxia Research Association.

References

Adhikary, S. and Eilers, M. (2005). "Transcriptional regulation and transformation by Myc proteins." *Nat Rev Mol Cell Biol* **6**(8): 635-45.

Ambrosetti, D. C., Basilico, C., et al. (1997). "Synergistic activation of the fibroblast growth factor 4 enhancer by Sox2 and Oct-3 depends on protein-protein interactions facilitated by a specific spatial arrangement of factor binding sites." *Mol Cell Biol* **17**(11): 6321-9.

Amit, M., Carpenter, M. K., et al. (2000). "Clonally derived human embryonic stem cell lines maintain pluripotency and proliferative potential for prolonged periods of culture." *Dev Biol* **227**(2): 271-8.

Amit, M., Shariki, C., et al. (2004). "Feeder layer- and serum-free culture of human embryonic stem cells." *Biol Reprod* **70**(3): 837-45.

Androutsellis-Theotokis, A., Leker, R. R., et al. (2006). "Notch signalling regulates stem cell numbers in vitro and in vivo." *Nature* **442**(7104): 823-6.

Armstrong, L., Hughes, O., et al. (2006). "The role of PI3K/AKT, MAPK/ERK and NFkappabeta signalling in the maintenance of human embryonic stem cell pluripotency and viability highlighted by transcriptional profiling and functional analysis." *Hum Mol Genet* **15**(11): 1894-913.

Assou, S., Le Carrour, T., et al. (2007). "A meta-analysis of human embryonic stem cells transcriptome integrated into a web-based expression atlas." *Stem Cells* **25**(4): 961-73.

Atlasi, Y., Mowla, S. J., et al. (2008). "OCT4 spliced variants are differentially expressed in human pluripotent and nonpluripotent cells." *Stem Cells* **26**(12): 3068-74.

Avery, K., Avery, S., et al. (2008). "Sphingosine-1-phosphate mediates transcriptional regulation of key targets associated with survival, proliferation, and pluripotency in human embryonic stem cells." *Stem Cells Dev* **17**(6): 1195-205.

Avilion, A. A., Nicolis, S. K., et al. (2003). "Multipotent cell lineages in early mouse development depend on SOX2 function." *Genes Dev* **17**(1): 126-40.

Balzer, E. and Moss, E. G. (2007). "Localization of the developmental timing regulator Lin28 to mRNP complexes, P-bodies and stress granules." *RNA Biol* **4**(1): 16-25.

Beattie, G. M., Lopez, A. D., et al. (2005). "Activin A maintains pluripotency of human embryonic stem cells in the absence of feeder layers." *Stem Cells* **23**(4): 489-95.

Bendall, S. C., Stewart, M. H., et al. (2007). "IGF and FGF cooperatively establish the regulatory stem cell niche of pluripotent human cells in vitro." *Nature* **448**(7157): 1015-21.

Besser, D. (2004). "Expression of nodal, lefty-a, and lefty-B in undifferentiated human embryonic stem cells requires activation of Smad2/3." *J Biol Chem* **279**(43): 45076-84.

Boyer, L. A., Lee, T. I., et al. (2005). "Core transcriptional regulatory circuitry in human embryonic stem cells." *Cell* **122**(6): 947-56.

Brandenberger, R., Wei, H., et al. (2004). "Transcriptome characterization elucidates signaling networks that control human ES cell growth and differentiation." *Nat Biotechnol* **22**(6): 707-16.

Brimble, S. N., Sherrer, E. S., et al. (2007). "The cell surface glycosphingolipids SSEA-3 and SSEA-4 are not essential for human ESC pluripotency." *Stem Cells* **25**(1): 54-62.

Brons, I. G., Smithers, L. E., et al. (2007). "Derivation of pluripotent epiblast stem cells from mammalian embryos." *Nature* **448**(7150): 191-5.

Burdon, T., Chambers, I., et al. (1999). "Signaling mechanisms regulating self-renewal and differentiation of pluripotent embryonic stem cells." *Cells Tissues Organs* **165**(3-4): 131-43.

Burdon, T., Smith, A., et al. (2002). "Signalling, cell cycle and pluripotency in embryonic stem cells." *Trends Cell Biol* **12**(9): 432-8.

Burdon, T., Stracey, C., et al. (1999). "Suppression of SHP-2 and ERK signalling promotes self-renewal of mouse embryonic stem cells." *Dev Biol* **210**(1): 30-43.

Cadigan, K. M. and Liu, Y. I., (2006). "Wnt signaling: complexity at the surface." *J Cell Sci* **119**(Pt 3): 395-402.

Cartwright, P., McLean, C., et al. (2005). "LIF/STAT3 controls ES cell self-renewal and pluripotency by a Myc-dependent mechanism." *Development* **132**(5): 885-96.

Chambers, I., Colby, D., et al. (2003). "Functional expression cloning of Nanog, a pluripotency sustaining factor in embryonic stem cells." *Cell* 113(5): 643-55.

Chambers, I., Silva, J., et al. (2007). "Nanog safeguards pluripotency and mediates germline development." *Nature* **450**(7173): 1230-4.

Chan, K. K., Zhang, J., et al. (2009). "KLF4 and PBX1 Directly Regulate NANOG Expression in Human Embryonic Stem Cells." *Stem Cells* **27**(9): 2114-25.

Charron, J., Malynn, B. A., et al. (1992). "Embryonic lethality in mice homozygous for a targeted disruption of the N-myc gene." *Genes Dev* **6**(12A): 2248-57.

Chen, X., Xu, H., et al. (2008). "Integration of external signaling pathways with the core transcriptional network in embryonic stem cells." *Cell* **133**(6): 1106-17.

Cheon, S. H., Kim, S. J., et al. (2005). "Defined Feeder-Free Culture System of Human Embryonic Stem Cells." *Biol Reprod* **74**(3): 611.

Chew, J. L., Loh, Y. H., et al. (2005). "Reciprocal transcriptional regulation of Pou5f1 and Sox2 via the Oct4/Sox2 complex in embryonic stem cells." *Mol Cell Biol* **25**(14): 6031-46.

Chun, J., Goetzl, E. J., et al. (2002). "International Union of Pharmacology. XXXIV. Lysophospholipid Receptor Nomenclature." *Pharmacol Rev* **54**(2): 265-9.

Claassen, D. A., Desler, M. M., et al. (2009). "ROCK inhibition enhances the recovery and growth of cryopreserved human embryonic stem cells and human induced pluripotent stem cells." *Mol Reprod Dev* **76**(8): 722-32.

D'Amour, K. A., Agulnick, A. D., et al. (2005). "Efficient differentiation of human embryonic stem cells to definitive endoderm." *Nat Biotechnol* **23**(12): 1534-41 .

Daheron, L., Opitz, S. L., et al. (2004). "LIF/STAT3 signaling fails to maintain self-renewal of human embryonic stem cells." *Stem Cells* **22**(5): 770-8.

Damoiseaux, R., Sherman, S. P., et al. (2008). "Integrated Chemical Genomics Reveals Modifiers of Survival in Human Embryonic Stem Cells." *Stem Cells* 27(3): 533-42.

Darr, H. and Benvenisty N. (2009). "Genetic analysis of the role of the reprogramming gene LIN-28 in human embryonic stem cells." *Stem Cells* **27**(2): 352-62.

Darr, H., Mayshar, Y., et al. (2006). "Overexpression of NANOG in human ES cells enables feeder-free growth while inducing primitive ectoderm features." *Development* **133**(6): 1193-201.

Davidson, K. C., Jamshidi, P., et al. (2007). "Wnt3a regulates survival, expansion, and maintenance of neural progenitors derived from human embryonic stem cells." *Mol Cell Neurosci* **36**(3): 408-15.

Davis, A. C., Wims, M., et al. (1993). "A null c-myc mutation causes lethality before 10.5 days of gestation in homozygotes and reduced fertility in heterozygous female mice." *Genes Dev* **7**(4): 671-82.

Delrieu, I. (2000). "The high molecular weight isoforms of basic fibroblast growth factor (FGF-2): an insight into an intracrine mechanism." *FEBS Lett* **468**(1): 6-10.

Diecke, S., Quiroga-Negreira, A., et al. (2008). "FGF2 signaling in mouse embryonic fibroblasts is crucial for self-renewal of embryonic stem cells." *Cells Tissues Organs* **188**(1-2): 52-61.

Dravid, G., Ye, Z., et al. (2005). "Defining the Role of Wnt/{beta}-Catenin Signaling in the Survival, Proliferation, and Self-Renewal of Human Embryonic Stem Cells." *Stem Cells* **23**(10): 1489-1501.

Dvorak, P., Dvorakova, D., et al. (2005). "Expression and potential role of fibroblast growth factor 2 and its receptors in human embryonic stem cells." *Stem Cells* **23**(8): 1200-11.

Eilers, M. and Eisenman, R. N. (2008). "Myc's broad reach." *Genes Dev* **22**(20): 2755-66.

Ellis, P., Fagan, B. M., et al. (2004). "SOX2, a persistent marker for multipotential neural stem cells derived from embryonic stem cells, the embryo or the adult." *Dev Neurosci* **26**(2-4): 148-65.

Ema, M., Mori, D., et al. (2008). "Kruppel-like factor 5 is essential for blastocyst development and the normal self-renewal of mouse ESCs." *Cell Stem Cell* **3**(5): 555-67.

Evans, P. M. and Liu, C., (2008). "Roles of Krupel-like factor 4 in normal homeostasis, cancer and stem cells." *Acta Biochim Biophys Sin* (Shanghai) **40**(7): 554-64.

Feng, B., Ng, J. H., et al. (2009). "Molecules that promote or enhance reprogramming of somatic cells to induced pluripotent stem cells." *Cell Stem Cell* **4**(4): 301-12.

Fong, H., Hohenstein, K. A., et al. (2008). "Regulation of self-renewal and pluripotency by Sox2 in human embryonic stem cells." *Stem Cells* **26**(8): 1931-8.

Ghaleb, A. M., Nandan, M. O., et al. (2005). "Kruppel-like factors 4 and 5: the yin and yang regulators of cellular proliferation." *Cell Res* **15**(2): 92-6.

Ginis, I., Luo, Y., et al. (2004). "Differences between human and mouse embryonic stem cells." *Dev Biol* **269**(2): 360-80.

Gotoh, N. (2009). "Control of stemness by fibroblast growth factor signaling in stem cells and cancer stem cells." *Curr Stem Cell Res Ther* **4**(1): 9-15.

Guo, Y., Costa, R., et al. (2002). "The embryonic stem cell transcription factors Oct-4 and FoxD3 interact to regulate endodermal-specific promoter expression." P*roc Natl Acad Sci* U S A **99**(6): 3663-7.

Harb, N., Archer, T. K., et al. (2008). "The Rho-Rock-Myosin signaling axis determines cell-cell integrity of self-renewing pluripotent stem cells." *PLoS ONE* **3**(8): e3001.

Hasegawa, K., Fujioka, T., et al. (2006). "A method for the selection of human embryonic stem cell sub-lines with high replating efficiency after single cell dissociation." *Stem Cells* **24**(12): 2649-60.

Hatano, S. Y., Tada, M., et al. (2005). "Pluripotential competence of cells associated with Nanog activity." *Mech Dev* **122**(1): 67-79.

Heng, B. C. (2009). "Effect of Rho-associated kinase (ROCK) inhibitor Y-27632 on the post-thaw viability of cryopreserved human bone marrow-derived mesenchymal stem cells." *Tissue Cell* **41**(5): 376-80.

Hohenstein, K. A., Pyle, A. D., et al. (2008). "Nucleofection mediates high-efficiency stable gene knockdown and transgene expression in human embryonic stem cells." *Stem Cells* **26**(6): 1436-43.

Humphrey, R. K., G. M. Beattie, et al. (2004). "Maintenance of pluripotency in human embryonic stem cells is STAT3 independent." *Stem Cells* **22**(4): 522-30.

Hyslop, L., Stojkovic, M., et al. (2005). "Downregulation of NANOG induces differentiation of human embryonic stem cells to extraembryonic lineages." *Stem Cells* **23**(8): 1035-43.

Inniss, K. and Moore, H., (2006). "Mediation of apoptosis and proliferation of human embryonic stem cells by sphingosine-1-phosphate." *Stem Cells Dev* **15**(6): 789-96.

Itoh, N. and Ornitz, D. M. (2004). "Evolution of the Fgf and Fgfr gene families." *Trends Genet* **20**(11): 563-9.

Itsykson, P., Ilouz, N., et al. (2005). "Derivation of neural precursors from human embryonic stem cells in the presence of noggin." *Mol Cell Neurosci* **30**(1): 24-36.

Ivanova, N., Dobrin, R., et al. (2006). "Dissecting self-renewal in stem cells with RNA interference." *Nature* **442**(7102): 533-8.

James, D., Levine, A. J., et al. (2005). "TGFbeta/activin/nodal signaling is necessary for the maintenance of pluripotency in human embryonic stem cells." *Development* **132**(6): 1273-82.

Jiang, J., Chan, Y. S., et al. (2008). "A core Klf circuitry regulates self-renewal of embryonic stem cells." *Nat Cell Biol* **10**(3): 353-60.

Kang, H. B., Kim, J. S., et al. (2005). "Basic fibroblast growth factor activates ERK and induces c-fos in human embryonic stem cell line MizhES1." *Stem Cells Dev* **14**(4): 395-401.

Katoh, M. (2006). "CER1 is a common target of WNT and NODAL signaling pathways in human embryonic stem cells." *Int J Mol Med* **17**(5): 795-9.

Kendall, S. D., Adam, S. J., et al. (2006). "Genetically engineered human cancer models utilizing mammalian transgene expression." *Cell Cycle* **5**(10): 1074-9.

Kim, J., Chu, J., et al. (2008). "An extended transcriptional network for pluripotency of embryonic stem cells." *Cell* **132**(6): 1049-61.

Klimanskaya, I., Chung, Y., et al. (2005). "Human embryonic stem cells derived without feeder cells." *Lancet* **365**(9471): 1636-41.

Knoepfler, P. S., Zhang, X. Y., et al. (2006). "Myc influences global chromatin structure." *EMBO J* **25**(12): 2723-34.

Kondoh, H., Uchikawa, M., et al. (2004). "Interplay of Pax6 and SOX2 in lens development as a paradigm of genetic switch mechanisms for cell differentiation." *Int J Dev Biol* **48**(8-9): 819-27.

Kopp, J. L., Ormsbee, B. D., et al. (2008). "Small increases in the level of Sox2 trigger the differentiation of mouse embryonic stem cells." *Stem Cells* **26**(4): 903-11.

Krawetz, R. J., Li, X., et al. (2009). "Human embryonic stem cells: caught between a ROCK inhibitor and a hard place." *Bioessays* **31**(3): 336-43.

Kunath, T., Saba-El-Leil, M. K., et al. (2007). "FGF stimulation of the Erk1/2 signalling cascade triggers transition of pluripotent embryonic stem cells from self-renewal to lineage commitment." *Development* **134**(16): 2895-902.

Kuroda, T., Tada, M., et al. (2005). "Octamer and Sox elements are required for transcriptional cis regulation of Nanog gene expression." *Mol Cell Biol* **25**(6): 2475-85.

Lee, J., Kim, H. K., et al. (2006). "The human OCT-4 isoforms differ in their ability to confer self-renewal." *J Biol Chem* **281**(44): 33554-65.

Letamendia, A., Labbe, E., et al. (2001). "Transcriptional regulation by Smads: crosstalk between the TGF-beta and Wnt pathways." *J Bone Joint Surg Am* **83-A** Suppl 1(Pt 1): S31-9.

Levenstein, M. E., Ludwig, T. E., et al. (2006). "Basic FGF Support of Human Embryonic Stem Cell Self-Renewal." *Stem Cells* **24**(3): 568-74.

Li, J., Pan, G., et al. (2007). "A dominant-negative form of mouse SOX2 induces trophectoderm differentiation and progressive polyploidy in mouse embryonic stem cells." *J Biol Chem* **282**(27): 19481-92.

Li, J., Wang, G., et al. (2007). "MEK/ERK signaling contributes to the maintenance of human embryonic stem cell self-renewal." *Differentiation* **75**(4): 299-307.

Li, M., Pevny, L., et al. (1998). "Generation of purified neural precursors from embryonic stem cells by lineage selection." *Curr Biol* **8**(17): 971-4.

Li, X., Krawetz, R., et al. (2009). "ROCK inhibitor improves survival of *cryopreserved serum/feeder-free single human embryonic stem cells." Hum Reprod* **24**(3): 580-9.

Li, X., Meng, G., et al. (2008). "The ROCK inhibitor Y-27632 enhances the survival rate of human embryonic stem cells following cryopreservation." *Stem Cells Dev* **17**(6): 1079-85.

Li, Y., McClintick, J., et al. (2005). "Murine embryonic stem cell differentiation is promoted by SOCS-3 and inhibited by the zinc finger transcription factor Klf4." *Blood* **105**(2): 635-7.

Liu, L., Leaman, D., et al. (1997). "Silencing of the gene for the alpha-subunit of human chorionic gonadotropin by the embryonic transcription factor Oct-3/4." *Mol Endocrinol* **11**(11): 1651-8.

Liu, L. and Roberts, R. M., (1996). "Silencing of the gene for the beta subunit of human chorionic gonadotropin by the embryonic transcription factor Oct-3/4." *J Biol Chem* **271**(28): 16683-9.

Lu, B., P. Pang, T., et al. (2005). "The yin and yang of neurotrophin action." *Nat Rev Neurosci* **6**(8): 603-14.

Ludwig, T. E., Levenstein, M. E., et al. (2006). "Derivation of human embryonic stem cells in defined conditions." *Nat Biotechnol* **24**(2):185-7.

Masui, S., Nakatake, Y., et al. (2007). "Pluripotency governed by Sox2 via regulation of Oct3/4 expression in mouse embryonic stem cells." *Nat Cell Biol* **9**(6): 625-35.

Matin, M. M., Walsh, J. R., et al. (2004). "Specific knockdown of Oct4 and beta2-microglobulin expression by RNA interference in human embryonic stem cells and embryonic carcinoma cells." *Stem Cells* **22**(5): 659-68.

Mayshar, Y., Rom, E., et al. (2008). "Fibroblast growth factor 4 and its novel splice isoform have opposing effects on the maintenance of human embryonic stem cell self-renewal." *Stem Cells* **26**(3): 767-74.

McConnell, B. B., Ghaleb, A. M., et al. (2007). "The diverse functions of Kruppel-like factors 4 and 5 in epithelial biology and pathobiology." *Bioessays* **29**(6): 549-57.

McLean, A. B., D'Amour, K. A., et al. (2007). "Activin a efficiently specifies definitive endoderm from human embryonic stem cells only when phosphatidylinositol 3-kinase signaling is suppressed." *Stem Cells* **25**(1): 29-38.

Mitsui, K., Tokuzawa, Y., et al. (2003). "The homeoprotein Nanog is required for maintenance of pluripotency in mouse epiblast and ES cells." *Cell* **113**(5): 631-42.

Miyazawa, K., Shinozaki, M., et al. (2002). "Two major Smad pathways in TGF-beta superfamily signalling." *Genes Cells* **7**(12): 1191-204.

Moss, E. G., Lee, R. C., et al. (1997). "The cold shock domain protein LIN-28 controls developmental timing in C. elegans and is regulated by the lin-4 RNA." *Cell* **88**(5): 637-46.

Nakagawa, M., Koyanagi, M., et al. (2008). "Generation of induced pluripotent stem cells without Myc from mouse and human fibroblasts." *Nat Biotechnol* **26**(1): 101-6.

Nakatake, Y., Fukui, N., et al. (2006). "Klf4 cooperates with Oct3/4 and Sox2 to activate the Lefty1 core promoter in embryonic stem cells." *Mol Cell Biol* **26**(20): 7772-82.

Naz, R. K., Kumar, G., et al. (1994). "Expression and role of c-myc protooncogene in murine preimplantation embryonic development." *J Assist Reprod Genet* **11**(4): 208-16.

Nichols, J., Zevnik, B., et al. (1998). "Formation of pluripotent stem cells in the mammalian embryo depends on the POU transcription factor Oct4." *Cell* **95**(3): 379-91.

Nishimoto, M., Fukushima, A., et al. (1999). "The gene for the embryonic stem cell coactivator UTF1 carries a regulatory element which selectively interacts with a complex composed of Oct-3/4 and Sox-2." *Mol Cell Biol* **19**(8): 5453-65.

Nishimoto, M., Miyagi, S., et al. (2005). "Oct-3/4 maintains the proliferative embryonic stem cell state via specific binding to a variant octamer sequence in the regulatory region of the UTF1 locus." *Mol Cell Biol* **25**(12): 5084-94.

Niwa, H., Miyazaki, J., et al. (2000). "Quantitative expression of Oct-3/4 defines differentiation, dedifferentiation or self-renewal of ES cells." *Nat Genet* **24**(4): 372-6.

Niwa, H., Toyooka, Y., et al. (2005). "Interaction between Oct3/4 and Cdx2 determines trophectoderm differentiation." *Cell* **123**(5): 917-29.

Okamoto, K., Okazawa, H., et al. (1990). "A novel octamer binding transcription factor is differentially expressed in mouse embryonic cells." *Cell* **60**(3): 461-72.

Okuda, A., Fukushima, A., et al. (1998). "UTF1, a novel transcriptional coactivator expressed in pluripotent embryonic stem cells and extra-embryonic cells." *EMBO J* **17**(7): 2019-32.

Paria, B. C., Dey, S. K., et al. (1992). "Antisense c-myc effects on preimplantation mouse embryo development." *Proc Natl Acad Sci U S A* **89**(21): 10051-5.

Patel, J. H., Loboda, A. P., et al. (2004). "Analysis of genomic targets reveals complex functions of MYC." *Nat Rev Cancer* **4**(7): 562-8.

Pebay, A., Wong, R. C., et al. (2005). "Essential roles of sphingosine-1-phosphate and platelet-derived growth factor in the maintenance of human embryonic stem cells." *Stem Cells* **23**(10): 1541-8.

Pera, M. F., Andrade, J., et al. (2004). "Regulation of human embryonic stem cell differentiation by BMP-2 and its antagonist noggin." *J Cell Sci* **117**(Pt 7): 1269-80.

Pera, M. F., Andrade, J., et al. (2004). "Regulation of human embryonic stem cell differentiation by BMP-2 and its antagonist noggin." *J Cell Sci* **117**(Pt 7): 1269-80.

Pera, M. F., Reubinoff, B., et al. (2000). "Human embryonic stem cells." *J Cell Sci* **113** (Pt 1): 5-10.

Pesce, M. and Scholer, H. R., (2001). "Oct-4: gatekeeper in the beginnings of mammalian development." *Stem Cells* **19**(4): 271-8.

Peter, M. E. (2009). "Let-7 and miR-200 microRNAs: guardians against pluripotency and cancer progression." *Cell Cycle* **8**(6): 843-52.

Pitson, S. M. and Pebay, A., (2009). "Regulation of stem cell pluripotency and neural differentiation by lysophospholipids." *Neurosignals* **17**(4): 242-54.

Polesskaya, A., Cuvellier, S., et al. (2007). "Lin-28 binds IGF-2 mRNA and participates in skeletal myogenesis by increasing translation efficiency." *Genes Dev* **21**(9): 1125-38.

Pyle, A. D., Lock, L. F., et al. (2006). "Neurotrophins mediate human embryonic stem cell survival." *Nat Biotechnol* **24**(3): 344-50.

Reissmann, E., Jornvall, H., et al. (2001). "The orphan receptor ALK7 and the Activin receptor ALK4 mediate signaling by Nodal proteins during vertebrate development." *Genes Dev* **15**(15): 2010-22.

Reubinoff, B. E., Pera, M. F., et al. (2000). "Embryonic stem cell lines from human blastocysts: somatic differentiation in vitro." *Nat Biotechnol* **18**(4): 399-404.

Rho, J. Y., Yu, K., et al. (2006). "Transcriptional profiling of the developmentally important signalling pathways in human embryonic stem cells." *Hum Reprod* **21**(2): 405-12.

Richards, M., Tan, S. P., et al. (2004). "The transcriptome profile of human embryonic stem cells as defined by SAGE." *Stem Cells* **22**(1): 51-64.

Rodda, D. J., Chew, J. L., et al. (2005). "Transcriptional regulation of nanog by OCT4 and SOX2." *J Biol Chem* **280**(26): 24731-7.

Rosner, M. H., Vigano, M. A., et al. (1990). "A POU-domain transcription factor in early stem cells and germ cells of the mammalian embryo." *Nature* **345**(6277): 686-92.

Rowland, B. D., Bernards, R., et al. (2005). "The KLF4 tumour suppressor is a transcriptional repressor of p53 that acts as a context-dependent oncogene." *Nat Cell Biol* **7**(11): 1074-82.

Rowland, B. D. and Peeper, D. S., (2006). "KLF4, p21 and context-dependent opposing forces in cancer." *Nat Rev Cancer* **6**(1): 11-23.

Sato, N., Meijer, L., et al. (2004). "Maintenance of pluripotency in human and mouse embryonic stem cells through activation of Wnt signaling by a pharmacological GSK-3-specific inhibitor." *Nat Med* **10**(1): 55-63.

Sato, N., Sanjuan, I. M., et al. (2003). "Molecular signature of human embryonic stem cells and its comparison with the mouse." *Dev Biol* **260**(2): 404-13.

Schlessinger, J. (2004). "Common and distinct elements in cellular signaling via EGF and FGF receptors." *Science* **306**(5701): 1506-7.

Scholer, H. R., Balling, R., et al. (1989). "Octamer binding proteins confer transcriptional activity in early mouse embryogenesis." *EMBO J* **8**(9): 2551-7.

Segre, J. A., Bauer, C. et al. (1999). "Klf4 is a transcription factor required for establishing the barrier function of the skin." *Nat Genet* **22**(4): 356-60.

Shi, Y. and Massague, J. (2003). "Mechanisms of TGF-beta signaling from cell membrane to the nucleus." *Cell* **113**(6): 685-700.

Shimozaki, K., Nakashima, K., et al. (2003). "Involvement of Oct3/4 in the enhancement of neuronal differentiation of ES cells in neurogenesis-inducing cultures." *Development* **130**(11): 2505-12.

Sperger, J. M., Chen, X., et al. (2003). "Gene expression patterns in human embryonic stem cells and human pluripotent germ cell tumors." *Proc Natl Acad Sci U S A* **100**(23): 13350-5.

Sridharan, R., Tchieu, J., et al. (2009). "Role of the murine reprogramming factors in the induction of pluripotency." *Cell* **136**(2): 364-77.

Stachowiak, M. K., Fang, X., et al. (2003). "Integrative nuclear FGFR1 signaling (INFS) as a part of a universal "feed-forward-and-gate" signaling module that controls cell growth and differentiation." *J Cell Biochem* **90**(4): 662-91.

Stanton, B. R., Perkins, A. S., et al. (1992). "Loss of N-myc function results in embryonic lethality and failure of the epithelial component of the embryo to develop." *Genes Dev* **6**(12A): 2235-47.

Sumi, T., Tsuneyoshi, N., et al. (2007). "Apoptosis and differentiation of human embryonic stem cells induced by sustained activation of c-Myc." *Oncogene* **26**(38): 5564-76.

Suzuki, A., Raya, A., et al. (2006). "Nanog binds to Smad1 and blocks bone morphogenetic protein-induced differentiation of embryonic stem cells." *Proc Natl Acad Sci U S A* **103**(27): 10294-9.

Takahashi, K., Tanabe, K., et al. (2007). "Induction of pluripotent stem cells from adult human fibroblasts by defined factors." *Cell* **131**(5): 861-72.

Takahashi, K. and Yamanaka, S., (2006). "Induction of pluripotent stem cells from mouse embryonic and adult fibroblast cultures by defined factors." *Cell* **126**(4): 663-76.

Takeda, J., Seino, S., et al. (1992). "Human Oct3 gene family: cDNA sequences, alternative splicing, gene organization, chromosomal location, and expression at low levels in adult tissues." *Nucleic Acids Res* **20**(17): 4613-20.

Takuwa, Y., Takuwa, N., et al. (2002). "The edg family g protein-coupled receptors for lysophospholipids: their signaling properties and biological activities." *J Biochem (Tokyo)* **131**(6): 767-71.

Thomson, J. A., Itskovitz-Eldor, J., et al. (1998). "Embryonic stem cell lines derived from human blastocysts." *Science* **282**(5391): 1145-7.

Tokuzawa, Y., Kaiho, E., et al. (2003). "Fbx15 is a novel target of Oct3/4 but is dispensable for embryonic stem cell self-renewal and mouse development." *Mol Cell Biol* **23**(8): 2699-708.

Tomioka, M., Nishimoto, M., et al. (2002). "Identification of Sox-2 regulatory region which is under the control of Oct-3/4-Sox-2 complex." *Nucleic Acids Res* **30**(14): 3202-13.

Vallier, L., Alexander, M., et al. (2005). "Activin/Nodal and FGF pathways cooperate to maintain pluripotency of human embryonic stem cells." *J Cell Sci* **118**(Pt 19): 4495-509.

Vallier, L., Reynolds, D., et al. (2004). "Nodal inhibits differentiation of human embryonic stem cells along the neuroectodermal default pathway." *Dev Biol* **275**(2): 403-21.

Vallier, L., Touboul, T., et al. (2009). "Early cell fate decisions of human embryonic stem cells and mouse epiblast stem cells are controlled by the same signalling pathways." *PLoS One* **4**(6): e6082.

Varelas, X., Sakuma, R., et al. (2008). "TAZ controls Smad nucleocytoplasmic shuttling and regulates human embryonic stem-cell self-renewal." *Nat Cell Biol* **10**(7): 837-48.

Vermeulen, K., Berneman, Z. N., et al. (2003). "Cell cycle and apoptosis." *Cell Prolif* **36**(3): 165-75.

Viswanathan, S. R., Daley, G. Q., et al. (2008). "Selective blockade of microRNA processing by Lin28." *Science* **320**(5872): 97-100.

Walsh, J. and Andrews, P. W., (2003). "Expression of Wnt and Notch pathway genes in a pluripotent human embryonal carcinoma cell line and embryonic stem cell." *Apmis* **111**(1): 197-210; discussion 210-1.

Wang, G., Zhang, H., et al. (2005). "Noggin and bFGF cooperate to maintain the pluripotency of human embryonic stem cells in the absence of feeder layers." *Biochem Biophys Res Commun* **330**(3): 934-42.

Wang, J., Rao, S., et al. (2006). "A protein interaction network for pluripotency of embryonic stem cells." *Nature* **444**(7117): 364-8.

Wang, L., Li, L., et al. (2005). "Human embryonic stem cells maintained in the absence of mouse embryonic fibroblasts or conditioned media are capable of hematopoietic development." *Blood* **105**(12): 4598-603.

Watanabe, K., Ueno, M., et al. (2007). "A ROCK inhibitor permits survival of dissociated human embryonic stem cells." *Nat Biotechnol* **25**(6): 681-6.

Wernig, M., Meissner, A., et al. (2008). "c-Myc is dispensable for direct reprogramming of mouse fibroblasts." *Cell Stem Cell* **2**(1): 10-2.

Wong, R. C., Tellis, I., et al. (2007). "Anti-apoptotic effect of sphingosine-1-phosphate and platelet-derived growth factor in human embryonic stem cells." *Stem Cells Dev* **16**(6): 989-1001.

Xiao, L., Yuan, X., et al. (2006). "Activin A maintains self-renewal and regulates FGF, Wnt and BMP pathways in human embryonic stem cells." *Stem Cells* **24**(6): 1476-86.

Xu, B., Zhang, K., et al. (2009). "Lin28 modulates cell growth and associates with a subset of cell cycle regulator mRNAs in mouse embryonic stem cells." *RNA* **15**(3): 357-61.

Xu, C., Inokuma, M. S., et al. (2001). "Feeder-free growth of undifferentiated human embryonic stem cells." *Nat Biotechnol* **19**(10): 971-4.

Xu, C., Rosler, E., et al. (2005). "Basic fibroblast growth factor supports undifferentiated human embryonic stem cell growth without conditioned medium." *Stem Cells* **23**(3): 315-23.

Xu, R. H., X. Chen, et al. (2002). "BMP4 initiates human embryonic stem cell differentiation to trophoblast." *Nat Biotechnol* **20**(12): 1261-4.

Xu, R. H., Peck, R. M., et al. (2005). "Basic FGF and suppression of BMP signaling sustain undifferentiated proliferation of human ES cells." *Nat Methods* **2**(3): 185-90.

Xu, R. H., Sampsell-Barron, T. L., et al. (2008). "NANOG is a direct target of TGFbeta/activin-mediated SMAD signaling in human ESCs." *Cell Stem Cell* **3**(2): 196-206.

Yao, S., Chen, S., et al. (2006). "Long-term self-renewal and directed differentiation of human embryonic stem cells in chemically defined conditions." *Proc Natl Acad Sci U S A* **103**(18): 6907-12.

Ying, Q. L., Nichols, J., et al. (2003). "BMP induction of Id proteins suppresses differentiation and sustains embryonic stem cell self-renewal in collaboration with STAT3." *Cell* **115**(3): 281-92.

Yu, J., Vodyanik, M. A., et al. (2007). "Induced pluripotent stem cell lines derived from human somatic cells." *Science* **318**(5858): 1917-20.

Yuan, H., Corbi, N., et al. (1995). "Developmental-specific activity of the FGF-4 enhancer requires the synergistic action of Sox2 and Oct-3." *Genes Dev* **9**(21): 2635-45.

Zaehres, H., Lensch, M. W., et al. (2005). "High-efficiency RNA interference in human embryonic stem cells." *Stem Cells* **23**(3): 299-305.

Zeineddine, D., Papadimou, E., et al. (2006). "Oct-3/4 dose dependently regulates specification of embryonic stem cells toward a cardiac lineage and early heart development." *Dev Cell* **11**(4): 535-46.

Zhao, S., Nichols, J., et al. (2004). "SoxB transcription factors specify neuroectodermal lieage choice in ES cells." *Mol Cell Neurosci* **27**(3): 332-42.

In: Pluripotent Stem Cells
Editors: D.W. Rosales et al, pp. 81-112
ISBN: 978-1-60876-738-0

Chapter 3

GENERATION OF CLINICALLY RELEVANT "INDUCED PLURIPOTENT STEM" (iPS) CELLS

Corey Heffernan, Huseyin Sumer and Paul J. Verma*
Reprogramming and Stem Cell Laboratory, Monash Institute of Medical Research, Monash University, 27-31 Wright St., Clayton, VIC, 3168, Australia

Abstract

Proviral expression of early development genes Oct4 and Sox2, in concert with cMyc and Klf4 or Nanog and Lin28, can induce differentiated cells to adopt morphological and functional characteristics of pluripotency indistinguishable from embryonic stem cells. Termed induced pluripotent stem (iPS) cells, in mice the pluripotency of these cells was confirmed by altered gene/surface antigen expression, remodeling of the epigenome, ability to contribute to embryonic lineages following blastocyst injection and commitment to all three germ layers in teratomas and liveborn chimeras. Importantly, *in vitro* directed differentiation of iPS cells yield cells capable of treating mouse models of humanized disease. Despite these impressive results, iPS cell conversion is frustratingly inefficient. Also, the unpredictable and random mutagenesis imposed on the host cell

* E-mail address: paul.verma@med.monash.edu.au. Tel: 61 3 9594 7000, Fax: 61 3 9594 7100. Corresponding author: Paul J. Verma Ph.D.; c/o Reprogramming and Stem Cell Laboratory, Centre for Reproduction and Development, Level 2, Monash Institute of Medical Research, Monash University, 27-31 Wright Street, Clayton, VIC 3168, Australia.

genome, inherent with integrative viral methodologies, continues to hamper use of these cells in a therapeutic setting. This has initiated exploration of non-integrating strategies for generating iPS cells. Here, we review mechanisms that drive conversion of somatic cells to iPS cells and the strategies adopted to circumvent integrative viral strategies. Finally, we discuss practical, ethical and legal considerations that require addressing before iPS cells can realize their potential as patient-specific cells for treatment of degenerative disease.

1. Introduction: Generation of Induced Pluripotent Stem (iPS) Cells

The process of reversing the genetic program of a somatic cell to one characteristic of embryonic cells, so elegantly demonstrated by cloning of *Dolly* the sheep by somatic cell nuclear transfer (SCNT), is referred to as 'nuclear reprogramming' (Wilmut et al., 1997). The subsequent excitement in the possibility of deriving patient-specific stem cells for autologous cell replacement therapy was counterbalanced with moral ethical concerns surrounding oocyte donation and embryo destruction. The search for alternative methodologies that successfully induce pluripotency in differentiated somatic cells lead to the development of ES-somatic cell fusion, and treatment of somatic cells with cell extracts (for review, see Hochedlinger & Jaenisch, 2007). Takahashi & Yamanaka (2006) invigorated the reprogramming field when they successfully reprogrammed somatic cells by retroviral delivery and forced expression of four key transcription factors Oct4, Sox2, cMyc and Klf4. These cells were coined 'induced pluripotent stem' (iPS) cells. The reversal of the biological safeguards maintaining the stability of lineage committed cells to pluripotent, colony-forming iPS cells was confirmed collectively by gene/surface antigen expression, epigenetic remodeling, contribution to embryonic lineages in liveborns following diploid and tetraploid blastocyst injection and commitment to all three germ layers in teratomas generated in SCID mice (Takahashi & Yamanaka, 2006; Takahashi et al., 2007; Wernig et al., 2007; Maherali et al., 2007; Okita et al., 2008; Kang at el., 2009; Zhao et al., 2009). Originally demonstrated in mouse, iPS cells have been generated in rat (Li et al., 2008), rhesus monkey (Liu et al., 2008[a]) and pig (Esteban et al., 2009; Ezashi et al., 2009), as well as from a range of human cells including keratinocytes (Aasen et al., 2008; Maherali et al., 2008), dermal fibroblasts (Maherali et al., 2008) and peripheral blood (Loh et al., 2009). Interestingly, mouse sequences for the four reprogramming factors can effectively reprogram human somatic cells (Woltjen et al., 2008). Subsequent to the original reports from the Yamanaka lab, a reprogramming cocktail similarly incorporating

Oct4 and Sox2, with two alternative factors Nanog and Lin28 was shown to reprogram human cells to pluripotency (Yu et al., 2007). However, low efficiency of conversion from somatic to iPS cells continues to hamper either methodology.

1.1. The Mainstays of the Reprogramming Cocktail: Oct4 & Sox2

Collectively, Oct4 and Sox2 play crucial roles in maintaining pluripotency and self-renewal in ES cells *in vivo* and *in vitro*, and in inducing pluripotency in somatic cells (Takahashi & Yamanaka, 2006; Yu et al., 2007). Expression of the POU domain transcription factor Oct4 from the *POU5F1* locus is a well documented feature of early embryogenesis and ES cells *in vitro.* Oct4 incorporates a POU specific domain (POU_s) and POU homeobox domain (POU_h) coupled by a variable linker sequence (reviewed Pan et al., 2002). The POU_s domain of Oct4 interacts with one of at least two known (sequence dependent) binding sites in the HMG domain of Sox2, an SRY-related HMG domain-box transcription factor (Remenyi et al., 2003). The proximity of POU and HMG DNA recognition sequences, which often reside immediately adjacent to or in close proximity to each other, may dictate assembly of distinct structural confirmations of the Oct4/Sox2 dimer at individual genomic loci, thus mediating diverse regulatory affects of numerous target genes (Tomioka et al., 2002; Remenyi et al., 2003; Catena et al., 2005; Chew et al., 2005; Rodda et al., 2005). However, recent experimental evidence questions the essential nature of Sox2 in Oct4/Sox2 enhancer function. Although Sox2 null ES cells repress Oct4 expression and differentiate into trophectoderm, forced expression of Oct4 in these cells reinstates the ability to contribute to all germ layers of mid-gestation chimeras (Masui et al., 2007). In addition, Nanog expression is maintained in (differentiating) Sox2 null ES cells and Oct4-rescued, Sox2 null ES cells. Surprisingly, Sox2 may regulate Oct4 expression indirectly through regulation of several Oct4 enhancer- and promoter-binding factors, namely nuclear receptor family proteins (Masui et al., 2007). Despite binding regulatory elements as a monomer, Sox2 primarily regulates target genes in concert with co-factor binding. Indeed, DNA binding of Sox2 is enhanced through HMG/POU domain interactions (Remenyi et al., 2003). In contrast to other Octomer family members, fluctuations of Oct4 expression beyond critical upper or lower thresholds induce differentiation into endoderm and mesoderm, or trophectoderm, respectively (Niwa et al., 2000). Intriguingly, recent reports highlight non-transcriptional roles for Oct4 in female cells, primarily X-X chromosome pairing and binding of accessory factors for random X chromosome deactivation (Donohue et al., 2009).

In ES cells, transcriptional repression of genes elicited by binding of the Oct4/Sox2 ternary complex is relieved upon detachment of the complex at initiation of differentiation (Boyer et al., 2005). Unsurprisingly, Oct4 and Sox2 null embryos die through lack of ES cell maintenance.

1.2. Alternative Reprogramming Factors: cMyc & Klf4

cMyc is a proto-oncogene with an expanding list of genomic target genes. This factor influences cell proliferation through (i) transcriptional control through co-factor binding or localized chromatin modification, and (ii) pre-replication fork assembly/DNA replication during the G1/S transition (Dominguez-Sola et al., 2007; Martinato et al., 2008; reviewed Eilers & Eisenman, 2009). Myc exerts a combinatorial affect on cell growth; it readily heterodimerizes with the bHLHZ protein Max on *E-box* recognition sequence, (CACGTG)-containing DNA to promote metabolism, translation and mitochondrial processes. Recruitment of cMyc to regulatory elements by Myc-interacting zinc-finger protein (Miz-1) represses expression of factors involved in cell cycle arrest, eg. cyclin-dependent kinase inhibitors; a process that is reversed by TGFβ (Seoane et al., 2001; reviewed Eilers & Eisenman, 2009). Occupancy of cMyc at target promoters results in major, localized chromatin modifications, namely recruitment of histone methyltranferases and acetylases for assembly of regulatory histone marks, and exchange of regular histones for euchromatic histone variants at Myc target promoters (Martinato et al., 2008). In mES cells, Myc occupies one-fifth of all promoters and target gene expression occurs regardless of co-binding with Oct4, Sox2 or Klf4 (Liu et al., 2008[c]). Interestingly, cMyc is the only factor in the cocktail that can't autoregulate in ES cells (Liu et al., 2008[c]).

Structurally, family members of the Kruppel-like transcription factors (Klf) share a C-terminal, zinc finger coupled with a conserved linker sequence. In particular, Klf4 is a tumor-suppressor that can perform transcriptional co-activator or repressor functions in a number of embryonic and adult tissues. The considerable functional redundancy of Kruppel-like factors in ES cell self-renewal perhaps highlights this gene family's importance in maintenance of pluripotency (Jiang et al., 2008). Simultaneous knockdown of Klf2, Klf4 and Klf5 in ES cells initiates loss of pluripotency and upregulation of a number of differentiation genes, including the trophectoderm marker *Cdx2* (an antagonist of Oct4 expression; Jiang et al., 2008). Although these three Klf family members collectively bind a DNA recognition sequence in the Nanog distal enhancer to upregulate its activity, loss of any individual protein can be compensated for by the remaining Klf family members. iPS cells can be induced in neural stem cells with Klf4 omitted from the reprogramming cocktail, however formation of reporter gene$^+$ colonies is delayed compared to four factor, and three factor (Myc omitted) induction (Kim et al., 2008).

Occupancy of many transcriptional regulators at the promoters of transcriptionally active and silent genes in somatic and ES cells, leading to transcriptional initiation and interrupted transcript elongation, suggests a genetic program representative of pluripotency is potentially permissive to activation (Guenther et al., 2007). Collectively, the four Yamanaka factors regulate 16 developmental pathways in ES cells, including the *p53,* Wnt and TGF-β pathways (Liu et al., 2008[c]). Binding of individual factors, in the absence of co-binding with the other factors, more often elicits transcriptional repression; conversely, co-binding more often associates with transcriptional permissiveness (Liu et al., 2008[c]). Interestingly, excess concentrations of all reprogramming factors are not required to kickstart the reprogramming process; forced expression of Oct4 and Sox2 to levels comparable to that observed in ES cells are sufficient to mediate reprogramming (Carey et al., 2009).

Deciphering levels of cMyc and Klf4 required for reprogramming is more challenging given considerable expression of these factors in many somatic cells (Nakagawa et al., 2007; Segre et al., 1999). Similarly for Oct4 and Sox2, collective exogenous and endogenous cMyc expression that exceeds required concentrations may be detrimental to the specificity of reprogramming, a notion supported by a greater proportion of reporter gene positive colonies in cells reprogrammed with cMyc omitted (Nakagawa et al., 2007). However, augmentation of the Oct4/Sox2/Nanog regulatory network is more rapidly established when cMyc is expressed (Wernig et al., 2008). Future experiments inducing pluripotency in cMyc null somatic cells, or malignant/transformed cells over-expressing cMyc, may elucidate the role this factor has in the reprogramming process.

Despite sharing a conserved Octomer binding motif, Oct4 is not functionally redundant with Octomer family members in an iPS setting, perhaps due to protein stability (Nakagawa et al., 2007). However, Oct4 can be replaced with application of a chemical agent, albeit at the expense of reprogramming efficiency (Shi et al., 2008[a]; Shi et al., 2008[b]; discussed later). However, cMyc can be substituted with (i) less teratogenic Myc family members N-Myc and L-Myc, (ii) a cMyc mutant or (iii) even an alternative transcriptional coactivator, the latter even resulting in markedly increased reprogramming efficiency (Nakagawa et al., 2007; Blelloch et al., 2007; Zhao et al., 2008[b]).

1.3. Alternative Reprogramming Factors: Nanog & Lin28

Klf4 (±Myc) is functionally redundant to Nanog and Lin28, perhaps in part reflective of the many shared regulatory targets of Nanog and Klf4, and potential upregulation of Nanog expression through Klf4-mediated p53 transcriptional repression (Yu et al., 2007; Takahashi & Yamanaka, 2006; Rowland et al., 2005). Nanog is a homeobox domain protein expressed in embryonic lineage committed cells of the morula and ES blastocyst (Mitsui et al., 2003). Nanog expression can maintain pluripotency in the absence of LIF/gp130/Stat3 pathway. Although overexpression of Nanog is beneficial for cell fusion-based reprogramming (Silva et al., 2006), targeted ablation of Nanog in ES cells initiates expression of endoderm transcription factors, parietal and visceral endoderm (Mitsui et al., 2003). Lin28 is highly expressed in ES cells, binding cytosolic RNA to regulate mechanisms such as RNA translation and stability, and cell proliferation. Forced expression or knockdown of Lin28 exerts corresponding affects on cell proliferation. Knockdown of Lin28 in ES cells retards cell proliferation (Xu et al., 2009). During S-phase, the different cell-specific demand for individual core histone monomers is regulated by Lin28 at the RNA level, either by enhancing translation or through RNA stabilization (Xu et al., 2009). Yu et al., (2007) demonstrated reprogramming of human fibroblasts from lentiviral expression of Oct4, Sox2, Nanog and Lin28. Considerable reductions in colony number result from omission of Nanog and/or Lin28 from the reprogramming cocktail, with total loss of colony formation with individual omission of Oct4 or Sox2 (Yu et al., 2007; Nakagawa et al., 2007).

1.4. Early Events in iPS Reprogramming

iPS experiments utilizing somatic cells harboring antibiotic-responsive promoters that drive expression of each reprogramming factor have proved an invaluable tool in revealing the temporal and sequential molecular events that regulate derivation of iPS cells (Stadtfeld et al., 2008; Mikkelsen et al., 2008; Brambrink et al., 2008). To date, experiments investigating the mechanisms of iPS-based reprogramming have focused on those induced by the 'Yamanaka' factors, with little known of the mechanisms that direct Nanog/Lin28-mediated reprogramming.

iPS cell derivation commences with progressive down-regulation of lineage associated genes (eg. Thy1.1, Col5a2, Fibrillin2 in fibroblasts), a phenomenon primarily coordinated directly or indirectly by cMyc ± Klf4 (Stadtfeld et al., 2008;

Sridharan et al., 2009; Heffernan et al., manuscript in preparation). Three days of exclusive cMyc expression initiates upregulation of genes implicated in metabolism, translational control, RNA splicing, cell cycle and energy production, whilst repressing collagens, signaling and organ development (Sridharan et al., 2009). In concert with the other 3 reprogramming factors, expression of alkaline phosphatase (AP), an indicator of early reprogramming and marker of stem cells, becomes evident in 3-4% of cells after three days of induction. Although a direct link between cMyc and AP expression has not been demonstrated, the critical role played by cMyc in the initial days of reprogramming is highlighted by reductions in the frequency of alkaline phosphatase $(AP)^+$ colonies when cMyc expression is extinguished at three days post-induction (Sridharan et al., 2009), and may also explain reductions in reprogramming efficiency when cMyc is omitted from the reprogramming cocktail (Nakagawa et al., 2007). The progressive increase in AP expression to almost half of all cells after 12 days of induction renders it an unreliable prospective indicator of cells destined for complete conversion to the iPS phenotype, or marker for late-stage/fully reprogrammed cells (Brambrink et al., 2008). Indeed, a screen of over 150 AP-positive hiPS colonies at day 17-post infection revealed considerable heterogeneity in their transcriptional profile (Masaki et al., 2008). Nanog-driven drug selection is possible many days before Nanog-driven GFP expression is observed (Okita et al., 2007). Interestingly, expression of Fbx15, an Oct4 downstream target gene, is detectable a number of days preceding detectable Oct4 expression (Stadtfeld et al., 2008), in contrast to Oct4 representing an initial activator of transcriptional cascade in pluripotent ES cells *in vivo*. Since minimal improvement in AP^+ colonies results from cMyc expression past the initial 5 days of reprogramming, and well documented links between cMyc and chromatin modification and proliferative responses, the primary role of cMyc appears to be deactivating expressed lineage genes and preparation for initiation of the embryonic genetic program, through resetting of histone marks (Nakagawa et al., 2007; Sridharan et al., 2009).

1.5. The Partially Reprogrammed Phenotype

A transitional period between days 5-12 days post infection/induction in mouse demarks the partially reprogrammed cell phenotypically lineage gene $(Thy1)^-$ $/AP^+$/stage specific embryonic antigen-1 $(SSEA1)^+$. Partially reprogrammed cells account for between 5-10% of a previously homogenous $Thy1^+$ population (Stadtfeld et al., 2008; Brambrink et al., 2008). The majority of partially reprogrammed cells remain partially reprogrammed, never converting to a fully reprogrammed phenotype. Although genes associated with ES cell self-renewal and maintenance are reactivated in partially reprogrammed cells, genes strictly associated with pluripotency are incompletely activated (Mikkelsen et al., 2008). Seemingly, repression of the host cell expression profile is more readily accomplished than activation of silenced genes, with only cells capable of undertaking both progressing to a fully reprogrammed phenotype. Notably, histone methylation at the promoters of OSK targets is partially reset in the transitional/partially reprogrammed cell. Partially reprogrammed cells appear incapable of reactivating the silent X chromosome in female cells and inept at reactivating Nanog, both characteristic of the ES cells (Sridharan et al., 2009). Incomplete silencing of transgenes may be a feature of partially reprogrammed cells; indeed, expression of the four factors is 3-8-fold higher in partially reprogrammed cells than iPS or ES cells (Sridharan et al., 2009). Also, ES specific metabolic regulators are more completely reprogrammed than transcriptional regulators (Sridharan et al., 2009). Partially reprogrammed cells express a defined panel of genes and remain hypermethylated at loci for pluripotency genes (Mikkelsen et al., 2008). Promoter binding profiles are less conserved between (i) partially reprogrammed cells and (ii) fully reprogrammed iPS or ES cells, particularly in genes co-bound by Oct4, Sox2 and Klf4 with is largely lacking in partially reprogrammed cells. Genes lacking ES-like binding are more often targets of Nanog, a feature that is unsurprising since partially reprogrammed cells lack Nanog expression (Sridharan et al., 2009).

1.6. The Fully Reprogrammed Phenotype

The conversion to a fully reprogrammed mouse iPS cell state occurs between 1-2 weeks from induction/infection, and requires 10-16 days of transgene expression to be fully realized (Stadtfeld et al., 2008; Brambrink et al., 2008). In comparison to partially reprogrammed cells, fully reprogrammed iPS cell lines undergo reactivation of the silent X chromosome (in case of female cells), promoter de-methylation and expression of endogenous Oct4 and Nanog loci (confirmed by knock-in reporter gene expression), widespread resetting of histone methylation marks, mTert activation (albeit with a heterogeneous pattern of expression) and endogenous Sox2 expression (Maherali et al., 2007; Stadtfeld et al., 2008; Sridharan et al., 2009). Activation of endogenous Oct4 and Nanog is temporally correlated with down-regulation of the reprogramming transgenes (Wernig et al., 2007; Brambrink et al., 2008). DNA methyltransferase expression increases over the reprogramming period, with maximal expression in Oct4-GFP expressing cells late in the reprogramming process, and is speculated to mediate gradual ransgene silencing (Stadtfeld et al., 2008). However, specific knockdown of Dnmt1, or *de novo* demethylation with a chemical agent at defined periods of transgene expression, presumably leading to demethylation of the Oct4 and Nanog promoter, increases reprogramming efficiency (Mikkelsen et al., 2008).

ES cells and iPS cells share demethylation of pluripotency gene promoters, high expression of pluripotent and self renewal genes and low expression of some, but not all, lineage specific genes (Mikkelsen et al., 2008). Both cell types self-renew, give rise to germ layers in teratomas and contribute to chimeric development. Genome wide analysis of promoter binding and expression shows strong overlap in iPS cells and ES cells (Sridharan et al., 2009); two-thirds of genes in ES cells co-bound by three or four iPS factors binds the same loci in iPS cells. It is noteworthy that very few promoters co-bound by 3 or 4 factors in ES cells are not bound by any key factor in iPS cells (Sridharan et al., 2009). In loci bound by 1 or 2 factors, the similarity between ES cells and iPS cells increases to 87%. However, some genes are bound by fewer factors in iPS than ES cells, although differences may be insignificant to affect transcription. Total Oct4 and Nanog protein expression in numerous iPS cell lines are comparable to ES cells by qRT-PCR and Western Blot (Wernig et al., 2007). In addition, bivalent histone lysine methylation is noted in iPS cell lines, a characteristic of ES cells that are lacking in somatic cells. Although proviral expression of Oct4, Sox2, and Klf4 is sufficient to mediate upregulation of telomerase activity to similar levels as each other and ES cells, iPS cells also expressing viral cMyc comprise longer telomeres (Marion et al., 2009).

Conceptually, initiation/reactivation of transcriptionally silent genes in terminally differentiated cells during iPS induction is possible since most genes in ES and somatic cells experience transcriptional initiation and suspended elongation regardless of transcriptional status (Guenther et al., 2007). Transcriptionally permissive histone methyl and acetyl marks and occupancy of RNA polymerase II at most promoters initiate transcription, although only a subset of genes produces full-length transcript. However, translated protein levels are likely to be crucial for successful iPS conversion, particularly in the case of Oct4. As discussed, over- and under-expression of Oct4 in ES cells leads to differentiation, and is at least partially regulated by optimal levels of Sox2 (Masui et al., 2007). The majority of Oct4 targets in ES cells are targets of Nanog and Sox2, therefore activation of endogenous Nanog expression is a likely prerequisite for reprogramming progression and may explain low efficiency (Boyer et al., 2005). Perhaps differential expression levels of all factors applicable to viral technologies ensure a cohort of cells will have the right combination of factors at desired concentrations. Knowledge of precise levels of each factor would benefit protein delivery strategies and potentially improve reprogramming efficiency. From 16 days of induction, a small proportion of $SSEA1^+$ cells/colonies express endogenous Oct4 and/or Nanog, however $Nanog^+$ hiPS cells are heterogeneous for numerous ES associated genes (Brambrink et al., 2008; Masaki et al., 2008).

Comparisons of the *temporal efficiency*, ie length of time to reverse the epigenotype and phenotype of the somatic genome, and the *reprogramming efficiency*, ie number of fully reprogrammed cells as a proportion of the starting cells, are difficult to elucidate between the various reprogramming methods due to differences in starting cell populations, mechanism of reprogramming, cell proliferation rates and outcomes. In the case of SCNT, the time from transfer of the donor nucleus to harvest of ES cells is constrained by the temporal requirements of embryonic development to blastocyst, typically 5-7 days for many mammals. Although conversion of murine somatic cells to full pluripotency by iPS technology occurs within similar a timeframe, antibiotic selection driven by Nanog has been demonstrated as early as three days post-infection, although there is a delay in observable GFP expression from the same promoter (Okita et al., 2007). Somatic Oct4 reporter gene expression in mES-thymocyte hybrids is observable much sooner (<48 hours from hybridization; Tada et al., 2001), suggesting complete erasure of the somatic cell epigenotype and reactivation of pluripotency markers is possible within shorter timeframes than that observed with SCNT and iPS induction. Viral reprogramming in human cells, and reprogramming with non-viral methods (eg. protein delivery), is more protracted. It should be remembered that the pluripotent partner in SCNT and hybrids, namely the oocyte and ES cell respectively, delivers the entire compliment of factors to induce pluripotency in the somatic cell, whereas iPS technology takes a minimalist approach in respect to number of factors utilized. In addition, the reprogramming efficiency of SCNT continues to be low, where initially 440 oocyte manipulations were required to generate just 29 sheep blastocysts (Wilmut et al., 1997). Similarly, initial iPS experiments could convert only 0.02% of infected human fibroblasts to a pluripotency phenotype (Takahashi & Yamanaka., 2007). Suggestions that differential integrations within a population of infected cells account for the low reprogramming efficiency were dispelled when no improvement in reprogramming efficiency was achieved in iPS experiments utilizing clonal lines of somatic cells harboring inducible transgenes of each key reprogramming factor at identical loci (Brambrink et al., 2008).

Lentivirus, adenovirus and transient plasmid transfection circumvent the requirement of target somatic cells to proliferate for virally-delivered, transgene integration (Stadtfeld et al., 2008[b]; Okita et al., 2008; discussed later). Nonetheless, 80% retroviral infection efficiency (as judged by GFP transgene integration and expression) equates to estimations of 40% of cells receiving all four factors. This method assumes that 20% of cells that are permissive to infection and receive one factor fail to receive one additional factor. Hence, this method is likely to underestimate the number of cells that receive all four factors since cells permissive for viral integration would conceivably receive atleast one copy of all factors during the infection period, generally overnight or 24hours in duration.

2. Explored / Proposed Alternative Strategies to Viral Delivery of Key Factors

The unpredictable and random modifications to the host cell genome inherent with retroviral and lentiviral infection methodologies hamper use of these cells in a therapeutic setting and provoked exploration of non-mutagenic expression strategies (figure 1C-G; Carey et al., 2009; Kaji et al., 2009; Woltjen et al., 2009). Although reprogramming factors expressed from monkey moloney leukemia viral (MMLV) promoters are highly expressed in fibroblast, and selectively silenced in ES cells, insertional mutagenesis could activate oncogenes or silence/disrupt key genes. Efforts have also been directed towards improving the poor reprogramming efficiency documented thus far. Alternative reprogramming methods include (i) substituting key factors with chemical agents known to upregulate endogenous loci of key factors, or chromatin modifiers that enhance reprogramming efficiency (Shi et al., 2008[a]; Shi et al., 2008[b]; Huangfu et al., 2008[a]; Huangfu et al., 2008[b]), (ii) use of cells that naturally express combinations of the key iPS factors (Kim et al., 2008; Eminli et al.2008; Kim et al., 2009[a]), (iii) use of excisable transgenes (Kaji et al., 2009; Woltjen et al., 2009), (iv) delivery of protein of each reprogramming factor (Zhou et al., 2009; Kim et al., 2009[b]), and (v) delivery and expression of microRNA to compliment viral-mediated reprogramming or microRNA to knockdown specific factors (Judson et al., 2009; Zhao et al., 2008[b]). Each of these approaches is outlined diagrammatically in figure 1 and further described in the text below.

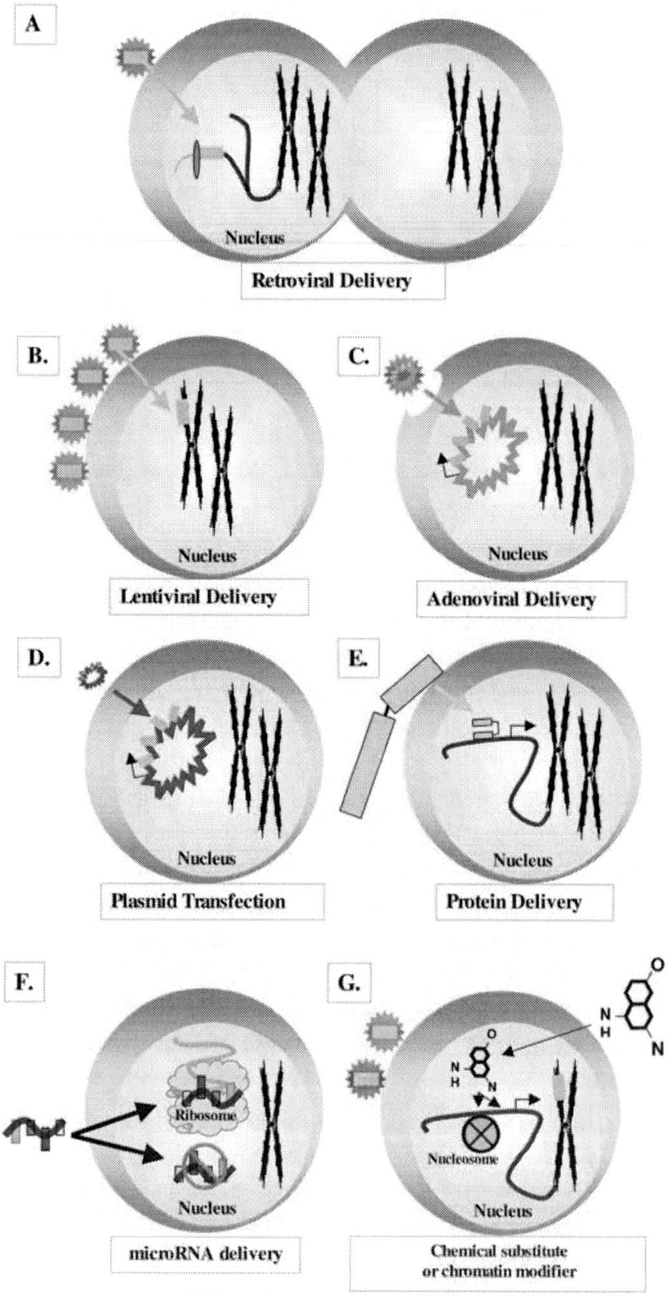

Figure 1. Continued on next page.

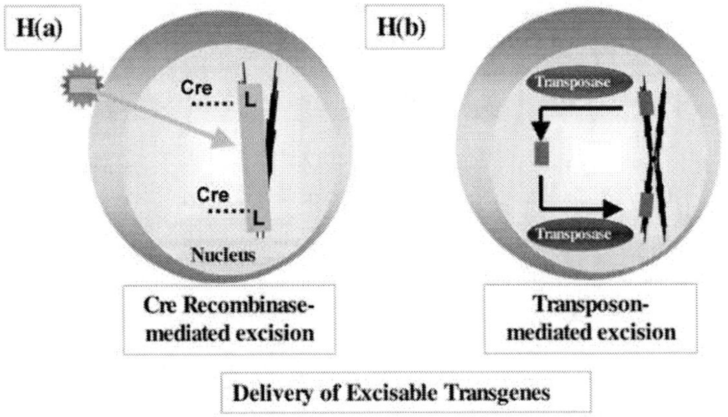

(A) Retroviral Delivery: retrovirus can deliver DNA sequence for each reprogramming factor to proliferating cells where they integrate into target cell DNA, **(B)** Lentiviral Delivery: the lentiviral pre-integration complex can transduce across the plasma membrane of proliferating and non-proliferating cells to deliver transgenes for each reprogramming factor before integrating into host DNA, **(C)** Adenoviral Delivery: adenoviral attachment to the host cell initiates invagination of the membrane and packaging into endocytotic vesicles for release into the cytosol. Expression of each reprogramming factor from episomal expression can induce pluripotency before being diluted from the cell population, **(D)** Plasmid Transfection: plasmids carrying each reprogramming factor can be directly transfected to target cells to drive reprogramming, **(E)** Protein Delivery: Recombinant proteins incorporating each of reprogramming factor and a plasma membrane transduction domain can transduce to the nuclei of target cells to drive target gene expression, **(F)** microRNA: microRNA can be delivered to target cells to induce expression of factors favorable to reprogramming, or to knockdown RNA's in the host cell to improve reprogramming efficiency, **(G)** Chemical Substitute or Chemical Modifier: chemical agents that upregulate endogenous loci of key reprogramming factors, or modify histone or DNA methyl and acteyl patterns, can be added to target cell culture media to improve reprogramming efficiency or replace integrative viral transgenes, **(H)** Delivery of Excisable Transgenes: *(a)* Cre Recombinase-mediated excision: floxed, integrated transgenes can be excised from genomic DNA with the application or expression of Cre-recombinase before DNA recombination, L: lox-P site flanking proviral sequences, *(b)* Transposase-mediated excision: transposase enzyme can integrate and excise transposon DNA elements comprising the reprogramming factors, followed by recombination of the host DNA.

Figure 1. The Numerous Methods for Deriving "Inducing Pluripotent Stem" iPS Cells.

2.1. Treatment of Target Cells with Chemical Agents: (i) to Replace Individual Transgenes, or (ii) Used in Concert with Viral Strategies to Improve Reprogramming Efficiency

The application of chemical agents that activate expression of endogenous loci of key factors (thus eliminating these individual factors from the reprogramming cocktail) remains an attractive alternative to viral-based iPS strategies (figure 1G). Although chemical inducers are readily reversible and allow temporal control over target gene regulation (Xu et al., 2008), chemicals that activate individual reprogramming factors, with minimal secondary affects on other factors or processes, are rare. Since Octamer family members are not functionally redundant and expression of Oct4 is rare in somatic cells, finding a suitable chemical substitute for Oct4 is imperative. Oct4 deactivation in differentiating ES cells is mediated by the histone methyltransferase G9a through direct methylation of histone lysines, or successive recruitment of epigenetic modifiers to chromatin (Tachibana et al., 2002; Feldman et al., 2005; Ikegami et al., 2006; Esteve et al., 2006). Unsurprisingly, G9a is expressed at significantly higher levels in somatic cells than ES cells. Chemical inhibition of G9a with BIX-01294 (BIX) eases the antagonism on histone 3, lysine 9 methylation (H3K9me)-mediated Oct4 expression and can fully substitute virally-delivered Oct4 for derivation of iPS cells from neural progenitor cells (in concert with proviral expression of remaining factors), albeit with dramatically reduced efficiency (Shi et al., 2008[a]). Short-hairpin RNA (shRNA) knockdown of G9a in adult NSC results in demethylation of Oct4 promoter and partial reactivation (~10% of ES cells) of Oct4 expression Ma et al., 2008). Addition of BIX compliments Oct4 and Klf4 retroviral reprogramming in NPC and maintains colony formation efficiency in NPC to four factor levels (Shi et al., 2008[a]). Interestingly, this implies that permanent Oct4 deactivation in differentiated cells is an active and not a permanently static process which can be disrupted some time after terminal differentiation. In concert with BIX, addition of an L-channel calcium agonist (Bayk8644) can substitute for Sox2 and cMyc in fibroblasts, cells that do not express appreciable levels of any reprogramming factor (Shi et al., 2008[b]). However, this compound exerts little affect in the absence of BIX. As noted for ES cells, inhibition of extracellular regulated kinase (ERK) signaling by chemically inhibiting ERK-activating (MEK) enzymes, seven to nine days after Oct4/Klf4 infection to NPC (and continually for 5 days) results in enhanced growth of reprogrammed iPS colonies with higher Oct4 expression (Burdon et al., 1999; Shi et al., 2008[a]). Extracellular Wnt3a can stimulate β–catenin-mediated induction of endogenous cMyc expression in target cells, producing a dramatic improvement in reprogramming efficiency (Marson et al., 2008). These results are not surprising considering Oct4, Sox2 and Nanog collectively activate components of Wnt signalling (Boyer et al., 2005). Another possible and undocumented substitute for cMyc is Okadaic acid (OA), a potent inhibitor of protein serine/threonine phosphatase 2A (PP2A). PP2A dephosphorylates specific serine residues in cMyc and targets it for rapid ubiquitin-regulated degradation. PP2A repression results in accumulated cMyc through upregulation of RNA production and protein sythesis (Zhang et al., 2007). OA also elicits increased Klf4, which in turn binds OA-responsive elements in the cMyc promoter eliciting upregulation of cMyc gene expression (Zhang et al., 2007). OA's additional inhibitory effect on translation, through repression of EIFα, may lead to an initial accumulation of mRNA transcript and subsequent delivery of bolus amounts of translated protein upon OA withdrawal. Replacement of Klf4 with Kenpaullone, a broad spectrum protein kinase inhibitor, to Oct4/Sox2/cMyc retrovirus expressing MEF generates Oct4 selectable iPS cells (albeit at reduced efficiency) able to contribute to germline-competent chimeras (Lyssiotis et al., 2009). Despite these impressive results, deriving iPS cells exclusively through chemical treatment, eg. BIX± Bayk8644+PD0325901+Wnt3a+Kenpaullone, may prove challenging due to only modest induction of target genes, and numerous potential secondary affects due to their broad spectrum of affects.

Treatment with chemical chromatin modifiers, disrupting methyl or acetyl patterns to core histones or DNA, that compliment viral iPS strategies can enhance reprogramming efficiency. High expression of jumonji-domain containing H3K9 demethylase Jhdm2a in ovum and early embryo reflects a critical role in pluripotency and reprogramming (Ma et al., 2008). Reflective of fold-differences between ES cells and somatic cells, overexpression of Jhdm2a in NSC caused global loss of H3K9me and promotes ES-NSC fusion based reprogramming (Ma et al., 2008). Deacetylation of N-terminal histone residues, associated with transcriptional deactivation, can be chemically inhibited to promote transcriptional permissiveness. Indeed, histone deacetylase (HDAC) inhibitor trichostatin A (TSA) increases cloning efficiency by SCNT (Kishigami et al., 2006). One hundred-fold improvements in iPS reprogramming efficiency of murine fibroblasts to (4 viral factor) iPS cells have been observed through chemical inhibition of histone deacetylase activity (Huangfu et al., 2008[a]; 2008[b]). Huangfu et al., (2008[a]; 2008[b]) tested a suite of HDAC inhibitors and found Valproic acid to improve reprogramming efficiency of 2,3 and 4 factor iPS. SCNT cloning efficiency can be improved using somatic cell nuclei genetically deficient in Dnmtl (Blelloch et al., 2007). It is therefore of little surprise that transient, *de novo* DNA demethylation following retroviral infection increases numbers of AP^+

colonies and/or proportion of reporter gene[+] colonies (Mikkelsen et al., 2008; Huangfu et al., 2008; Shi et al., 2008[b]). Dnmt inhibition can also enhance reprogramming of Oct4/Klf4 mediated reprogramming in the presence of BIX (Shi et al., 2008[b]).

2.2. Elimination of Transgenes by Utilizing Somatic Cells that (i) Express High Concentrations of the Key iPS Factors from Endogenous Loci, or (ii) are Readily Accessible

Sox2, cMyc and Klf4 are each expressed from endogenous loci in a number of somatic cell types. Utilizing somatic cell populations that express high levels of these factors for iPS conversion enables elimination of individual, or combinations, of transgenes. Since endogenous Oct4 expression occurs rarely in adult tissues, it remains the single factor most difficult to substitute or omit. When used as nuclear donors for SCNT, neural stem cells increase the rate of blastocyst formation compared with terminally differentiated neural cells (Blelloch et al., 2007). The unusually high expression of Sox2 and cMyc, as well as pluripotency related factors alkaline phosphatase and SSEA1, in cranial neural progenitor cells (NPC) can be exploited to generate iPS cell viral delivery of Oct4 alone, or in concert with Klf4 (Kim et al., 2008; Eminli et al.2008; Kim et al., 2009[a]). Expression of OSMK from endogenous loci is comparable to that of ES cells in Oct4/Klf4 induced iPS cells by qRT-PCR (Kim et al., 2008). However, differences in Oct4 and Nanog promoter methylation were noted between Oct4 alone, NPC-derived iPS cell and (i) ES cells, and (ii) iPS cells generated from Oct4/Kf4 infection (Kim et al., 2008; Kim et al., 2009[a]). Endogenous Sox2 in NPC is higher than most cells but insufficient to reprogram in the absence of Oct4 (substituted with BIX; Shi et al., 2008[a]). Omission of Sox2 and cMyc from the reprogramming cocktail in NPC doesn't delay conversion to iPS cell as compared to four factor controls (Shi et al., 2008). Addition of BIX with Oct4/Klf4 maintains reprogramming efficiency as observed in four factor reprogramming (Shi et al., 2008a), and reprogrammed cells still commit to the germline in chimeras. However, since NPC's are harvested from crude brain cell extracts, they are not ideal for generating human iPS cells in a therapeutic setting.

Human foreskin represents an abundant source of cells for generating male iPS cells (Yu et al., 2007; Maherali et al., 2008). Human epidermal cells are not only readily accessible, they express high levels of Klf4, are similarly infectable as human interstitial fibroblasts whilst having less viral integrations (Segre et al., 1999; Aasen et al., 2008). Furthermore, human keratinocytes (from human hair follicles) express endogenous Klf4 and cMyc and readily reprogram in less time than other human cells, however improvements in reprogramming efficiency have not been achieved to date (Aasen et al., 2008; Maherali et al., 2008). However, when differentiated, fibroblastic outgrowths from plated hiPS-derived embryoid bodies were picked and re-induced, 'secondary' $Oct4^{+}/Tra\text{-}1\text{-}81^{+}$ iPS cells were derived at 100-fold greater efficiency with reduced background iPS-like colonies (Maherali et al., 2008).

2.3. Non-Integrating Virus, Self-cleaving/Excisable Constructs and Direct Transfection of Plasmid to Target Somatic Cells

Random, insertional mutagenesis is neither required nor desirable for reprogramming (Stadfeld et al., 2008[b]). The particular site of retroviral and lentiviral integration could possibly disrupt host genes, influence proviral silencing and/or disrupt host gene expression. In addition, basal proviral expression suspends development of reprogramming cells in a partially reprogrammed phenotype. To facilitate, transient expression of key genes from transient and largely non-integrative adenoviral and plasmid transfection is markedly less likely to result in genomic integration (figure 1C&D). Adenoviral infection of mouse fibroblast, fetal liver and hepatocytes generated iPS cells with high degree chimerism in newborns following blastocyst injection (Stadfeld et al., 2008[b]). However, the markedly reduced efficiency could at least in part be due to reduced infectability. Although episomal adenovirus does integrate rarely (Harui et al., 1999), viral vectors progressively dilute as resultant iPS cells proliferate. Although high degree chimeras can form without evidence of tumour formation, a high incidence (almost a quarter) of tetraploidy has been noted in reprogrammed cells, through unpredictable cell fusion or selective infection of tetraploid cells in original population (Stadtfeld et al., 2008[b]).

Expression of all four factors simultaneously from polycistronic expression cassettes, incorporating 'self-cleaving' 2A peptides, causes 'ribosomal skipping' to enable comparable expression of each factor from a single promoter (Sommer et al., 2008; Carey et al., 2009). With an IRES sequence separating pairs of factors, infected MEF and tail-tip fibroblasts (TTF) expressed a Sox2/GFP reporter and required only 1-3 copies of each factor for complete reprogramming (Sommer et al., 2008). Carey et al., (2009) subsequently constructed doxycycline-inducible factors separated by self-cleaving 2A peptides, without IRES technology. Induced expression of Oct4 and Sox2 from a single polycistronic construct was comparable to that in ES cells and, in addition to Myc and Klf4 expression, sufficient to reprogram murine fibroblast and postnatal human fibroblasts. Reprogramming efficiency of MEF was estimated at 0.0001%, a reduction when compared to alternative viral methods (Carey et al., 2009).

DNA transposons are genetic elements that are excised and re-integrated throughout the genome by specific 'transposase' enzymes, a phenomenon referred to a transposition. *piggyBac* is one such transposon capable of harboring a multiple-gene payload that preferentially inserts in transcriptional DNA units harboring TTAA sequences (Ding et al., 2005). Induction of individual or polycistronic, doxycycline-inducible constructs, delivered to murine and human fibroblasts by transposase-mediated integration and subsequent excision, generated iPS cells exhibiting all the hallmarks of pluripotency, including contribution to mid-gestation embryos by tetraploid complementation assay (figure 1Hb; Woltjen et al., 2009). Although the efficiency of transgene excision by transient transposase expression was variable, proficient recombination of insertion sites to wild type resulted following excision and endogenous pluripotency genes continued to be expressed.

Additionally, floxed proviral constructs can be excised through subsequent infection with transient Cre-recombinase expressing adenovirus (figure Ha; Kaji et al., 2009). Recombined MEF convert to AP^+ colonies 9 days post-infection and undergo endogenous gene expression and demethylation of Nanog and Oct4 promoters. A single insertion of multi-expression cassette was enough to induce complete reprogramming. Concurrent and repeated plasmid transfection of two polycistronic plasmids expressing (i) Oct4, Sox2, Klf4, and (ii) cMyc to mouse embryonic fibroblasts also induced pluripotency and produced chimeras, however reprogramming efficiency was compromised compared to retroviral methodologies (Okita et al., 2008). Plasmid construction of the polycistronic plasmid appeared to alter reprogramming efficiencies in some clones, suggesting unexpected and differential expression levels of each factor. This approach is further hampered by rare integration events in some clones (although not detected in chimeras), and a 10-fold reduction in efficiency when cMyc is not transfected with the major construct. In addition, integrative technologies may express higher levels of each factor.

2.4. Protein Delivery as an Alternative to Viral Strategies

Like use of small molecule compounds, protein delivery is an attractive approach to iPS cell generation due to its reversibility (figure 1E). However, the hydophobicity of the cellular lipid bilayer core represents a significant barrier to passive movement of proteins from surrounding milieu to the cellular interior. The inevitable progression to non-viral, non-DNA delivery was first demonstrated by Zhou et al., (2009)[c]. Expressed in *E.coli* and subsequently purified, recombinant proteins incorporating a poly-arginine targeting sequence linked to the four human iPS factors were capable of converting MEF to protein-iPS (piPS) cells with global gene expression patterns similar to ES cells. It should be noted that modifying host cell histone aceytlation patterns was required to yield stable cell lines, and contrary to viral strategies, omission of cMyc protein induced colony formation without reporter gene expression. These results were soon extrapolated to human cells, although this study expressed proteins in transfected human cells and applied whole protein extracts to targets cells without purification (Kim et al., 2009[b]). Importantly, supplementation with chemical agent/s was not required. In addition to being the first demonstration of non-DNA mediated iPS reprogramming, these reports highlight some interesting points. Efficiencies in retroviral reprogramming are calculated on assumptions that around half of the infected cells receive all four viral factors. Yet immunocytochemical stains confirm nuclear localization of each fusion protein in treated cells (Zhou et al., 2009[c]; C.Heffernan, manuscript in preparation). Significant improvements in reprogramming efficiency did not result from protein delivery, regardless of histone deacetylation modulation. Protein delivery circumvents the lag in transcription and translation of critical factors to levels required for reprogramming, yet ES-like colonies were observed much later than in viral strategies. It is unclear whether the thresholds of Oct4 expression that are critical in maintaining pluripotency in ES cells are also applicable in somatic cell conversion to iPS cells.

An arginine-rich basic domain (^{49}**RKKRRQRRR**^{57}) of trans-activating transcriptional-activator (TAT) of HIV binds heparan sulfate proteoglycans before trans-membrane import through caveolar ('lipid raft') endocytosis (Green & Loewenstein, 1988; Frankel & Pabo, 1988; Rusnati et al., 1999; Tyagi et al., 2001; Fittipaldi et al., 2003). Over 60 TAT-fusion proteins have been used to delivery proteins to nucleus (Becker-Hapak et al., 2001). This domain also mediates importin-independent translocation to the nuclear compartment (Efthymiadis et al., 1998). The rapid (in the order of minutes; Fittipaldi et al., 2003) and efficient translocation to the nuclear compartment renders TAT an ideal fusion partner for delivery of recombinant transcriptional activators to nuclear chromatin (Efthymiadis et al., 1998; Yun et al., 2008). Due to their wide range of biological functions and ligands, heparan sulfate proteoglycans are ubiquitously expressed within and between cell populations, a feature that could be exploited for future experimental and therapeutic applications in piPS.

2.5. RNA Delivery Strategies

Introduction of either (i) miRNA transcripts that mimic those expressed in ES cells, or (ii) siRNAs that interfere with expression of endogenous factors, are both approaches that can be applied to derive iPS cells (figure 1F; Mikkelsen et al., 2008; Zhao et al., 2008[b]; Judson et al., 2009). ES cell-specific cell cycle-regulating (ESCC) miRNA's of the miR290 cluster are expressed in ES cells and accelerate transition through G1/S. Hence, cMyc and nMyc both target mIR-290 cluster, and Oct4 binds five known promoters for miRNA in ES cells (Boyer et al., 2005). Since the miR-290 cluster is a target of cMyc, it is perhaps unsurprising that transfection of miR-294 on days 0 and 6 post-retroviral infection can replace cMyc to 75% efficiency, but not enhance 4 factor iPS (Judson et al., 2009). However, it is noteworthy that replacement of cMyc with miR-294 yielded a greater proportion of Oct4-GFP^{+} colonies (Judson et al., 2009).

siRNA knockdown of Dnmt1 can aid cells transgress from partially to fully reprogrammed and increase reprogramming efficiency (Mikkelsen et al., 2008). Similarly, short-hairpin RNA (shRNA) knockdown of G9a, a histone methyltransferase involved in Oct4 deactivation in post-implantation embryos *in vivo*, results in demethylation of the Oct4 promoter and partial reactivation (Feldman et al., 2005; Ma et al., 2008). Addition of p53 siRNA to adult human fibroblasts, in concert with Oct4/Sox2/Klf4 infection, increased efficiency to varying degrees, alone or in combination with additional treatments (Zhao et al., 2008[b]).

3. Experimental Application of iPS Cells for Therapy

Original reports demonstrating induction of iPS cells in human cells confirmed their potential to be differentiated into a number of cell types (Takahashi et al., 2007). Since the therapeutic potential of human differentiated iPS cells cannot be ascertained *in vivo*, mouse models of humanized disease represent an invaluable resource in exploring therapeutic applicability of iPS technology. Hanna et al., (2007) infected adult mouse cells harboring a defective human sickle hemoglobin allele with retrovirus for OSK plus lentivirus for floxed cMyc cDNA. Following adenoviral expression of Cre recombinase and excision of the cMyc sequence, one clone engrafted to peripheral blood and rescued the disease phenotype in the absence of tumor formation (Hanna et al., 2007).

For experimental iPS technology to be translated into therapeutic application, diseased and aged donor cells firstly need to readily convert to iPS cells (Dimos et al., 2008; Soldner et al., 2009). Dimos et al., (2008) was first to demonstrate the feasibility of generating iPS cells in aged, amyotrophic lateral sclerois (ALS) sufferers. Embryoid bodies actively differentiated into glia and neural cells, cell types defective in ALS sufferers. In addition, lentiviral integration of floxed reprogramming factors to fibroblasts from Parkinsons disease sufferers, followed by Cre recombinase-mediated excision of transgenes, generates iPS cells that display molecular signatures closer to ES cells than non-excised iPS cells (Soldner et al., 2009). Dopaminergic neuronal-marker positive neural cells could be derived from these cells by directed differentiation. However, systemic genetic polymorphisms will require correction prior to transplantation, either in the pluripotent state or potentially in the post-iPS differentiated cell. To facilitate, Zou et al., (2009) elegantly demonstrated sequence-specific DNA targeting of a non-specific endonuclease domain in hES and hiPS cells. Digestion of DNA with subsequent homologous recombination can be utilized for gene deletion, or site-specific insertion of wild-type gene sequences.

4. Applicability of iPS in Therapeutic Setting

It is now indisputable that iPS cells acquire many morphological and functional characteristics reminiscent of ES cells. iPS technology enables retrospective study of disease, once pathology has been identified in sufferers, instead of studying cells of expected sufferers of known pedigree (Nishikawa et al., 2008). Although stem cells generated by nuclear transfer and iPS technology are autologous for donor nuclear DNA, only iPS cells are homoplasmic for mitochondrial DNA (Condic & Rao, 2008). This is an important point when considering the transmission of numerous mitochondrial dysfunctions due to the inherent mixing of mitochondria in NT-derived cells. Thankfully, the US President's Council of Bioethics states "there would seem to be nothing to object to ethically if procedures were developed to turn somatic cells into pluripotent stem cells, non-embryonic functional equivalents of embryonic stem cells", and "...no obstacle to, or reason to oppose, federal funding of research on dedifferentiation of somatic cells" (White Paper: Alternative Sources of Pluripotent Stem Cells, http://www. bioethics.gov/reports/ white_ paper/text.html).

However, despite circumventing the concerns associated with SCNT and animal/human hybrids, significant practical, legal and ethical concerns will impede a smooth transition of iPS cells from lab-bench to clinic. With the recent development of non-integrative methods of iPS generation, it seems timely to consider (i) practical issues associated with generating iPS cells, and (ii) the legal and ethical considerations for using these cells for therapy. Due to familiarity, we focus on regulations under USA and Australian law. Alternative sources of autologous, differentiated cells for therapy are also outlined below.

4.1. Practical Pitfalls of iPS Cells for Human Therapy

From the outset, it was evident that integrating viral-based generation of autologous cells was undesirable for human therapeutic applications. Now, micromolar concentrations of recombinant protein transduced into somatic cells is sufficient to reverse their development fate (Zhou et al., 2009[c]; Kim et al., 2009[b]). In the absence of reporter gene expression, we require stringent criteria for selection of desirable clones from human iPS cultures (Blelloch et al., 2007; Meissner et al., 2007). Although serum starvation of reprogrammed (murine) cells reportedly accelerates reprogramming and also aids selection of desirable clones (Blelloch et al., 2007), such success has not been demonstrated in human iPS. Hence, partially reprogrammed, colony forming units that share many characteristics with fully reprogrammed cells require exclusion from the transplantable cell pool. We need to ensure a homogenously differentiated population of cells is transplanted, and cells remain differentiated following transplantation. Mouse iPS cells initiate tumor formation as prevalent as ES cells when transplanted to brains of immune suppressed mice (Miura et al., 2009). When transplanted to mice following differentiation into neural cells, tumorgenicity is depended on the original cells used for reprogramming and all tumors examined contained variable levels of undifferentiated cells. It is noteworthy that considerably higher tumor formation was observed when adult cells were used. Interestingly, tumor formation occurrence did not correlate with retroviral cMyc expression (Miura et al., 2009).

Since pluripotent cells are inherently teratogenic *in vivo*, complete and universal differentiation of a pool of pluripotent cells to the desired cell type is required for transplantation. It remains an important consideration when potentially treating non-life threatening injury such as spinal cord injury in young sufferers, who are likely to benefit from such a procedure. Will/should spinal cord injury patients accept risks of malignancy with untimely and premature death for greater mobility? The inefficient and protracted isolation, derivation and expansion of iPS cells also limits the swift treatment required of a spinal cord injury, not to mention the related regulatory approval of patient-specific iPS cell lines (Cyranoski, 2008).

Due to differential expression patterns, the cells able to be reprogrammed with the fewest reprogramming factors are perhaps the least accessible in therapeutic settings (Kim et al., 2008; Kim et al., 2009[a]). Indeed, standard protocols for human iPS include two extra factors for reprogramming (Park et al., 2008). In light of results shown in the mouse, a logical step forward will be to generate iPS cells in cranial NPC with Oct4 recombinant protein alone. Although impressive in an experimental sense, is it really therapeutically relevant due to their relatively inaccessibility? Isolation of neural progenitors from olfactory mucosa may be more applicable due to greater accessibility, however generation of iPS cell from this cell population has yet to be demonstrated (Murrell et al., 2008). Although hES-like colonies appear 21-30 days post-infection and demonstrate many of hallmarks of ES cells, long term studies are required to ensure malignancy doesn't result from this transient, intracellular over-expression of reprogramming factors. Importantly, dysregulation of each individual iPS factor is causative, or a feature of, malignancy (Liu, 2008).

4.2. Legal and Ethical Considerations of iPS Cells for Human Therapy

In the absence of a universal pluripotent cell line for therapy, each individual iPS cell line would likely be classified a "Class 4 *in vitro* device (IVD)" under Australia Federal law, of "high public health risk ... intended to be used to screen for transmissible agents ... or transplantation (Australian Government Department of Health and Aging, Therapeutic Goods Administration http://www.tga.gov.au/ivd/overview.htm). The American equivalent would be Code of Federal Regulations (CFR) governing transplantation of laboratory processed human cells and tissues (Condic & Rao, 2008). Class 4 IVD materials are subject to numerous *in vitro* testing and evaluation before transplantation, a point that may render iPS cells cost inhibitive for many people if not subsidized by Governmental Agencies. Since long term culture of converted iPS cells are almost universally reliant on culture on irradiated fibroblast feeder layer, regulatory authorities are likely to insist on feeder layer-free technologies to eliminate possibility of cross-species or allogenic contamination. Also, random genomic recombination events following (*Cre*-mediated) excision of polycistronic expression cassettes, are likely to attract attention from regulatory authorities, and non-excisable remnants still render the resultant cells genetically modified (Kaji et al., 2009). Although *piggyBac* transposon/transposase based excision of expression cassettes is reportedly 'seamless (Woltjen et al., 2009), similar concerns surrounding unpredictable recombination events in the resultant cell still apply. Incomplete conversion of the epigenome to that of the adopted transplantable cell (from iPS to desired differentiated cell type) may result in regression of transplanted cells to iPS cell *in vivo* or even to that of the original cell type (Miura et al., 2009). These issues will need to be addressed and satisfied for regulatory body approval of such technologies.

Without strict authoritative guidelines, the simplicity of iPS cell derivation may also be its ethical downfall; renegade practitioners may easily undertake transplantation in vulnerable human patients without approval. Consensus will need to be reached between the scientific and lay-communities on what is deemed acceptable. Do the notable differences between iPS cells and ES cells preclude them from being utilized in the clinic? Do we really need to generate iPS cells that are identical, or near identical, to ES cells? Or should the ultimate criteria be direct comparisons between differentiated iPS cells and their *in situ* equivalents?

The use of aged fibroblasts for iPS conversion and subsequent gamete production and IVF could potentially pass on imprinting and DNA damage acquired over time to offspring, and also challenges sensitivities surrounding reproduction for infertile couples (Cyranoski, 2008; Condic & Rao, 2008). However, sperm require a Y-chromosome to form, therefore lesbian couples would be unable to produce genetically-related offspring. Such concerns even provoked Yamanaka himself to lobby for regulation (Cyranoski, 2008). In a therapeutic sense, is it ethically sound to risk the potential teratogenicity of cell transplantation to treat more imminent disease, eg. Parkinson's or Alzheimer's diseases, if death is imminent?

4.3. Potential Alternatives to iPS Cells

The lineage commitment of *in vivo* progenitor cells can be re-directed down a related, but alternative, developmental lineage. Referred to as transdetermination (TDE), this differs from transdifferentiation (TDI) whereby somatic cells substitute their differentiated genetic program with an unrelated other. Utilizing either method for the derivation of cells for therapy circumvents the requirement of a pluripotent intermediate, and represents a possible alternative to the two stage iPS method.

Transdetermination of permissive, hepatic progenitor cells to islet cells can be achieved through transfer of a single transcription factor (Yechoor et al., 2009). Furthermore, adenovirus expressing single pancreatic transcription factor re-directs differentiation to insulin expressing cells (Ferber et al., 2000).

Alternatively, TDI has now demonstrated in mesoderm and endoderm lineage cells (Zhou et al., 2008[a]; Takeuchi & Bruneau, 2009). A screen of lineage regulators identified factors that directing pancreatic development *in vivo* (Zhou et al., 2008). Pancreatic exocrine cells derive from pancreatic endoderm. Directed adenoviral delivery of three key factors to pancreatic exocrine cells to immune deficient adult mice *in* vivo resulted in >20% conversion to insulin+ cells. As shown in iPS, one factor can be replaced with alternative factor with accompanying loss in efficiency. Resultant cells were functionally similar to endogenous insulin-secreting β–cells and remained throughout assessment period. They express and suppress relevant markers and recruit vasculature to the local milieu. Adenoviral infection of mice chemically rendered diabetic by ablation of β–cell population caused reprogramming to islet cells and resulted in improved glucose tolerance and serum insulin after 8 weeks. Transgene expression was extinguished within 2 months (Zhou et al., 2008).

Cultured mouse embryos transiently transfected with two transcription factors (Gata4 and Tbx5) and a chromatin modifier (Baf60c) transformed non-cardiac mesoderm to beating cardiomyocytes (Takeuchi & Bruneau, 2009). This pattern is reflective of 4 factor iPS cells, if you consider cMyc a chromatin modifier allowing expression of repressed genes, and experiments using chemical chromatin modifier. As for iPS, redundancy with Gata and Baf family members reduced efficiency. Cardiac gene expression can be induced with Gata4 and Baf60c alone, but Tbx5 is required to achieve beating tissue in half of embryos. Importantly, converted cells did not arise from specific targeting of undifferentiated $Isl1^+$ progenitor cells. Although this study demonstrates conversion of non-cardiac mesoderm to myocytes, it remains conversion of lineages in the same germ layer.

TDE and TDI represents a preferable method for cell derivation; reprogramming can be achieved with minimal number of factors (Takeuchi & Bruneau, 2009), alleviation of the teratogenicity associated with pluripotent cells, and rapid conversion of intra-lineage cells, suggested to be a result of less epigenetic remodeling (Zhou et al., 2008). Such rapidity of conversion may be attractive for treatment of spinal cord injury, provided suitable methods for trans-differentiating between neural cells *in vitro* are developed. Although demonstrated *in vivo*, efficiency of TDI is reportedly many orders of magnitudes higher that iPS conversion (Zhou et al., 2008), and alleviates the requirement for pre-transplantation, *in vitro* differentiation protocols. Although TDE can be achieved with transfection with a one or two exogenous factor (Ferber et al., 2000; Yechoor et al., 2009), a related progenitor (lineage committed but partially differentiated) cell pool is required which may not be possible or accessible for all cell types/lineages.

Finally, HLA antigen null hES cells could conceivably constitute a 'universal' cell for widespread therapy (Vogel, 2002). These cells could be differentiated in numerous cell types for transplantation and would evade detection of any host immune system due its $HLA^{-/-}$ status. Obvious advantages include (i) evasion of concerns surrounding iPS and alternative technologies, (ii) alleviates the continued derivation of donor cells from each patient, (iii) cells would not have pre-existing mutations or be aged cells, and (iv) and only an initial approval from FDA/TGA agencies before widespread use. However, attempts have proved as yet unsuccessful as HLA molecules are represented by multiple genetic loci. In addition, unpredictable transformations in the transplanted cells would similarly evade detection by the host immune system and may continue unheeded.

5. Brief Conclusion

A considered approach should be employed before clinical trials initiate to avoid the adverse publicity following adverse outcomes of gene therapy trials (Raper et al., 2003). Even if the aforementioned concerns are insurmountable, this methodology is no less revolutionary and remains a radical change in thinking for cellular reprogramming. Indeed, application of iPS-based approaches has initiated development of alternative technologies for cellular therapy, namely transdifferentiation. Whether iPS, transdifferentiation or transdetermination translate to the therapeutic arena remain to be determined.

References

Aasen et al., (2008). Efficient and rapid generation of induced pluripotent stem cells from human keratinocytes. *Nat Biotech*. **26**: 1272-1284

Becker-Hapak et al., (2001). TAT-mediated protein transduction into mammalian cells. *Methods*. **24**:247-256.

Blelloch et al., (2007). Generation of induced pluripotent stem cells in the absence of drug selection. *Cell Stem Cell*. **1**: 245-247

Boyer et al., (2005). Core transcriptional regulatory circuitry in human embryonic stem cells. *Cell*. **122**: 947-956

Brambrink et al., (2008). Sequential expression of pluripotency markers during direct reprogramming of mouse somatic cells. *Cell Stem Cell.* **2**: 151-159.

Burdon et al., (1999). Suppression of SHP-2 and ERK signalling promotes self-renewal of mouse embryonic stem cells. *Dev. Biol.* **210**: 30-43.

Carey et al., (2009). Reprogramming of murine and human somatic cells using a single polycistronic vector. *PNAS.* **106**(1): 157-162

Catena et al., (2004). Conserved POU binding DNA sites in the Sox2 upstream enhancer regulate gene expression in embryonic and neural stem cells. *J. Biol. Chem.* **279**(40): 41846-41857

Chew et al., (2005). Reciprocal trasncriptional regulation of Pou5f1 and Sox2 via the Oct4/Sox2 complex in embryonic stem cells. *Mol. Cell Biol.* **25**(14): 6031-6046.

Condic ML. & Rao M. (2008). Regulatory issues for personalized pluripotent cells. *Stem Cells.* **26**(11): 2753-2758

Cyranoski, D. (2008). Stem Cells: 5 Things to know before jumping on the iPS bandwagon. *Nature.* **452**(7186): 406-408.

Dimos et al., (2008). Induced pluripotent stem cells generated from patients with ALS can be differentiated into motor neurons. *Science.* **321**:1218-1221

Ding et al., (2005). Efficient transposition of the piggyBac (PB) transposon in mammalian cells and mice. *Cell.* **122**:473-483.

Dominguez-Sola et al., (2007). Non-transcriptional control of DNA replication by c-Myc. *Nature.* **448**: 445-452.

Donohue et al., (2009). The pluripotency factor Oct4 interacts with Ctcf and also controls X-chromosome pairing and counting. *Nature.* In press.

Efthymiadis et al., (1998). The HIV-1 Tat nuclear localization sequence confers novel nuclear import properties. *J Biol.Chem.* **273**(3): 1623-1628.

Eilers & Eisenman (2009). Myc's broad reach. *Genes Dev.* **22**(20): 2755-2766.

Ema et al., (2008). Kruppel-like factor 5 is essential for blastocyst development and the normal self-renewal of mouse ESCs. *Cell Stem Cell.* **3**: 555-567.

Esteban et al., (2009). Generation of induced pluripotent stem cell lines from Tibetan miniature pig. *J.Biol.Chem.* **284**(26): 17634-17640.

Esteve et al., (2006). Direct interaction between DNMT1 and G9a coordinates DNA and histone methylation during replication. *Genes Dev.* **20**: 3089-3103.

Ezashi et al., (2009). Derivation of induced pluripotent stem cells from pig somatic cells. *PNAS.* **106**(27): 10993-10998

Feldman et al., (2005). G9a-mediated irreversible epigenetic inactivation of Oct3/4 during early embryogenesis. *Nat. Cell Biol.* **8**(2): 188-194.

Ferber et al., (2000). Pancreatic and duodenal homeobox gene 1 induces expression of insulin genes in liver and ameliorates streptozotocin-induced hyperglycemia. *Nat Med.* **6**(5): 568-572.

Fittipaldi et al., (2003). Cell membrane lipid rafts mediate caveolar endocytosis of HIV Tat fusion proteins. *J. Biol. Chem.* **278**(36): 34141-34149.

Frankel & Pabo, (1988). Cellular uptake of the Tat protein from human immunodeficiency virus. *Cell.* **55**:1189-1193.

Green & Loewenstein, (1988). Autonomous functional domains of chemically synthesized human immunodeficiency virus tat trans-activator protein. *Cell.* **55**(6): 1179-88.

Guenther et al., (2007). A chromatin landmark and transcription initiation at most promoters in human cells. *Cell Stem Cell.* **130**: 77-88

Hanna et al., (2007). Treatment of sickle cell anemia mouse model with iPS cells generated from autologous skin. *Science.* **318**(5858): 1920-1923.

Harui et al., (1999). Frequency and stability of chromosomal integration of adenovirus vectors. *J Virol.* **73**: 6141-6146

Hochedlinger & Jaenisch. (2007). Nuclear reprogramming and pluripotency. *Nature.* 441: 1061-1067

Huangfu et al., (2008)[a]. Induction of pluripotent stem cells by defined factors is greatly improved by small-molecule compounds. *Nat Biotech.* **26**(7): 795-797.

Huangfu et al., (2008)[b]. Induction of pluripotent stem cells from primary human fibroblasts with only Oct4 and Sox2. *Nat Biotech.* **26**(11): 1269-1275.

Ikegami et al., (2006). Genome-wide and locus-specific DNA hypomethylation in G9a deficient mouse embryonic stem cells. *Genes to Cells.* **12**(1): 1-11.

Jiang et al., (2008). The core Klf circuitry regulates self-renewal of embryonic stem cells. *Nat Cell Biol.* **10**(3): 353-360.

Judson et al., (2009). Embryonic stem cell-specific microRNAs promote induced pluripotency. *Nat. Biotech.* **27**(5): 459-461.

Kaji et al., (2009). Virus-free induction of pluripotency and subsequent excision of reprogramming factors. *Nature.* **458**(7239): 771-775.

Kang et al., (2009). iPS cells can support full-term development of tetraploid blastocyst-complemented embryos. *Cell Stem Cell.* **5**: in press.

Kim et al., (2008). Pluripotent stem cells induced from adult neural stem cells by reprogramming with two factors. *Nature.* **454**(7204): 646-650.

Kim et al., (2009)[a]. Oct4-induced pluripotency in adult neural stem cells. *Cell.* **136**(3): 411-419.

Kim et al., (2009)[b]. Generation of human induced pluripotent stem cells by direct delivery of reprogramming proteins. *Cell Stem Cells.* **4**: 472-476.

Kishigami et al., (2006). Significant improvement of mouse cloning technique by treatment with trichostatin A after somatic nuclear transfer. *Biochem. Biophys. Res. Commun.* **340**(1): 183-189.

Li et al., (2008). Generation of rat and human induced pluripotent stem cells by combining genetic reprogramming and chemical inhibitors. *Cell Stem Cell.* **4**:16-19.

Liu et al., (2008)[a]. Generation of induced pluripotent stem cells from adult rhesus monkey fibroblasts. *Cell Stem Cell.* **3**:587-590

Liu, (2008): iPS cells: a more critical review. *Stem Cell Dev.* **17**(3): 391-397.

Liu et al., (2008)[c]. Yamanaka factors critically regulate the developmental signaling network in mouse embryonic stem cells. *Cell Res.* **18**:1177-1189

Loh et al., (2009). Generation of induced pluripotent stem cells from human blood. *Blood.* **113**(22): 5476-5479.

Lyssiotis et al., (2009). Reprogramming of murine fibroblasts to induced pluripotent stem cells with chemical complementation of Klf4.*PNAS.* **106**(22): 8912-8917.

Ma et al., (2008). G9a and Jhdm2a regulate embryonic stem cell fusion-induced reprogramming of adult neural stem cells. *Stem Cells.* **26**(8): 2131-2141.

Maherali et al., (2007). Directly reprogrammed fibroblasts show global epigenetic remodeling and widespread tissue contribution. *Cell Stem Cell.* **1**:55-70.

Maherali et al., (2008). A high-efficiency system for the generation and study of human induced pluripotent stem cells. *Cell Stem Cell.* **3**(3):340-345.

Marion et al., (2009). Telomeres acquire embryonic stem cell characteristics in induced pluripotent stem cells. *Cell Stem Cell.* **4:** 141-154.

Marson et al., (2008). Wnt signalling promotes reprogramming of somatic cells to pluripotnecy. *Cell Stem Cell.* **7**: 132-135.

Martinato et al., (2008). Analysis of Myc-induced histone modifications on target chromatin. *PLoS ONE.* **3**(11): e3650

Masaki et al., (2008). Heterogeneity of pluripotent marker gene expression in colonies generated in human iPS cell induction culture. *Stem Cell Res.* **1**: 105-115

Masui et al., (2007). Pluripotency governed by Sox2 via regulation of Oct3/4 expression in mouse embryonic stem cells. *Nat Cell Biol.* **9**(6): 625-635

Meissner et al., (2007). Direct reprogramming of genetically unmodified fibroblasts into pluripotent stem cells. *Nature Biotech.* **25**(10): 1177-11

Mikkelsen et al., (2008). Dissecting direct reprogramming through integrative genomic analysis. *Nature.* **454**: 49-55.

Mitsui et al., (2003). The homeoprotein Nanog is required for maintenance of pluripotency in mouse epiblast and ES cells. *Cell.* **113**:631-642

Miura et al., (2009). Variation in the safety of inducd pluripotent stem cell lines. *Nat. Biotech.* In press.

Murrell et al., (2008). Olfactory mucoase is a potential source for autologous stem cell therapy for parkinson's disease. *Stem Cells.* **26**: 2183-2192.

Nakagawa et al., (2007). Generation of induced pluripotent stem cells without Myc from mouse and human fibroblasts. *Nat. Biotech.* **26**(1): 101-106.

Nishikawa et al., (2008). The promise of human induced pluripotent stem cells for research and therapy. *Nat Rev. Mol Cell. Biol.* **9**(9): 725-729.

Niwa et al., (2000). Quantitative expression of Oct3/4 defines differentiation, dedifferentiation or self-renewal of ES cells. *Nat Genet.* **24**: 372-376

Okita et al., (2007). Generation of germline-competent induced pluripotent stem cells. *Nature.* **448**(7151): 313-317.

Okita et al., (2008). Generation of mouse induced pluripotent stem cells without viral vectors. *Science.* **322**: 949-953.

Pan et al., (2002). Stem cell pluripotency and transcription factor Oct4. *Cell Res.* **12**(5-6):.321-329.

Park et al., (2008). Generation of human-induced pluripotent stem cells. *Nat. Protocols.* **7:** 1180-1186.

Raper et al. (2003). Fatal systemic inflammatory response syndrome in a orthinine transcarbamylase deficient patient following adenoviral gene transfer. *Mol. Genet. Metab.* **80**: 148–58.

Remenyi et al., (2003). Crystal structure of a POU/HMG/DNA ternary complex suggests differential assembly of Oct4 and Sox2 on two enhancers. *Genes Dev.* **17**: 2048-2059.

Rodda et al., (2005). Transcriptional regulation of Nanog by Oct4 and Sox2. *J. Biol. Chem.* **280**(26): 24731-24737

Rowland et al., (2005). The Klf4 tumour suppressor is a transcriptional repressor of p53 that acts as a context-dependent oncogene. *Nat. Cell Biol.* **7**(11): 1074-82.

Rusnati et al., (1999). Multiple interactions of HIV-1 Tat protein with size-defined heparin oligosaccharides. *J. Biol. Chem.* **274**(40): 28198-28205.

Segre et al., (1999). Klf4 is a transcription factor required for establishing the barrier function of the skin. *Nat Genetics.* **22**: 356-360.

Seoane et al., (2001). TGF influences Myc, Miz-1 and Smad to control the CDK inhibitor $p15^{INK4b}$. *Nat Cell. Biol.* **3**:400-408.

Shi et al., (2008)[a]. A combined chemical and genetic approach for the generation of induced pluripotent stem cells. *Cell Stem Cell.* **2**: 525-528.

Shi et al., (2008)[b]. *I*nduction of pluripotent stem cells from mouse embryonic fibroblasts by Oct4 and Klf4 with small-molecule compounds. *Cell Stem Cell.* **3:** 568-574.

Silva et al., (2006). Nanog promotes transfer of pluripotency after cell fusion. *Nature*. **441**(7096): 997-1001.

Soldner et al., (2009). Parkinson's disease patient-derived induced pluripotent stem cells free of viral reprogramming factors. *Cell*. **136**: 964-977.

Sommer et al., (2008). iPS cell generation using a single lentiviral stem cell cassette. *Stem Cells*. **27**(3): 543-549.

Sridharan et al., (2009). Role of the murine reprogramming factors in the induction of pluripotency. *Cell*. **136**:364-377

Stadtfeld et al., (2008)[a]. Defining molecular cornerstones during fibroblast to iPS cell reprogramming in mouse. *Cell Stem Cell*. **2**: 230-240.

Stadtfeld et al., (2008)[b]. Induced pluripotent stem cells generated without viral integration. *Science*. **322**(5903): 945-949.

Tachibana et al., (2002). G9a histone methyltransferase plays a dominant role in euchromatic histone H3 lysine 9 methylation and is essential for early embryogenesis. *Genes Dev*. **16**: 1779-1791.

Tada et al., (2001). Nuclear reprogramming of somatic cells by in vitro hybridization with ES cells. *Curr. Biol*. **11**(19): 1553-1558

Takahashi & Yamanaka, (2006). *I*nduction of pluripotent stem cells from mouse embryonic and adult fibroblasts by defined factors. *Cell*. 126:1-14.

Takahashi et al., (2007). Induction of pluripotent stem cells from adult human fibroblasts by defined factors. *Cell*. **131**:861-872.

Takeuchi & Bruneau, (2009). Directed transdifferentiation of mouse mesoderm to heart tissue by defined factors. *Nature*. **459**(7247): 708-711.

The President's Council on Bioethics. *White Paper: Alternative Sources of Human Pluripotent Stem Cells*. In. Washington, D.C.; 2005.

Tomioka et al., (2002). Identification of Sox-2 regulatory region which is under control of Oct3/4-Sox2 complex. *Nuc. Acids Res*. **30**(14): 3202-3213.

Tyagi et al., (2001). Internalization of HIV-1 tat requires cell surface heparan sulfate proteoglycans. *J.Biol.Chem*. **276**(5): 3254-3261.

Vogel, (2002). *In the Midwest, pushing back the stem cell frontier. Science*. **295**: 1818-1820.

Wilmut et al., (1997). Viable offspring derived from fetal and adult mammalian cells. *Nature*. **385**: 810-813

Wernig et al., (2007). In vitro reprogramming of fibroblasts into a pluripotent ES-cell-like state. *Nature*. **448**: 318-324.

Wernig et al., (2008). c-Myc is dispensible for direct reprogramming of mouse fibroblasts. *Cell Stem Cell.* **2**:10-12.

Woltjen et al., (2009). piggyBac transposition reprograms fibroblasts to induced pluripotent stem cells. *Nature.* **458**(7239): 766-770

Xu et al., (2008). A chemical approach to stem-cell biology and regenerative medicine. *Nature.* **453**: 338-344.

Xu et al., (2009). Histone H2a mRNA interacts with Lin28 and contains a Lin28-dependent posttranscriptional regulatory element. *Nuc. Acids.* Res. In press.

Yechoor et al., (2009). Neurogenin 3 is sufficient for transdetermination of hepatic progenitor cells into neo-islets in vivo but not transdifferentiation of hepatocytes. *Dev. Cell.* **16**: 358-373.

Yu et al., (2007). Induced pluripotent stem cell lines derived from human somatic cells. *Science.* **318**:1917-1920

Yu et al., (2009). Human induced pluripotent stem cells free of vector and transgene sequences. *Science.* **324**(5928): 797-801.

Yun et al., (2008). Transduction of artificial transcriptional regulatory proteins into human cells. *Nuc. Acids. Res.* **36**(16): 103

Zhao et al., (2009). iPS cells produce viable mice through tetraploid complementation. *Nature.* In press.

Zhou et al., (2008)[a]. In vivo reprogramming of adult pancreatic exocrine cells to β–cells. *Nature.* **455**(7213): 627-632.

Zhou et al., (2008)[b]. Two supporting factors greatly improve the efficiency of human iPSC generation. *Cell Stem Cell.* **3**(5):475-479.

Zhou et al., (2009)[c]. Generation of induced pluripotent stem cells using recombinant proteins. *Cell Stem Cell.* **4**(5): 381-384.

In: Pluripotent Stem Cells
Editors: D.W. Rosales et al, pp. 113-135
ISBN: 978-1-60876-738-0

Chapter 4

AMNIOTIC FLUID AND PLACENTAL STEM CELLS

Emily C. Moorefield, Dawn M. Delo, Paolo De Coppi and Anthony Atala *

Wake Forest Institute for Regenerative Medicine,
Wake Forest University Health Sciences, Medical Center Boulevard,
Winston-Salem, NC 27157 USA

Abstract

Human amniotic fluid has been used in prenatal diagnosis for more than 70 years. It has proven to be a safe, reliable, and simple screening tool for a wide variety of developmental and genetic diseases. However, there is now evidence that amniotic fluid may be used as more than simply a diagnostic tool. It may be the source of a powerful therapy for a multitude of congenital and adult disorders. A subset of cells found in amniotic fluid and placenta has been isolated and found to be capable of maintaining prolonged undifferentiated proliferation as well as able to differentiate into multiple tissue types encompassing the three germ layers. It is possible that in the near future, we will see the development of therapies using progenitor cells isolated from amniotic fland and placenta for the treatment of newborns with congenital malformations, as well as adults with various disorders, using

* E-mail address: aatala@wfubmc.edu. Telephone: 336-716-5701, Fax: 336-716-0656, Corresponding author: W. Boyce Professor and Chair, Department of Urology, Director, Wake Forest Institute for Regenerative Medicine, Wake Forest University Health Sciences, Medical Center Boulevard, Winston-Salem, NC 27157 USA.

cryopreserved amniotic fluid and placental stem cells. In this chapter, we describe a number of experiments that have isolated and characterized pluripotent progenitor cells from amniotic fland and placenta. We also discuss various cell lines derived from amniotic fluid and placenta and future directions for this area of research.

Introduction

Amniotic fluid-derived progenitor cells can be obtained from a small amount of fluid during amniocentesis, a procedure that is already often performed in many pregnancies in which the fetus has a congenital abnormality. Placenta-derived stem cells can be obtained from a small biopsy of the chorionic villi. Observations of cell cultures from these two sources provide evidence that they may represent new sources for the isolation of cells with the potency to differentiate into different cell types, suggesting a new source of cells for research and treatment.

Amniotic Fluid and Placenta in Developmental Biology

Gastrulation is a major milestone in early postimplantation development (Snow and Bennett, 1978). At about embryonic day6.5 (E6.5), gastrulation begins in the posterior region of the embryo. Pluripotent epiblast cells are allocated to the three primary germ layers of the embryo (ectoderm, mesoderm, and endoderm) and germ cells, which are the progenitors of all fetal tissue lineages as well as the extraembryonic mesoderm of the yolk sac, amnion, and allantois (Downs and Harmann, 1997; Downs et al., 2004; Gardner and Beddington, 1988; Loebel et al., 2003). The latter forms the umbilical cord as well as the mesenchymal part of the labyrinthine layer in the mature chorioallantoic placenta (Downs and Harmann, 1997; Moser et al., 2004; Smith et al., 1994). The final positions of the fetal membranes result from the process of embryonic turning, which occurs around day 8.5 of gestation and ''pulls'' the amnion and yolk sac around the embryo (Kinder et al., 1999; Parameswaran and Tam, 1995). The specification of tissue lineages is accomplished by the restriction of developmental potency and the activation of lineage-specific gene expression (Parameswaran and Tam, 1995; Rathjen et al., 1999). This process is strongly influenced by cellular interactions and signaling (Dang et al., 2002; Li et al., 2004).

The amniotic sac is a tough but thin transparent pair of membranes that holds the developing embryo (and later, the fetus) until shortly before birth. The inner membrane, the amnion, contains the amniotic fluid and the fetus. The outer membrane, the chorion, contains the amnion and is part of the placenta (Kaviani et al., 2001; Kinder et al., 1999; Robinson et al., 2002). Amnion is derived from ectoderm and mesoderm, and as it grows itbegins to fill with a fluid composed mainly of water (Robinson et al., 2002). Originally, it is isotonic, containing proteins, carbohydrates, lipids and phospholipids, urea, and electrolytes. Later, urine excreted by the fetus increases its volume and changes the concentrations of these components (Bartha et al., 2000; Heidari et al., 1996; Sakuragawa et al., 1999; Srivastava et al., 1996). The fetus can breathe in the water, allowing normal growth and the development of lungs and the gastrointestinal tract. The fluid is swallowed by the fetus and passes via the fetal blood into the maternal blood. The amniotic fluid ensures symmetrical structural development and growth, cushions and protects the embryo, helps maintain consistent pressure and temperature, and permits freedom of fetal movement, which is important for proper musculoskeletal development and blood flow (Baschat and Hecher, 2004).

Different origins have been suggested for the mixture of cells within amniotic fluid (Medina-Gomez and del Valle, 1988). The heterogeneous cell population comprising the amniotic fluid has been reported to contain cells of all three germ layers (In 't Anker et al., 2003; Prusa et al., 2004). These cells are thought to be sloughed from the fetal amnion, skin, and alimentary, respiratory, and urogenital tracts. The cell population found within the amniotic fluid changes with time and reflects the changes in the developing fetus (Torricelli et al., 1993). In addition, observations of cells cultured from amniotic fluid as well as placenta provide evidence that some of the cells may represent new stem cell sources with the potential to differentiate into different cell types (Prusa and Hengstschlager, 2002 and DeCoppi et al., 2007). Interestingly, it has been demonstrated that a subpopulation of cells in amniotic fluid expresses high levels of Oct-4, a transcription factor that preserves the undifferentiated state and the pluripotency of ES cells (Prusa et al., 2003 and DeCoppi et al., 2007). Although research is still in early stages, these cells may be used to find treatments or even cures for many diseases in which irreplaceable cells are damaged.

Amniotic Fluid and Placenta for Cell Therapy

Pluripotent stem cells are ideal for regenerative medicine applications because they have the capability to differentiate in stages into a huge number of different types of human cells. Amniotic fluid cells can be obtained from a small amount of fluid during amniocentesis at the second trimester. This procedure is already performed in many pregnancies in which the fetus has a congenital abnormality and is used to determine characteristics such as sex (Hoehn et al., 1975). Kaviani and co-workers reported that just 2 milliliters of amniotic fluid can provide up to 20,000 cells, 80% of which are viable (Kaviani et al., 2001, 2003). Because many pregnant women already undergo amniocentesis to screen for fetal abnormalities, cells can be isolated from this test fluid and saved for future use. Amniotic fluid cells will double in number in about 20 to 24 h, which is faster than umbilical cord stem cells (28 to 30 h) and bone marrow stem cells (more than 30 h) (Tsai et al., 2004). This phenomenon is important and suggests amniotic fluid stem cells might be a better choice for treatment of urgent medical conditions in the future.

In addition, while scientists have been able to isolate and differentiate, on average, only 30% of the mesenchymal stem cells (MSCs) extracted from a child's umbilical cord shortly after birth, the success rate for amniotic fluid-derived MSCs is close to 100% (In 't Anker et al., 2003; Tsai et al., 2004; DeCoppi et al., 2007). Another advantage of extracting cells from amniotic fluid or placenta is that it allows for autologous reimplantation, effectively bypassing the problems associated with a technique called donor-recipient HLA matching and minimizing the chances of cell rejection (Tsai et al., 2004). An additional characteristic which makes AFS cells an ideal candidate for cell therapy is their ability to readily take up retroviral, lentiviral, adenoviral and baculoviral vectors without altering the differentiation potential of the cells (DeCoppi et al., 2007, Grisafi et al., 2008 and Liu et al., 2009). This aids in the ability to track cells both *in vitro* and *in vivo* by infecting cells with a viral vector carrying a GFP or LacZ tag, and it also suggests that the cells could eventually be used in cell-based gene therapy applications.

Isolation and Characterization of Progenitor Cells

Amniotic fluid progenitor cells are isolated by centrifugation of amniotic fluid obtained via amniocentesis. Placental cells are isolated from single chorionic villi under light microscopy. Amniotic fluid cells and placental cells are allowed to proliferate *in vitro* and are maintained in culture for 4 weeks. The culture medium consists of modified alpha-modified Earl's medium (18% Chang medium B, 2% Chang medium C with 15% embryonic stem cell certified fetal bovine serum, antibiotics, and L-glutamine) (DeCoppi et al, 2007).

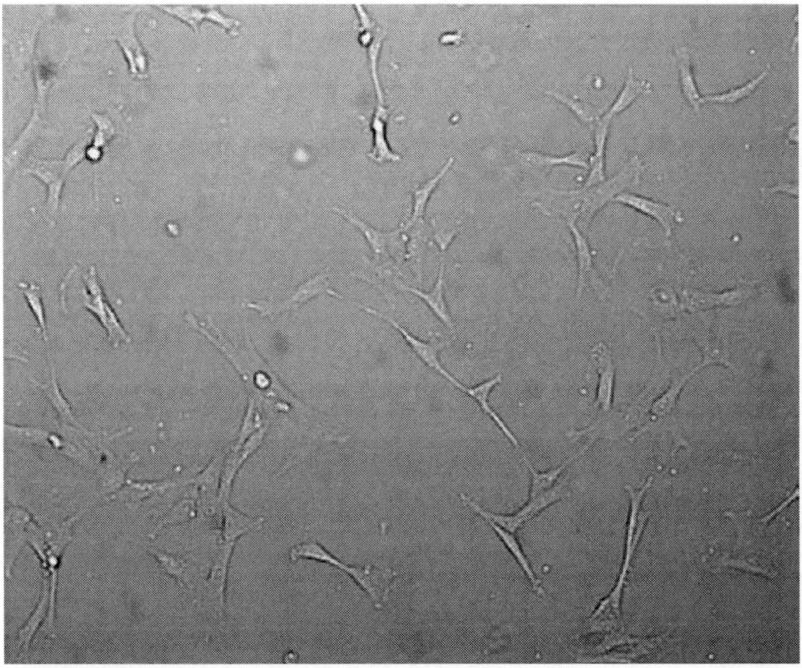

Figure 1. Morphology of amniotic fluid-derived stem cells (AFSCs) in culture.

A pluripotential subpopulation of progenitor cells present in the amniotic fluid and placenta can be isolated through positive selection for cells expressing the membrane receptor c-kit (CD117) (Figure 1) (DeCoppi et al., 2007; DeCoppi, 2001; Siddiqui and Atala, 2004). C-kit is a protein tyrosine-kinase receptor that specifically binds to the ligand stem cell factor (SCF) and it is this complex which has critical functions in gametogenesis, melanogenesis and hematopoiesis (Chabot et al., 1988; Fleischman et al., 1993). In addition, c-kit is expressed on a variety of stem cells including embryonic stem (ES) cells (Hoffman et al., 2005), primordial germ cells and many somatic stem cells (Guo et al., 1997 and Crane et al., 2006). About 0.8 to 1.4% of cells present in amniotic fluid and placenta have been shown to be c-kit positive in analysis by fluorescence-activated cell sorting (FACS) (DeCoppi et al., 2007). Progenitor cells maintain a round shape for 1 week post isolation when cultured in nontreated culture dishes. In this state, they demonstrate low proliferative capability. After the first week the cells begin to adhere to the plate and change their morphology, becoming more elongated and proliferating more rapidly, reaching 80% confluence and a need for passage every 48 to 72 h (DeCoppi et al., 2007). The doubling time of the undifferentiated cells under growth conditions is 36 h, with little variation with passages. No feeder layers are required for maintenance or expansion. The progenitor cells show a high self-renewal capacity with over 250 population doublings. This far exceeds Hayflick's limit, which is defined as 50 doublings for most cultured somatic cells (DeCoppi et al., 2007).

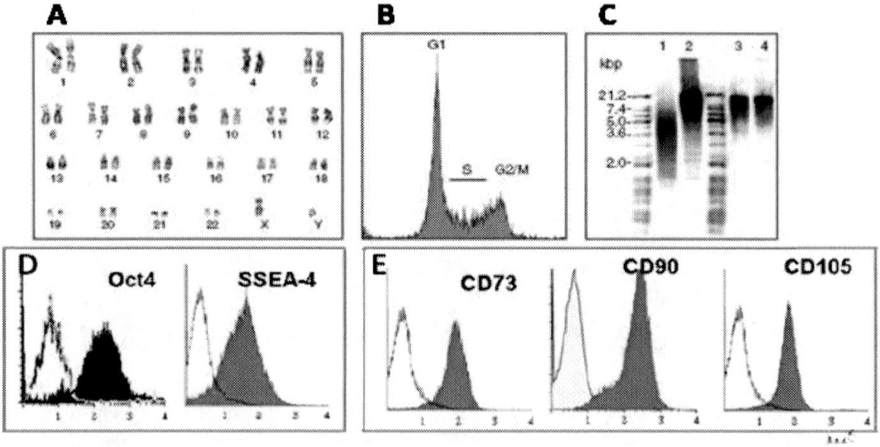

Figure 2. Consistent phenotype of hAFSCs in long term culture. A. Clonal human AFS cells maintain a normal karyotype after 250 pds. B. AFS cells passaged in culture show normal cell cycle control. C. Telomere length is conserved in AFS cells between early passage (20 p.d., lane 3) and late passage (250 p.d., lane 4). Lane 1: short length telomere standards, Lane 2: high length telomere standards. D. AFS cells express markers characteristic of ES cells, Oct4 and SSEA4. E. AFS cells express markers characterisitc of MSCs, CD73, CD90, CD105.

AFS cells have been shown to maintain a normal karyotype at late passages and display normal G1 and G2 cell cycle checkpoints (Figure 2A, 2B). They demonstrate telomere length conservation while in the undifferentiated state as well as telomerase activity even in late passages (Figure 2C). Analysis of protein expression shows that progenitor cells from amniotic fluid express human embryonic stage-specific marker SSEA-4, and the stem cell marker Oct-4, supporting the idea that these cells are able to maintain their pluripotentiality

(Figure 2D). Further surface marker analysis demonstrated the presence of the mesenchymal and/or neuronal markers CD29, CD44, CD73, CD90 and CD105 (Figure 2E). AFS cells are also characterized by the absence of a variety of surface molecules, including the hematopoetic lineage marker CD45, hematopoietic stem cell markers CD34, CD133 and ES cell markers SSEA3 and Tr 1-81. This expression profile is of interest as it demonstrates expression of e key markers of the embryonic stem cell phenotype, but not the full plement of markers expressed by ES cells. This indicates that these amniotic s are not quite as primitive as ES cells, yet they maintain greater potential than st adult stem cells.

Other behaviors showing similarities and differences between these nniotic fluid-derived cells and blastocyst-derived cells exist as well. For xample, amniotic fluid progenitor cells do form embryoid bodies *in vitro*, which stain positive for markers of all three germ layers. However, unlike ES cells, when implanted into immunodeficient mice *in vivo*, AFS cells do not form teratomas, an essential consideration for potential cell therapy (DeCoppi et al., 2007). AFS cells have a high clonal capacity based on a technique involving retrovirally tagged cells (DeCoppi et al., 2007). In this assay, a tagged single cell gave rise to a population that was able to be differentiated along six distinct lineages from all three germ layers: adipogenic, osteogenic, myogenic, endothelial, neurogenic and hepatic (DeCoppi et al., 2007). This broad differentiation capability, along with their high proliferation rate, gives AFS cells and placental derived stem cells a clear advantage over other known adult stem cell sources.

In Vitro Differentiation of Amniotic Fluid and Placenta Derived Progenitor Cells

Cell populations derived from amniotic fluid and placenta can be selected for c-kit expression, and the c-kit expressing cells are then cloned. The selected cells have been shown to be pluripotent and able to differentiate into osteogenic, adipogenic, myogenic, neurogenic, endothelial, hepatic and chondrocytic phenotypes *in vitro*. Each differentiation has been performed through proof of phenotypic and biochemical changes consistent with the differentiated tissue type of interest (Figure 3). We discuss each set of differentiations separately as reported in DeCoppi et al. (2007) unless otherwise noted.

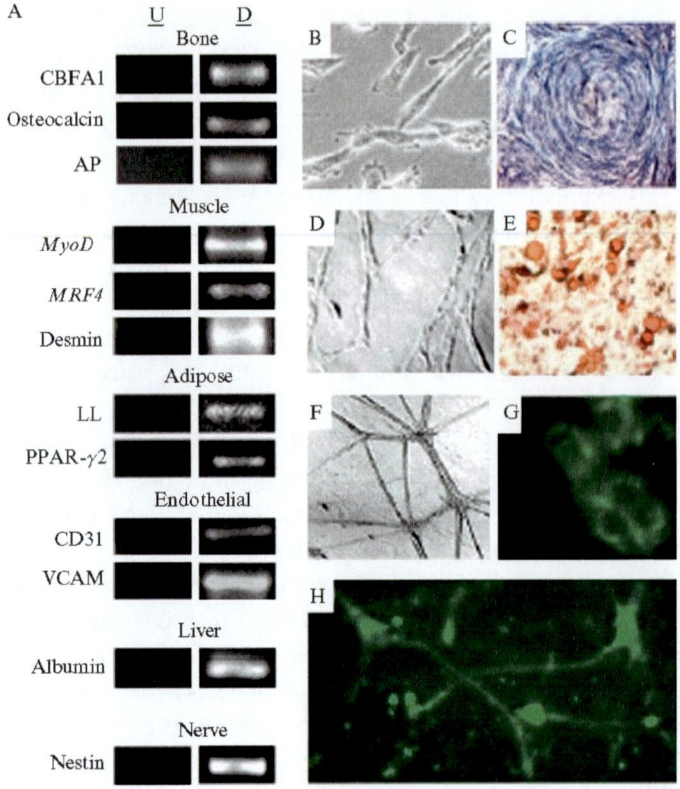

Figure 3. Multilineage differentiation of hAFSCs *in vitro*. (A) RT-PCR analysis of mRNA. Left: Control undifferentiated cells. Right: Cells maintained under conditions for differentiation to bone (8 days), muscle (8 days), adipocyte (16 days), endothelial (8 days), hepatic (45 days), neuronal (2 days) lineages. (B) Phase-contrast microscopy of control, undifferentiated cells. (b–h) Differentiated progenitor cells. (C) Bone: Histochemical staining for alkaline phosphatase. (D) Muscle: Phase contrast microscopy showing fusion into multinucleated myotube-like cells. (E) Adipocyte: Staining with oil red O (day 8) shows intracellular oil aggregation. (F) Endothelial: Phase-contrast microscopy of capillary-like structures. (G) Hepatic: Fluorescent antibody staining (FITC, green) for albumin. (H) Neuronal: Fluorescent antibody staining of nestin (day 2).

Adipocytes

To promote adipogenic differentiation, progenitor cells can be induced in dexamethasone, 3-isobutyl-1-methylxanthine, insulin, and indomethacin. Progenitor cells cultured with adipogenic supplements change their morphology from elongated to round within 8 days. This coincides with the accumulation of intracellular droplets. After 16 days in culture, more than 95% of the cells have their cytoplasm filled with lipid-rich vacuoles. Adipogenic differentiation also induces the expression of peroxisome proliferation-activated receptor 2 (PPAR-2), a transcription factor that regulates adipogenesis, and of lipoprotein lipase, as measured by reverse transcription-polymerase chain reaction (RT-PCR) analysis (Cremer et al., 1981; Medina-Gomez and del Valle,1988). Expression of these genes is noted in progenitor cells under adipogenic conditions but not in undifferentiated cells.

Osteocytes

Osteogenic differentiation was induced in progenitor cells with the use of dexamethasone, beta-glycerophosphate, and ascorbic acid 2-phosphate (Jaiswal et al., 1997). Progenitor cells maintained in this medium demonstrated phenotypic changes within 4 days, including a loss of spindle-shape phenotype and development of an osteoblast-like appearance with finger-like excavations into the cytoplasm. At 16 days, the cells aggregated, showing typical lamellar bone-like structures. In terms of functionality, these differentiated cells demonstrate a major feature of osteoblasts, which is to precipitate calcium. Differentiated osteoblasts from the progenitor cells are able to produce alkaline phosphatase (AP) and to deposit calcium, consistent with bone differentiation. Undifferentiated progenitor cells lack this ability. Progenitor cells in osteogenic medium also express specific genes implicated in mammalian bone development [AP, core-binding factor A1 (CBFA1), and osteocalcin] in a pattern consistent with the physiological analog. In addition, cells grown in osteogenic medium show activation of the AP gene at each time point. Expression of CBFA1, a transcription factor specifically expressed in osteoblasts and hypertrophic chondrocytes and that regulates gene expression of structural proteins of the bone extracellular matrix, is highest in cells grown in osteogenic inducing medium on day 8 and decreases slightly on days 16, 24, and 32. Osteocalcin is expressed only in progenitor cells under osteogenic conditions at 8 days (Karsenty, 2000; Komori et al., 1997).

Endothelial Cells

Amniotic fluid progenitor cells can be induced to form endothelial cells through culture in endothelial basal medium on gelatin-coated dishes. Full differentiation is achieved by 1 month in culture; however, phenotypic changes are noticed within 1 week of initiation of the protocol. Human-specific endothelial cell surface marker (P1H12), factor VIII (FVIII), and kinase insert domain receptor (KDR) are specific for differentiated endothelial cells. Differentiated cells stain positively for FVIII, KDR, and P1H12. Progenitor cells do not stain for these endothelial-specific markers. Amniotic fluid progenitor-derived endothelial cells, once differentiated, are able to grow in culture and form capillary-like structures *in vitro*. These cells also express platelet endothelial cell adhesion molecule1 (PECAM-1 or CD31) and vascular cell adhesion molecule (VCAM), which are not detected in the progenitor cells on RT-PCR analysis.

Hepatocytes

For hepatic differentiation, progenitor cells are seeded on Matrigel or collagen-coated dishes at different stages and cultured in the presence of hepatocyte growth factor, insulin, oncostatin M, dexamethasone, fibroblast growth factor 4 and monothioglycerol for 45 days (Dunn et al., 1989; Schwartz et al., 2002). After 7 days of the differentiation process, cells exhibit morphological changes and shift from an elongated to a cobblestone-like appearance. The cells stain positively for albumin on day 45 post differentiation and also express the transcription factor hepatocyte nuclear factor 4 (HNF4), the c-Met receptor, the multidrug resistance (MDR) membrane transporter, albumin, and alpha-fetoprotein. RT-PCR analysis further supports albumin production. In addition, AFS cells differentiated to hepatocytes using this method were able to secrete urea, a characteristic liver-specific function that requires coordinated expression of several enzymes and specific mitochondrial amino acid transporters (Morris et al., 2002).

Myocytes

Myogenic differentiation is induced in amniotic fluid-derived progenitor cells by culture in medium containing horse serum and chick embryo extract on a thin coat of Matrigel (Rosenblatt et al., 1995). To initiate differentiation, the presence of 5-azacytidine in the medium for 24 h is necessary. Phenotypically, the cells tend to organize themselves into bundles that fuse to form multinucleated cells. These cells express sarcomeric tropomyosin and desmin, both of which are not expressed in the original progenitor population.

The development profile of cells differentiating into myogenic lineages interestingly mirrors a characteristic pattern of gene expression reflecting that seen with embryonic muscle development (Bailey et al., 2001; Rohwedel et al., 1994).

With this protocol, myogenic factor 6 (Myf6) is expressed on day 8 and suppressed on day 16. MyoD expression is detectable at 8 days and suppressed at 16 days in progenitor cells. Desmin expression is induced at 8 days and increases by 16 days in progenitor cells cultured in myogenic medium (Hinterberger et al., 1991; Patapoutian et al., 1995).

Neuronal Cells

For neurogenic induction, amniotic progenitor cells are cultured in dimethylsulfoxide (DMSO), butylated hydroxyanisole, and neuronal growth factor (Black and Woodbury, 2001; Woodbury et al., 2000). Progenitor cells cultured under neurogenic conditions change their morphology within the first 24 h. Two different cell populations become apparent: morphologically large flat cells and small bipolar cells. The bipolar cell cytoplasm retracts toward the nucleus, forming contracted multipolar structures. Over subsequent hours, the cells display primary and secondary branches and cone-like terminal expansions.

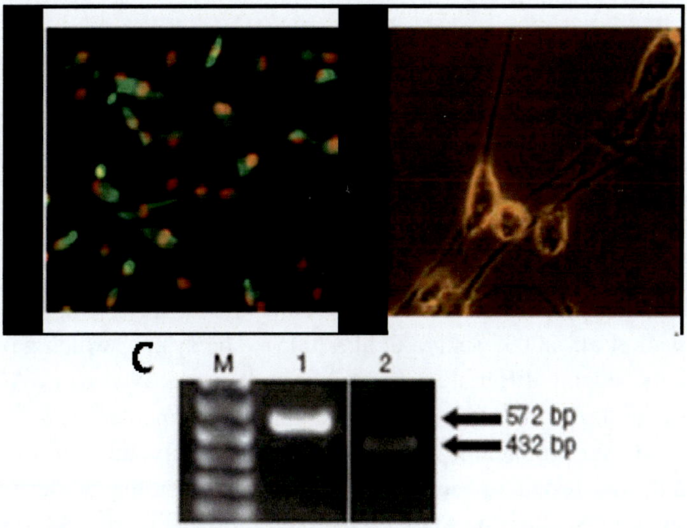

Figure 4. Neuronal differentiation of hAFS cells *in vitro* A. Immunocytochemical detection of nestin after 8 d in the first stage of dopaminergic neuron differentiation. B. Phase contrast image of pyramidal morphology of cells after the second stage of differentiation. C. RT-PCR analysis of cells at the end of the 2 stage dopaminergic neuron differentiation. M: size marker, lane 1: GAPDH, lane 2: GIRK2.

Induced progenitor cells show a characteristic sequence of expression of neural-specific proteins. At an early stage in differentiation conditions, AFS cells express high levels of the intermediate filament protein nestin, which is expressed in neuroepithelial stem cells. A 2-step process is utilized to differentiate AFS cells to dopaminergic neuron like cells. Induction begins with seeding cells onto fibronectin coated dishes and supplementing the culture medium with N2 and bFGF. During this stage, cells begin to express nestin and, by 8 days of induction, about 80 percent of the culture is positive for nestin protein (Figure 4A). At this stage the cells are then transferred to conditions that have been shown to bias toward the production of dopaminergic neurons (Perrier et al., 2004). Under these conditions a fraction of the cells begin to have a distinct pyramidal morphology (Figure 4B). In addition to the morphologic change, the cells also express a gene which is a member of the G-protein-gated inwardly rectifying potassium (GIRK) channel family, GIRK2, a known marker of dopaminergic neurons (Figure 4C).

Chondrocytes

Chondrogenic differentiation has been induced in progenitor cells *in vitro* by supplementing medium with members of the transforming growth factor-beta (TGF-β) superfamily in a three-dimensional culture system (Kolambkar et al., 2007). In this effort to test the chondrogenic potential of AFS cells in both pellet and hydrogel systems, many growth factors were tested including TGF-β1, TGF-β3, bone morphogenetic protein 2 (BMP2) and insulin-like growth factor 1 (IGF1), all of which have been previously shown to induce chondrogenic differentiation (Iwasaki eat al., 1993; Johnstone et al., 1998; Kramer et al., 2000; Awad et al., 2003; Sekiya et al., 2005). The system which gave the most robust chondrogenic differentiation of AFS cells as assayed by sGAG synthesis and type II collagen staining was the medium supplemented with TGF-β1. The amount of sGAG production is an indicator of the formation of a cartilaginous matrix and was tested by both biochemical and histological techniques at 3 week time points after the start of differentiation (Figure 5A). These recent experiments provide further evidence of the broad differentiation capabilities of AFS cells.

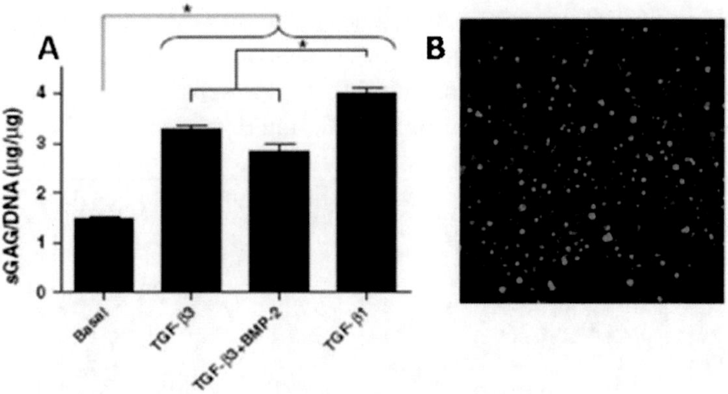

Figure 5. Chondrogenic differentiation of AFS cells *in vitro*. A. sGAG production normalized to the total amount of DNA present in pellet cultures under differentiation conditions after 21 days. B. Immunofluorescent staining for type II collagen deposited by AFS cells in alginate constructs at 21 days.

Preclinical Studies in Animal Models

More recent reports have examined the utility of progenitor cells within both *ex vivo* and *in vivo* environments. Undifferentiated c-kit selected and clonally derived AFS cells have been shown to contribute to renal and epithelial lung generation while partially differentiated AFS cells have the ability to contribute to the production of osteocytes and neurons. These important studies are significant for the long term clinical applications of these cells, including tissue engineering as well as gene therapy.

Bone Repair

In order to determine whether AFS cells have the ability to contribute to bone formation *in vivo,* cells were partially differentiated within a three dimensional scaffold and then implanted subcutaneously into immunodeficient mice (DeCoppi et al., 2007). Following the *in vitro* induction period as described above, the cells expressed genes consistent with the osteoblastic lineage and secreted alkaline phosphatase (AP), but did not yet show calcium deposition. After 8 weeks *in vivo,* the implanted constructs contained highly mineralized tissue as visualized by von Kossa's stain (Figure 6A). Micro CT scanning analysis of constructs at 18 weeks post implantation further confirmed the presence of hard tissue within the hAFSCseeded constructs (Figure 6B). Additionally, the density of the tissue-engineered bone found at the sites of implantation was found to be somewhat greater than that of mouse femoral bone, demonstrating that AFS cells do contribute to *in vivo* bone formation and may be a valuable tool in future therapies.

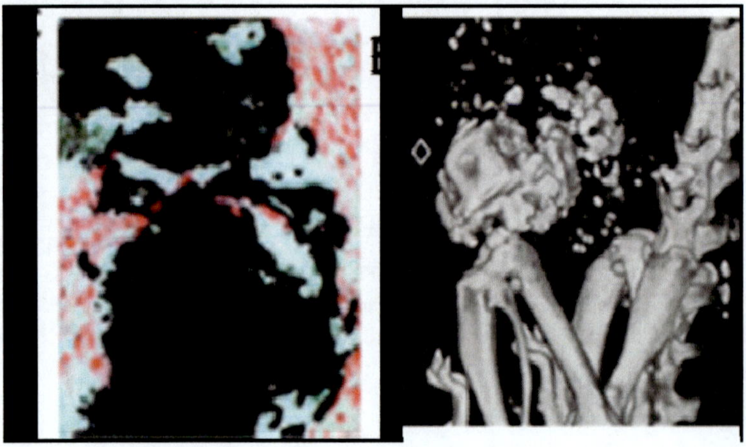

Figure 6. Production of tissue-engineered bone by AFS cells. A. von Kossa staining of AFS cell derived osteocyte seeded scaffold recovered 8 weeks after implantation, black staining indicates strong mineralization. C. Close up view of micro CT scan of seeded scaffold site in mouse 8 weeks post implantation.

Cardiac Repair

To examine the ability of these progenitor cells to integrate into and repair cardiac tissue, undifferentiated AFS cells shown to be capable of differentiation down the cardiomyocyte linage *in vitro* were injected directly into the wall of the heart in a rat model of myocardial infarction (Chiavegato et al., 2007). Myocardial infarction (MI) causes tissue death, and the ability to replace that lost myocardial tissue has previously been accomplished by transplanting stem cells from various sources (Davani et al., 2005). Surprisingly, transplantation of AFS cells into the heart wall of a xenogeneic host lead to an acute rejection of the cells within 15 days after injection, whether or not an MI had occurred (Chiavegato et al., 2007). This rejection is likely due to the recruitment of immune cells including CD4+ T cells, CD8+ T cells, B lymphocytes, NK cells and macrophages.

Renal Repair

Perin et al. (2007) have shown that AFS cells can contribute to renal development both *ex vivo* and *in vivo*. In their *ex vivo* experiment, labeled hAFS cells were injected into the primordia of the developing kidney, which was maintained in a transwell culture system for 2 to 10 days. Immediately after injection, the AFS cells could be found only at the injection site in the center of the murine embryonic kidney. After just 4 days of culture, however, the AFS cells had divided and spread throughout the organ. In addition, the AFS cells were shown by immunohistochemistry and *in situ* hybridization to have contributed to the embryonic tubular and glomerular structures (Figure 7A). After 9 days of culture, RT-PCR was performed and the expression of several human-specific kidney genes was detected, including Zona occludins-1, claudin, and glial-derived neurotrophic factor (GDNF) (Figure 7B). GDNF is a particularly important factor in renal development and is known to be expressed only in the earliest stages of renal development (Basson et al., 2006; Costantini and Shakya, 2006), so GDNF upregulation at day 9 suggests the initiation of renal differentiation by the AFS cells. To follow up on these results, the same group tested the AFS cells in a mouse model of acute tubular necrosis (ATN). One million labeled AFS cells were injected directly into the damaged kidney and allowed to incubate for 1 day to 6 months. Histological and molecular results suggest that AFS cells were not only able to survive in this environment, but they were also able to integrate into the damaged tubules.

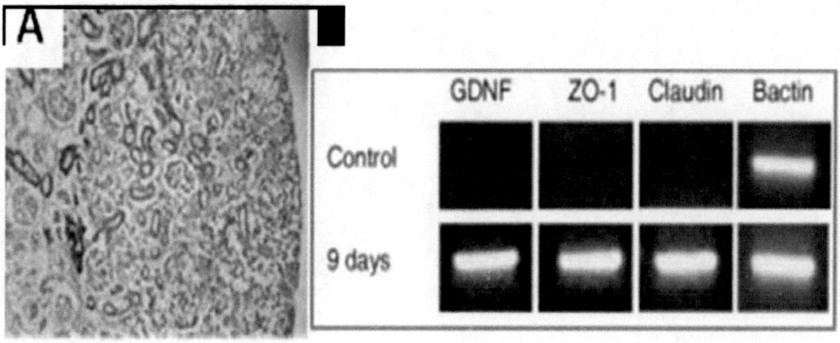

Figure 7. Undifferentiated human AFS cells are able to contribute to renal structures when injected into normal mouse kidneys. A. Chromogenic in situ hybridization for Y chromosome of male hAFS cells injected into a female mouse shows integration into embryonic kidney structures. B. Presence of early kidney markers is detected by RT-PCR 9 days after hAFS cell injection into mouse kidney.

Neural Repair

Survival and engraftment abilities of AFS cells within the rodent brain were also examined by DeCoppi et al. (2007). The *twitcher* mouse model of neurological disease, in which endogenous neurons undergo massive degeneration, was used in these studies. Neurogenic induction of AFS cells began *in vitro* by incubation with NGF, resulting in upregulation of the neural stem cell-related gene nestin. These cells were then implanted directly into the lateral ventricles of the developing brain of a newborn mouse in both normal and *twitcher* models, as had been done previously with neural stem cells (Taylor et al., 2006). Lateral ventricle implantation was selected to allow cell penetration into the subventricular zone, an area which contains endogenous, proliferating neural progenitors that have been shown to easily migrate into and integrate throughout the rest of the brain (Taylor and Snyder, 1997). Migration and integration of AFS cells were examined two months after implantation by immunohistochemistry (Figure 8). Both the normal and *twitcher* mice showed similar patterns of cell migration, suggesting that this process is not random. However, the number of cells that were able to engraft was dramatically different in the two groups, with the *twitcher* mice engrafting about 70% of the injected cells into the brain, while only about 30% of the injected cells engrafted in the normal mouse brain. These findings confirm that AFS cells are able to survive and integrate into the fetal mouse brain and may be a useful tool for future therapies for neurodegenerative disorders.

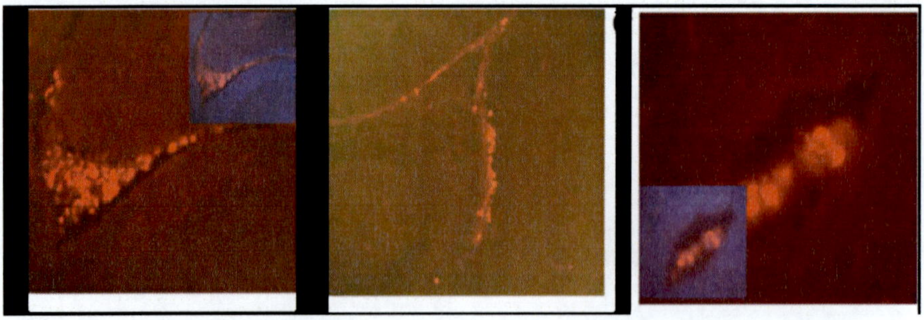

Figure 8. Neurogenically differentiated human AFS cells are able to integrate into the injured mouse brain. Immunohistochemistry performed on samples collected 1month after cell injection into *twitcher* mice. Red: human specific mitochondrial protein, Blue: DAPI. A. Lateral ventrical, B. Periventricular area and hippocampus, C. Olfactory bulb.

Repair of Lung Epithelium

Studies show that undifferentiated AFS cells have the ability to engraft into developing lung and injured lung tissues and to contribute to epithelial lung lineages (Carraro et al., 2008). *Ex vivo* injection of AFS cells into mouse embryonic lung demonstrated the ability of the cells to engraft and to express the early lung marker thyroid transcription factor 1(TTF1) within 1 week (Figure 9A). Further *in vivo* experimentation illustrated the ability of AFS cells injected into the mouse tail vein to home to the lung and differentiate into epithelial cells. AFS cells labeled with luciferase were injected into both normal and injured immunocompromised mice and their presence was detected 3 to 6 weeks later. In the absence of injury the cells were able to engraft into the recipient lung within 3 weeks after injection; however, no differentiation to epithelial cells was detected.

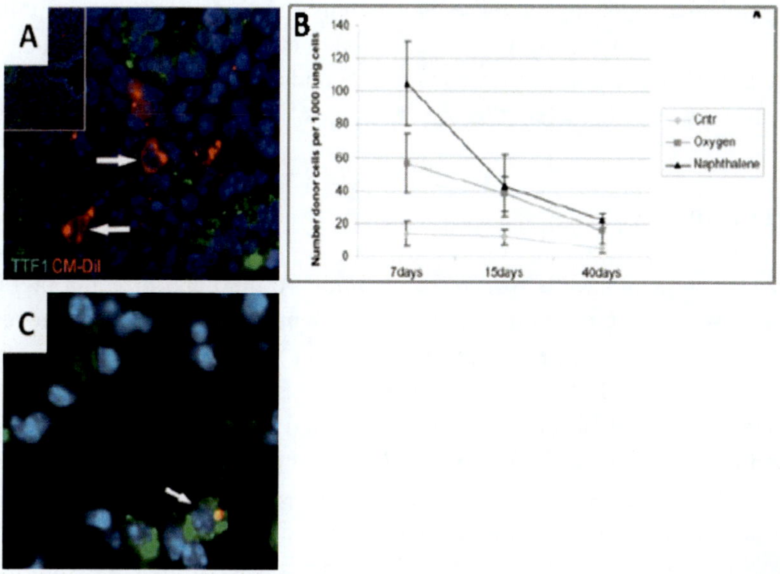

Figure 9. Undifferentiated hAFS cells can engraft and differentiate to epithelial cells in a mouse model of lung injury. A. hAFS cells injected into the embryonic lung ex vivo integrate into the lung epithelium and mesenchyme and express the early differentiation marker TTF1 7 days post injection, Red: CM-Dil-labeled hAFS cells, Green: TTF1, Blue: DAPI. B. Lung injury increases the degree of engraftment of hAFS within the mouse lung. C. Immunohistochemistry of lung 15 days after hAFS cell injection showing that cells can achieve a type II pneumocyte, Red: CM-Dil-labeled hAFS cell, Green: pro-SPC, Blue: DAPI.

The engraftment potential of hAFS cells was enhanced following lung injury induced either by hypoxia or the aromatic hydrocarbon naphthalene (Figure 9B). Integrated cells continued to show expression of TTF1 up to 7 months after injection as detected by RT-PCR and immunohistochemistry, suggesting the ability of the AFS cells to self-renew and preserve the expression of this early differentiation marker. Additionally, few engrafted cells expressed the mature type II pneumocyte lineage marker SPC as detected by immunohistochemistry. However gene expression was not detected by human specific RT-PCR. This evidence suggests that AFS differentiation to type II pneumocytes is a rare event *in vivo*.

The *in vivo* applications of fetally derived stem cells are still in the initial stages but based on these results, it appears that AFS cells are a pluripotential source of stem cells with the potential for alternative clinical treatment for a variety of diseases in the future. Importantly, AFS cells do not form teratomas when implanted into any of these *in vivo* environments. This fact is critically significant when considering future clinical applications and is an advantage over ES cells. AFS cells are at a stage between ES and adult stem cells, possessing the most advantageous characteristics of both groups.

Conclusion

Pluripotent progenitor cells isolated from amniotic fluid and placenta present an exciting possible contribution to the field of stem cell biology and regenerative medicine. These cells are an excellent source for research and therapeutic applications. The ability to isolate progenitor cells during gestation may also be advantageous for babies born with congenital malformations. Furthermore, progenitor cells can be cryopreserved for future self-use. Compared with embryonic stem cells, c-kit positive, cloned progenitor cells isolated from amniotic fluid have many similarities: they can differentiate into all three germ layers, they express common markers, and they preserve their telomere length. However, progenitor cells isolated from amniotic fluid and placenta have considerable advantages. They easily differentiate into specific cell lineages and they avoid the current controversies associated with the use of human embryonic stem cells. The discovery of these cells has been recent, and a considerable amount of work remains to be done to fully characterize these cells. In the future, cells derived from amniotic fluid and placenta may represent an attractive and abundant, noncontroversial source of cells for regenerative medicine.

References

Bailey, P., Holowacz, T. and Lassar, A. B. (2001). The origin of skeletal muscle stem cells in the embryo and the adult. *Curr.Opin.CellBiol.* **13**,679–689.

Bartha, J. L., Romero-Carmona, R., Comino-Delgado, R., Arce, F. and Arrabal, J. (2000). Alpha-Fetoprotein and hematopoietic growth factors in amniotic fluid. *Obstet.Gynecol.* **96**,588–592.

Baschat, A. A. and Hecher, K. (2004). Fetal growth restriction due to placental disease. *Semin.Perinatol.* **28**,67–80.

Basson, M. A., Watson-Johnson, J., Shakya, R., Akbulut, S., Hyink, D., Costantini, F. D., Wilson, P. D., Mason, I. J. and J. D. Licht. (2006). Branching morphogenesis of the ureteric epithelium during kidney development is coordinated by the opposing functions of GDNF and Sprouty1. *Dev.Biol.* **299**, 466–477.

Black, I. B. and Woodbury, D. (2001). Adult rat and human bone marrow stromal stem cells differentiate into neurons. *Blood Cells Mol.Dis.* **27**,632–636.

Carraro, G., Perin, L., Sedrakyan, S., Giuliani, S., Tiozzo, C., Lee, J., Turcatel, G., De Langhe, S. P., Driscoll, B., Bellusci, S., Minoo, P., Atala, A., De Filippo, R. E. and D. Warburton. (2008). Human amniotic fluid stem cells can integrate and differentiate into epithelial lung lineages. *Stem Cells.* **26**(11):2902-11.

Chabot, B., Stephenson, D. A., Chapman, V. M., Besmer, P. and Bernstein, A. (1988). The protooncogene c-kit encoding a transmembrane tyrosine kinase receptor maps to the mouse W locus. *Nature* 335, 88–89

Costantini F. and Shakya. R., (2006). GDNF/Ret signaling and the development of the kidney. *Bioessays* **28**, 117–127.

Crane, J. F. and Trainor, P. A. (2006). Neural crest stem and progenitor cells. Annu. Rev. *Cell Dev.Biol.* **22**, 267–286.

Cremer, M., Schachner, M., Cremer, T., Schmidt, W. and Voigtlander, T. (1981). Demonstration of astrocytes in cultured amniotic fluid cells of three cases with neural-tube defect. *Hum.Genet.* **56**,365–370.

Dang, S. M., Kyba, M., Perlingeiro, R., Daley, G. Q. and Zandstra, P. W. (2002). Efficiency of embryoid body formation and hematopoietic development from embryonic stem cells in different culture systems. *Biotechnol.Bioeng.* **78**,442–453.

Davani, S., Deschaseaux, F., Chalmers, F., Tiberghien P. and Kantelip. J. P. (2005). Can stem cells mend a broken heart? *Cardiovasc.Res.* **65**:305–16.

DeCoppi, P., Bartsch, G., Siddiqui, M. M., Xu, T., Santos, C. C., Perin, L., Mostoslavsky, G., Serre, A. C., Snyder, E. Y., Yoo, J. J., Furth, M. E., Soker,

S. and Atala, A. (2007). Isolation of amniotic stem cell lines with potential for therapy. *Nature Biotechnology* **25**, 100-106.

Downs, K. M. and Harmann, C. (1997). Developmental potency of the murine allantois. *Development* **124**,2769–2780.

Downs, K. M., Hellman, E. R., McHugh, J., Barrickman, K. and Inman, K. E. (2004). Investigation into a role for the primitive streak in development of the murine allantois. *Development* **131**,37–55.

Dunn, J. C., Yarmush, M. L., Koebe, H. G. and Tompkins, R. G. (1989). Hepatocyte function and extracellular matrix geometry: Long-term culture in a sandwich configuration. *FASEBJ.* **3**,174–177.

Fleischman, R. A. (1993). From white spots to stem cells: the role of the Kit receptor in mammalian development. *Trends Genet.* **9**, 285–290.

Gardner, R. L. and Beddington, R. S. (1988). Multi-lineage ''stem'' cells in the mammalian embryo. *J.CellSci.Suppl.***10**,11–27.

Grisafi, D. Piccoli, M., Pozzobon, M., Ditadi, A., Zaramella, P., Chiandetti, L., Zanon, G. F., Atala, A., Zacchello, F., Scarpa, M., De Coppi, P. and Tomanin, R. (2008). High transduction efficiency of human amniotic fluid stem cells mediated by adenovirus vectors. *Stem Cells Dev.* Oct;17(5):953-62.

Guo, C. S., Wehrle-Haller, B., Rossi, J. and Ciment, G. (1997). Autocrine regulation of neural crest cell development by steel factor. *Dev. Biol.* **184**, 61–69.

Heidari, Z., Isobe, K., Goto, S., Nakashima, I., Kiuchi, K. and Tomoda, Y. (1996). Characterization of the growth factor activity of amniotic fluid on cells from hematopoietic and lymphoid organs of different life stages. *Microbiol. Immunol.* **40**, 583–589.

Hinterberger, T. J., Sassoon, D. A., Rhodes, S. J. and Konieczny, S. F. (1991). Expression of the muscle regulatory factor MRF4 during somite and skeletal myofiber development. *Dev.Biol.* **147**,144–156.

Hoehn, H., Bryant, E. M., Fantel, A. G. and Martin, G. M. (1975). Cultivated cells from diagnostic amniocentesis in second trimester pregnancies. III. The fetal urine as a potential source of clonable cells. *Humangenetik.* **29**,285–290.

Hoffman, L. M. and Carpenter, M. K. (2005). Characterization and culture of human embryonic stem cells. Nat. *Biotechnol.* **23**, 699–708.In 't Anker, P. S., Scherjon, S. A., Kleijburg-van der Keur, C., Noort, W. A., Claas, F. H., Willemze, R., Fibbe, W. E. and Kanhai, H. H. (2003). Amniotic fluid as a novel source of mesenchymal stem cells for therapeutic transplantation. *Blood.* **102**, 1548–1549.

Jaiswal, N., Haynesworth, S. E., Caplan, A. I. and Bruder, S. P. (1997). Osteogenic differentiation of purified, culture-expanded human mesenchymal stem cells invitro. *J.Cell.Biochem.* **64**,295–312.

Karsenty, G. (2000). Role of Cbfa1 in osteoblast differentiation and function. Semin. *CellDev.Biol.* **11**,343–346.

Kaviani, A., Perry, T. E., Dzakovic, A., Jennings, R. W., Ziegler, M. M. and Fauza, D. O. (2001). The amniotic fluid as a source of cells for fetal tissue engineering. *J.Pediatr.Surg.* **36**,1662–1665.

Kaviani, A., Guleserian, K., Perry, T. E., Jennings, R. W., Ziegler, M. M. and Fauza, D. O. (2003). Fetal tissue engineering from amniotic fluid. *J.Am.Coll.Surg.* **196**,592–597.

Kinder, S. J., Tsang, T. E., Quinlan, G. A., Hadjantonakis, A. K., Nagy, A. and Tam, P. P. (1999). The orderly allocation of mesodermal cells to the extraembryonic structures and the anteroposterior axis during gastrulation of the mouse embryo. *Development* **126**,4691–4701.

Kolambkar, Y., K., Peister, A., Soker, S., Atala, A. and R. E. Guldberg. (2007). Chondrogenic differentiation of amniotic fluid-derived stem cells. *J Mol Hist* **38**:405–413

Komori, T., Yagi, H., Nomura, S., Yamaguchi, A., Sasaki, K., Deguchi, K., Shimizu, Y., Bronson, R. T., Gao, Y. H., Inada, M., Sato, M., Okamoto, R., Kitamura, Y., Yoshiki, S. and Kishimoto, T. (1997). Targeted disruption of Cbfa1 results in a complete lack of bone formation owing to maturational arrest of osteoblasts. *Cell.* **89**,755–764.

Li, L., Arman, E., Ekblom, P., Edgar, D., Murray, P. and Lonai, P. (2004). Distinct GATA6-and laminin-dependent mechanisms regulate endodermal and ectodermal embryonic stem cell fates. *Development* **131**,5277–5286.

Liu, Z. S., Xu, Y. F., Feng, S. W., Li, Y., Yao, X. L., Lu, X.L. and Zhang, C. Baculovirus-transduced mouse amniotic fluid-derived stem cells maintain differentiation potential. (2009). *Ann Hematol.* **88**(6):565-72.

Loebel, D. A., Watson, C. M., De Young, R. A. and Tam, P. P. (2003). Lineage choice and differentiation in mouse embryos and embryonic stem cells. *Dev.Biol.* **264**,1–14.

Medina-Gomez, P. and del Valle, M. (1988). The culture of amniotic fluid cells: An analysis of the colonies, metaphase and mitotic index for the purpose of ruling out maternal cell contamination. *Ginecol.Obstet.Mex.* **56**,122–126.

Moser, M., Li, Y., Vaupel, K., Kretzschmar, D., Kluge, R., Glynn, P. and Buettner, R. (2004). Placental failure and impaired vasculogenesis result in embryonic lethality for neuropathy target esterasedeficient mice. *Mol.Cell.Biol.***24**,1667–1679.

Morris, S. M., Jr. (2002). Regulation of enzymes of the urea cycle and arginine metabolism. *Annu. Rev. Nutr.* **22**, 87–105.

Parameswaran, M. and Tam, P. P. (1995). Regionalisation of cell fate and morphogenetic movement of the mesoderm during mouse gastrulation. *Dev.Genet.* **17**,16–28.

Patapoutian, A., Yoon, J. K., Miner, J. H., Wang, S., Stark, K. and Wold, B. (1995). Disruption of the mouse MRF4 gene identifies multiple waves of myogenesis in the myotome. *Development* **121**,3347–3358.

Perin, L., Giuliani, S., Jin, D., Sedrakyan, S., Carraro, G., Habibiat, R., Warburton, D.,Atala, A. and R. E. De Filippo. (2007). Renal differentiation of amniotic fluid stem cells. *Cell Prolif.* **40**, 936–948.

Perrier, A. L., Tabar, V., Barberi, T., Rubio, M.E., Bruses, J., Topf, N., Harrison, N. L. and L. Studer. (2004). Derivation of midbrain dopamine neurons from human embryonic stem cells. *Proc. Natl. Acad. Sci.* **101**, 12543–12548.

Prusa, A. R. and Hengstschlager, M. (2002). Amniotic fluid cells and human stem cell research: A new connection. *Med.Sci.Monit.* **8**,RA253–RA257.

Prusa, A. R., Marton, E., Rosner, M., Bernaschek, G. and Hengstschlager, M. (2003). Oct-4-expressing cells in human amniotic fluid: A new source for stem cell research? *Hum.Reprod.* **18**,1489–1493.

Prusa, A. R., Marton, E., Rosner, M., Bettelheim, D., Lubec, G., Pollack, A., Bernaschek, G. and Hengstschlager, M. (2004). Neurogenic cells in human amniotic fluid. *Am.JObstet.Gynecol.* **191**,309–314.

Rathjen, J., Lake, J. A., Bettess, M. D., Washington, J. M., Chapman, G. and Rathjen, P. D. (1999). Formation of a primitive ectoderm like cell population, EPL cells, from ES cells in response to biologically derived factors. *J.CellSci.* **112**,601–612.

Robinson, W. P., McFadden, D. E., Barrett, I. J., Kuchinka, B., Penaherrera, M. S., Bruyere, H., Best, R. G., Pedreira, D. A., Langlois, S. and Kalousek, D. K. (2002). Origin of amnion and implications for evaluation ofthe fetal genotype in cases of mosaicism. *Prenat.Diagn.* **22**,1076–1085.

Rohwedel, J., Maltsev, V., Bober, E., Arnold, H. H., Hescheler, J. and Wobus, A. M. (1994). Muscle cell differentiation of embryonic stem cells reflects myogenesis invivo: Developmentally regulated expression of myogenic determination genes and functional expression of ionic currents. *Dev.Biol.* **164**,87–101.

Rosenblatt, J. D., Lunt, A. I., Parry, D. J. and Partridge, T. A. (1995). Culturingsatellite cells from living single muscle fiber explants. *InVitroCellDev.Biol.Anim.* **31**,773–779.

Sakuragawa, N., Elwan, M. A., Fujii, T. and Kawashima, K. (1999). Possible dynamic neurotransmitter metabolism surrounding the fetus. *J.Child.Neurol.* **14**, 265–266.

Chiavegato, A., Bollini, S., Pozzobon, M., Callegari, A., Gasparotto, L., Taiani, J., Piccoli, M., Lenzini, E., Gerosa, G., Vendramin, I., Cozzi, E., Angelini, A., Iop, L., Zanon, G.F., Atala, A., DeCoppi, P. and S. Sartore. Human amniotic fluid-derived stem cells are rejected after transplantation in the myocardium of normal, ischemic, immuno-suppressed or immuno-deficient rat. (2007). *Journal of Molecular and Cellular Cardiology* **42**(4): 746–759.

Schwartz, R. E., Reyes, M., Koodie, L., Jiang, Y., Blackstad, M., Lund, T., Lenvik, T., Johnson, S., Hu, W. S. and Verfaillie, C. M. (2002). Multipotent adult progenitor cells from bone marrow differentiate into functional hepatocyte-like cells. *J.Clin.Invest.* **109**,1291–1302.

Siddiqui, M. J. and Atala, A. (2004). Amniotic fluid-derived pluripotentialcells. In''*Handbook of Stem Cells*,'' Vol. 2, pp. 175–179. Elsevier Academic Press, San Diego, CA.

Smith, J. L., Gesteland, K. M. and Schoenwolf, G. C. (1994). Prospective fate map of the mouse primitive streak at 7.5 days of gestation. *Dev.Dyn.* **201**,279–289.

Snow, M. H. and Bennett, D. (1978). Gastrulation in the mouse: Assessment of cell populations in the epiblast of tw18/tw18 embryos. *J.Embryol.Exp.Morphol.* **47**,39–52.

Srivastava, M. D., Lippes, J. and Srivastava, B. I. (1996). Cytokines of the human reproductive tract. *Am.J.Reprod.Immunol.* **36**,157–166.

Taylor, R. M. and Snyder, E. Y. (1997). Widespread engraftment of neural progenitor and stem-like cells throughout the mouse brain. *Transplant. Proc.* **29**, 845–847.

Taylor, R. M., Lee, J. P., Palacino, J. J., Bowker, K. A., Li, J., Vanier, M. T., Wenger, D. A., Sidman, R. L. and E. Y. Snyder. (2006). Intrinsic resistance of neural stem cells to toxic metabolites may make them well suited for cell non-autonomous disorders: evidence from a mouse model of Krabbe leukodystrophy. *J. Neurochem.* **97**, 1585–1599.

Tsai, M. S., Lee, J. L., Chang, Y. J. and Hwang, S. M. (2004). Isolation of human multipotent mesenchymal stem cells from second-trimester amniotic fluid using a novel two-stage culture protocol. *Hum.Reprod.* **19**,1450–1456.

Torricelli, F., Brizzi, L., Bernabei, P. A., Gheri, G., Di Lollo, S., Nutini, L., Lisi, E., Di Tomasso, M. and Cariati, E. (1993) Identification of hematopoietic progenitor cells in human amniotic fluid before the 12th week of gestation. Ital. *J. Anat. Embryol.* **98**:119-126.

Woodbury, D., Schwarz, E. J., Prockop, D. J. and Black, I. B. (2000). Adult rat and human bone marrow stromal cells differentiate into neurons. *J.Neurosci. Res.* **61**, 364–370.

In: Pluripotent Stem Cells
Editors: D.W. Rosales et al, pp. 137-154
ISBN: 978-1-60876-738-0

Chapter 5

EXPLORING A STEM CELL BASIS TO IDENTIFY NOVEL TREATMENT FOR HUMAN MALIGNANCIES

***Shyam A. Patel*[1,2] *and Pranela Rameshwar*[2,*]**
[1]Graduate School of Biomedical Sciences, University of Medicine and Dentistry of New Jersey, Newark, NJ, USA
[2]Department of Medicine – Division of Hematology/Oncology, New Jersey Medical School, University of Medicine and Dentistry of New Jersey, Newark, NJ, USA

Abstract

Research investigations on various sources of stem cells have been conducted for potential to exert tissue regeneration, reverse immune-enhancement, and protect against tissue insult. At a more distant goal, it is likely that stem cells could be applied to medicine via organogenesis. However, the field of stem cells is not new since immune replacement via bone marrow transplantation is considered a successful form of cell therapy. There is evidence that stem cell therapies are close for several disorders such as neurodegeneration, immune hyperactivity, and functional insufficiencies such as Type I diabetes mellitus. The field of stem cell biology is gaining a strong foothold in science and medicine as the molecular mechanisms underlying stem cell behavior are

* E-mail address: rameshwa@umdnj.edu. Tel. (973) 972-0625; Fax (973) 972-8854; Corresponding author: Pranela Rameshwar, Ph.D., UMDNJ-New Jersey Medical School, MSB, Rm. E-579, 185 South Orange Ave, Newark, NJ 07103.

gradually being unraveled. Although stem cells have tremendous therapeutic applicability in the aforementioned conditions, their uniqueness may also confer adverse properties, rendering them a double-edged sword. The discovery that stem cells have immortal and resilient characteristics has shed insight into the link between stem cells and tumorigenesis. Specifically, recent advancements in cancer research have implicated that a stem cell may be responsible for the refractoriness of cancers to conventional treatment such as chemotherapy and radiation. Here, we summarize the recent advancements in the cancer stem cell hypothesis and present the challenges associated with targeting resistant cancers in the context of stem cell microenvironments.

Traditional Views on Tumorigenesis

For years, cancer has been viewed as a stochastic process in which random genetic alterations lead to deregulation of cellular division [1]. Among the stochastic events a cell undergoes that ultimately lead to transformation include amplification or overexpression of proto-oncogenes, loss of function of tumor suppressors, and translocations of important cell cycle regulatory genes. In this model, genomic instability can predispose cells to attain mutations [2]. Furthermore, the model holds that all cancer cells from the same tumor are homogeneous and harbor equal malignant capabilities [3,4]. The underlying assumption of the traditional model is that any transformed cell can form new tumors limitlessly [5].

Although this non-hierarchal model is still accepted among scientists, it does not clearly explain the recurrence of cancer after years of disease-free or event-free survival. For example, approximately 30% of patients with breast cancer show micrometastatic foci in the bone marrow, and these sites may be able to serve as origins of relapse after many years from the time of diagnosis [6]. The original belief that that each transformed cell can form tumors indefinitely has been met with opposition on numerous occasions for many types of cancers [5]. For instance, malignant cells from Ewing's sarcoma fail to form tumors when serially transplanted into immunodeficient mice [5]. Therefore, the recurrence of cancer years following initial treatment has led to investigations into identifying resistant subpopulations of cells with indefinite tumor renewability. From these ideas arose the cancer stem cell hypothesis, which we will now discuss in detail.

Ambiguity about the Origin of Cancer Stem Cells

The cancer stem cell hypothesis, sometimes referred to as the tumor-initiating cell hypothesis, is based on a hierarchal model of cancer and holds that hematological and solid organ cancers arise from dysregulation of resident stem cells of normal tissue [4,7] (Figure 1). On the contrary, some groups believe that cancer stem cells arise first from transient amplifying cells that undergo de-differentiation while acquiring self-renewal characteristics [7,8] (Figure 1). It is likely that aspects of both of these theories are responsible for tumor initiation, drug and radiation resistance, dormancy, and recurrence of cancers. It is estimated that as few as 0.0001% of cells within heterogeneous tumors are stem-like in nature [9]. Common to most definitions of the cancer stem cell is that it must be able to self-renew and demonstrate multipotency [10]. Among the broader biological processes that are thought to be regulated by cancer stem cells are angiogenesis, invasion, and metastasis [11,12]. A hallmark of these cells is that they retain sphere-forming ability *in vitro* from single cells. The precise phenotype of tumor-initiating cells is unclear, but specific cluster designation (CD) markers have been attributed to particular tissues from which the cancer stem cells are thought to arise.

Although a functional definition of the cancer stem cell does not include drug resistance, this characteristic is well-recognized by many groups [13]. Normally, cancer treatment modalities such as chemotherapy and radiation can induce apoptosis in cancer cells in a p53-dependent manner [13]. Resistance has been attributed to many molecular events, such as the induction of xenobiotic transporters of the ATP-binding cassette family. This phenotype is discussed in the *Side Populations* section. In addition, although cellular quiescence is not a defining feature of stem cells, cells from tumor-initiating populations may harbor some degree of cell cycle arrest or slow-cycling ability [8].

Despite the unclear nature of the origin of cancer stem cells, it is commonly accepted that these cells have an indefinite ability to self-renew while giving rise to some cells with finite renewability [7]. The cells with finite renewal may include committed progenitors and transient amplifying populations [8]. Acute promyelocytic leukemia, for example, is thought to arise from committed progenitors that acquire self-renewal characteristics [14]. This phenomenon of asymmetric division appears to be partly responsible for resurgence of cancer after years of disease-free survival. Cancer stem cells appear to have limitless tumor-forming ability, unlike other cancer cells which fail to indefinitely repopulate tumors [7].

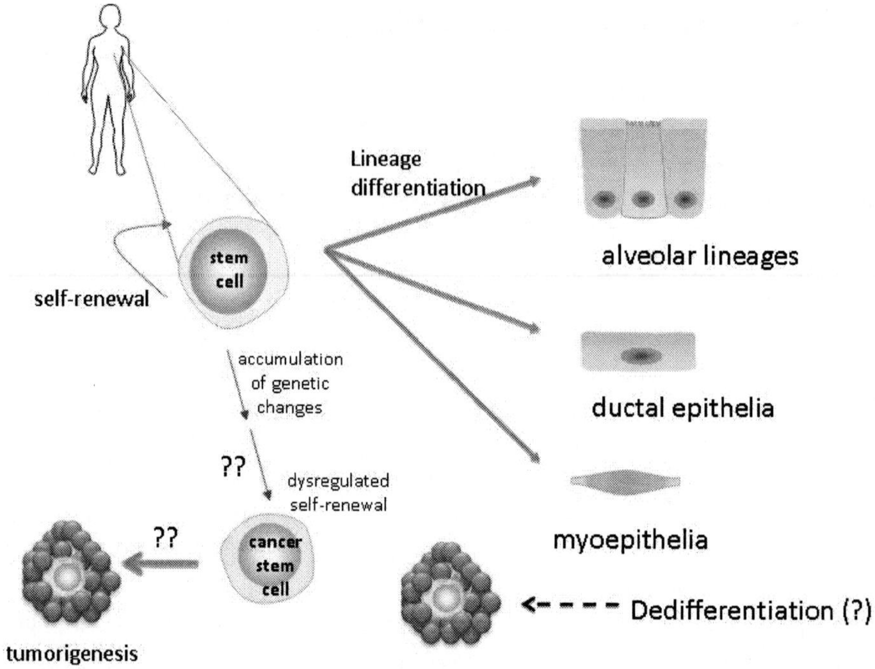

Figure 1. The cancer stem cell hypothesis. Shown is a normal mammary stem cell that differentiates along lineages to generate various epithelial types. Two hypotheses are shown. Firstly, genetic dysregulation can occur in mammary epithelial stem cells to form cancer stem cells, which then produce metastatic tumors through the formation of cancer progenitors (blue cells). Secondly, specialized cells can de-differentiate to form cancer stem cells, which similarly cause metastasis.

The Relevance of Epithelial-to-Mesenchymal Transition in Cancer Biology

During embryogenesis, unique phenomena occur at the cellular and molecular levels that permit the development of an intact organism [15]. Epithelial and mesenchymal morphologies predominate at different points in development, and both of these states may transition between one another [15]. The epithelial-to-mesenchymal transition is defined as the attainment of increased cellular invasiveness due to the acquisition of a fibroblast-like phenotype by differentiated epithelial cells [16]. In addition to morphological changes, the theory holds that junctional interactions between epithelial cells are lost [16]. Specifically, E-cadherin loss is a central feature of this dynamic process [17]. Cytoskeletal elements undergo re-organization to accommodate the mesenchymal appearance with loss of the apical-basal polarity [16]. These morphological changes have been suggested to underlie the tumor-initiating characteristics and cancer stem cell behavior, and this has been shown clearly for many carcinomas. The correlation between malignancy and the epithelial-to-mesenchymal transition is evident from data suggesting that a mesenchymal phenotype imparts increased motility to cells [15]. Differentiated epithelial cells do not possess invasive tendencies and rarely disseminate to distant sites [15]. Moreover, upon transition to a mesenchymal morphology, cells become less susceptible to apoptosis, a hallmark of tumor-initiating cells [15].

The stimuli for epithelial-to-mesenchymal transition in carcinomas have been investigated, and various growth factors such as transforming growth factor-β (TGF-β) are implicated. In pancreatic adenocarcinoma, TGF-β allows for loss of E-cadherin expression, thereby promoting increased invasiveness of these cancers [17]. This cytokine also promotes conversion to the spindle-shaped morphology [17]. Interestingly, TGF-β signaling is vital in breast cancer cell proliferation and embryogenesis, supporting the idea that undifferentiated cells may be driving tumor growth [18].

A few stem cell signaling pathways appear to mediate the events occurring in the epithelial-to-mesenchymal transition and may function in resistance of cancer to chemotherapy. Resistance to gemcitabine in advanced stage pancreatic adenocarcinoma has been attributable to Notch-2 signaling [16]. Increased expression of both the Notch-2 ligand and its receptor Jagged-1 has been reported in drug resistance cells [16]. Knockdown of Notch in pancreatic cancer appears to partially eliminate the epithelial-to-mesenchymal transition and reduce the invasiveness of pancreatic cancer [16]. The interaction between cancers and the underlying stroma likely plays a critical role in transition to a mesenchymal phenotype [15].

In colon adencarcinoma, the Wnt signaling pathway is important for induction of epithelial cells into a mesenchymal phenotype [19]. β-catenin-mediated gene transcription may be the reason for the dynamic changes in the epithelial-to-mesenchymal transition in these cancers [19]. Inhibitors of this pathway have been suggested for treatment of colon cancer, but the clinic has yet to experience success for these molecular targets. Hypoxia has also been suggested as a stimulus of the transition by some groups [15]. Nonetheless, the evidence is still somewhat ambiguous as most reports on cancer stem cells do not allude to the epithelial-to-mesenchymal transition [16].

As with any other theory, some scientists are wary of the validity of the epithelial-to-mesenchymal transition. Nonetheless, evidence from experiments on mesenchymal stem cells provides a foundation on which the theory may be based [20]. Mesenchymal stem cells have been consistently shown to harbor malignant potential when faced with environmental stressors [20]. Treatment of mesenchymal stem cells with low-dose ionizing radiation in the range representative of cancer radiotherapy has been shown to transform these cells. Irradiated mesenchymal stem cells demonstrate increased numbers of unbalanced translocations and loss of genomic integrity to the point of tumor development [20]. Among sarcomas, mesenchymal stem cells are thought to be the origin of tumors [21]. Fibrosarcoma and malignant histiocytomas are among the tumors with suspected mesenchymal stem cell origin based on recent reports [21] [22].

Tumor-Initiating Cells of the Breast

The idea that resident stem cells can undergo transformation arose not so long ago. Studies of the mammary gland from various specimens have indicated on multiple occasions that stem cells can become cancerous, contrary to the traditional belief that a terminally differentiated epithelial cell of the breast is the origin of tumors [23]. The seminal experiments on identification of the putative breast cancer stem cell demonstrated that the CD44+/CD24^{low}/lin- phenotype allows for the recapitulation of tumors in immunodeficient mice [6]. This subpopulation of cells is able to drive the growth of breast tumors far more successfully than other cancer cells of the breast, which have limited proliferation potential upon serial transplantation [6]. Nevertheless, there are limitations to accepting the CD44+/CD24^{low}/lin- phenotype as the profile for breast cancer stem cells. The phenotype does not correlate with prognosis and may only be applicable to certain type of breast cancers, such as hormone-resistant cancers of the basal type and cancers harboring the familial *BRCA1* mutation [24]. Hence, generalized judgments about breast cancer based on subtype-specific evidence should be cautioned [24].

Numerous ligand/receptor interactions have been suggested for breast cancer maintenance, such as the interaction between the TGF-β superfamily member Nodal and its receptor Cripto-1 [18]. This interaction is important for embryonic development [18]. The interaction between Notch-1 and survivin, a regulator of mitosis in cancer cells and stem cells, has been noted in estrogen receptor-negative basal breast cancers, which have worse prognoses than hormone-responsive cancers [25]. Notch-1 is becoming an important player in breast cancer in relation to the tumor-initiating cell phenotype [25].

Perhaps the most well-recognized ligand/receptor interaction involves chemokines of hematopoiesis. Chemokines involved in stem cell signaling have been implicated in cancer metastasis, especially stage IV breast cancer [26]. Elevated levels of stromal cell-derived factor 1 (SDF-1), the endogenous ligand for chemokine receptor 4 (CXCR4), have been found in metastatic breast cancer sites [27]. A positive correlation exists between CXCR4 expression and the aggressiveness of breast cancer [27]. Regarding highly aggressive breast cancer cells, the SDF-1/CXCR4 axis may be supporting a breast cancer stem cell niche in the bone marrow in addition to its endogenous role in hematopoiesis [28]. Aside from SDF-1/CXCR4 signaling, chemokine ligand 2 (CCL2) secretion by mesenchymal stem cells of the bone marrow also facilitates the homing of breast cancer cells towards osteoblasts [29]. Based on these findings, specific antagonists have been designed to target homing of cancer cells during stage IV breast cancer.

Clearly, determining the role of chemokines and growth factors in bone marrow stromal microenvironment is critical to understanding the behavior of invasive tumors [30]. The prospect of stem cell therapy for breast cancer has been brought forth recently by a study demonstrating the interactions between stroma and cancerous epithelia [31]. The current theory holds that the tumor stroma may be an impediment to the delivery of effective therapy [31]. Inducible expression of relaxin in hematopoietic stem cells has been proposed to cause degeneration of tumor stroma while promoting infiltration of beneficial immune cells that target the tumor [31]. This phenomenon emphasizes the role of the surrounding stroma in protecting tumors from immune effector mechanisms [31]. Hence, the use of stem cells, particular hematopoietic stem cells in this case, can serve as vehicle for delivery of anti-cancer genes to breast tumors.

The aforementioned evidence pertains mostly to ductal adenocarcinomas of the breast, which represent the most common types of breast cancers. There has been an upsurge of interest, however, in inflammatory breast cancer, which differs from ductal carcinoma in that it confers worse prognosis and invades the subdermal lymphatics [32]. Notch-3 signaling has been implicated in inflammatory breast cancer [32]. Emboli from this breast cancer subtype can obstruct lymphatic flow, and cells from the emboli have been found to possess stemness characteristics, although the existence of tumor-initiating cells from inflammatory breast cancers is not thoroughly supported to date [32].

Stemness Properties in Other Epithelial Malignancies

Cancers of the breast and prostate, although causing fewer deaths than carcinoma of the lung, are a significant cause of morbidity [33]. CD44 positivity is shared between both breast and neuroendocrine small cell carcinomas of the prostate tumor-initiating cells [33]. The normal function of CD44 is to help maintain cellular adhesions to adjacent cells and to the extracellular matrix [33]. Particular variants of CD44 have been correlated with increased invasiveness, even though CD44 is negatively correlated with invasive potential for many cases of prostate cancers [33,34]. Furthermore, a greater fraction of CD44+ cells in prostate cancer demonstrate aggressive behavior compared to CD44- cells, and they are more likely to form prostatospheres [34].

The commonality between breast and prostate tumors is that they are both modulated by hormonal activity: estrogen for breast cancer and androgens for prostate cancer. This prospect makes these two cancers unique from other malignancies and may explain the disparity in the phenotypes for organ-specific cancer stem cells. Recent studies in prostate cancer biology have shown that prostate tumor-initiating cells fail to express the androgen receptor and lineage-specific antigens [4]. Integrins are also thought to play a role in the prostate cancer stem cell phenotype [4]. Hormone sensitivity does not appear intact among CD44+ cells of the prostate, implying refractoriness of prostate cancer stem cells to treatment [34].

The most common cause of cancer-related death is carcinoma of the lung [35]. The reasons for sustenance and recurrence of lung cancer have been partially elucidated, yet the evidence is not as well-supported in comparison to other solid tumors [36]. Aldehyde dehydrogenase (ALDH1), a stem cell marker, has been found in lung carcinoma cells demonstrating stemness. The significance of this finding is that ALDH1 correlated positively with the tumor grade and stage, suggesting that ALDH1 may serve as a prognostic marker in these cancers [36] [37]. From these discoveries on the cancer stem cell hypothesis for epithelial cancers, it is reasonable to conclude that gaining insights into the molecular phenotypes of various cancers can lead to improvements in clinical decision-making [36].

The CD133 Phenotype: Growing Evidence among Central Nervous System Tumors

Tumors of the central nervous system have among the worst prognoses of all solid organ cancers and are refractory to conventional treatment in many cases [11]. Tumor-initiating cells of the central nervous system have received much attention in the recent years and are perhaps the most well-characterized cancer stem cells among solid organs.

The origin of brain tumor stem cells is also elusive, but current theories suggest that they may arise from either [1] dedifferentiation of committed glial progenitors or [2] transformed neural stem cells [38]. Medulloblastomas and glioblastomas have been shown to harbor stemness characteristics [39]. The presence of multiple distinct areas of differentiation among neurological tumors has helped support the brain tumor stem cell hypothesis [39]. Primary tissue from cancers of the central nervous system demonstrated stem-like properties before the findings were discovered in cell lines, but the evidence in human and rat glioma cell lines is gradually accruing [10,40]. The hallmark of sphere formation has been repeatedly demonstrated by the CD133+ phenotype [41].

The radiotherapy resistance of some medulloblastomas has prompted investigations into the reasons for this behavior. Among cerebellar medulloblastomas in children, radiation resistant stem cell compartments have been identified near blood vessels and have been shown to express the intermediate filament protein Nestin [13]. Nestin expression confers increased survivability through PI3K activation and p53-mediated cell cycle arrest [13]. Inhibition of components of the PI3K pathway results in re-establishment of radiosensitivity [13].

The putative phenotype for brain tumor-initiating cells involves CD133, also known as prominin-1, a well-known marker of hematopoietic stem cells, neural stem cells, and endothelial precursors [40]. CD133 positivity is not specific for cancer stem cells of neurological origin, however, as an important report on the characterization of stem cells from Ewing's sarcoma has delineated the role of CD133 in tumor-forming ability [5]. The repopulating ability of CD133+ cells is far superior to that of CD133- cells; the minimal threshold for tumor regeneration *in vivo* is two orders of magnitude less for CD133 positivity compared to negativity [40]. Similar findings have been associated with the putative breast tumor-initiating cell [3]. CD133 positivity is correlated with radiotherapy resistance in gliomblastoma and platinum-based chemotherapy resistance in ovarian cancer [42]. Surprisingly, CD133 has also been suggested to be the marker for pancreatic adenocarinoma stem cells and ovarian cancer stem cells [43,44]. CD133 positive cells have been shown to divide asymmetrically, producing both CD133+ cell daughter and a CD133- daughter, whereas parent cells lacking CD133 fail to produce any CD133+ progeny [44]. Thus, self-renewal has been demonstrated by these cells.

Evidence for Side Populations in Cancer

Side populations, defined by their ability to exclude DNA-binding dyes via ATP-dependent transporters, consist of early progenitors and their parent stem cells [45]. Side populations are also characteristic of endothelial cells [46]. Cells from side populations demonstrate increased ability to generate tumors compared to other cells [47]. The growth capacity of side population cells is superior to cells that are not from side populations, and they demonstrate higher levels of invasiveness [47]. Side populations are typically identified by flow cytometric analysis, and this technique is becoming an increasingly important tool for studying stem cells [48].

The key proteins that are characteristic of side populations are members of the ATP-binding cassette superfamily, such as the multidrug resistance transporter ABCB1 and the breast cancer resistance protein ABCG2. These transmembrane proteins function in ATP-dependent efflux of DNA-binding dyes such as Hoechst 33342 [45]. ATP-binding cassette transporters can be found on resident stem cells of various tissues [8]. ABCG2 expression in particular has been reported in both solid and hematological malignancies, including the lung cancer, prostate cancer, breast cancer, and leukemia [49]. Expression of a whole array of multidrug resistant transporters has been confirmed in a population of liver cell progenitors in patients with hepatocellular carcinoma [50]. The significance of these findings is that presence of particular transporters, such as the multidrug resistance-associated protein MRP1, is correlated with unfavorable prognosis in hepatocellular carcinoma [50]. Although these studies have not definitely demonstrated that a side population is responsible for the resistance of liver cancer to treatment, the possibility should be kept in mind as insights into the cancer stem cell hypothesis are gained.

Methods for the selection of cancer stem cells have been attempted and frequently involve the use of chemotherapeutic agents. In glioma, the alkylating agent temozolomide has been used to isolate a population of stem-like glioma cells [46]. Resistance in this population may be partly attributed to increased expression of O^6-methylguanine DNA methyltransferase. Temozolamide can also induce expression of ABCG2, thereby contributing to chemotherapy resistance [46]. In the case of osteogenic sarcoma, the use of the poly(A) polymerase inhibitor 3-aminobenzamide over a period of nearly four months allowed for the selection of transformed stem cells from these tumors [49]. The resultant population was heterogeneous and harbored the spindle-shaped appearance of mesenchymal stem cells [49]. Characterization of this population from osteosarcoma confirmed phenotypic and functional characteristics of stem cells, namely expression of Oct4 and Nanog and ability to efflux drugs via the ATP-binding cassette members [49].

Uroepithelial side populations have been isolated in cancers of the genitourinary tract based on Hoechst 33342 dye exclusion [48]. Cancers of the bladder, kidney, and prostate appear to entertain small populations of dye-excluding cells in the midst of large tumors. ABCG2 is the transporter responsible for dye exclusion in prostate cancer side populations [48].

Current efforts are geared towards identifying the link, if any, between side population characteristics and cancer quiescence. Some groups have suggested that tumor-initiating cells may be found within side populations, while other groups have shown distinct origins [17]. Side populations in pancreatic cancer may be enriched in cancer stem cells and cells with predilection to undergo the epithelial-to-mesenchymal transition [17]. In fact, both side populations and cells undergoing epithelial-to-mesenchymal transition have increased invasive capability compared to normal cells, and the bridge between these two populations may be closer than previously believed [17].

Future Insights

It has long been recognized that the efficacy of cancer treatment has been limited by resistance of cells to chemotherapy and radiation. Investigations in the recent years have culminated in the theory that a distinct subpopulation may be responsible for the maintenance and metastasis of tumors. Analysis of the integrity of the human genome in cancers is becoming an important factor in identifying resistant subpopulations [2]. The genomic stability of normal cells is maintained by various cellular repair processes and permits proper regulation of cellular division [2]. Maintenance of the genomic integrity of tumor-initiating cells, however, is not completely understood. Genomic instability has been suggested to promote heterogeneity in cancer as well as the development of cancer stem cells [2]. The origin of cancer stem cells and the underlying mechanisms that lead to development and sustenance of tumors have not been thoroughly explored and remain open to debate.

Differential gene expression may underlie the basis for the behavior of cancer stem cells in comparison to non-stem cancer cells and normal tissue [51]. Gene expression profiling has been proposed for identifying key players in the tumor-initiating populations [51]. Among the most important methods by which genomic profiles can be assessed is the use of microarray. For example, cDNA microarrays have been employed for comparison of high-grade astrocytomas with neural stem cells, and unique expression patterns have been identified in these cancers [38]. Identification of genes involves in tumor proliferation were specific to astrocytoma cells when compared with surrounding tissue, providing evidence for uniqueness of the putative astrocytoma stem cell population [38]. Such high-throughput studies can be followed by gene-specific and targeted studies; this approach may shed insight onto the molecular bases for the chemotherapeutic resistance and subsequent resurgence of cancer.

Only recently has the epithelial-to-mesenchymal transition been associated with the cancer stem cell phenotype, and much evidence is lacking on this dynamic process. Nonetheless, the data appears to support a stem cell basis for cancer. With further investigations into the cellular changes that confer resistance to chemotherapy and radiation, the link between cancer stem cells and epithelial-to-mesenchymal transition may be elucidated.

As scientists gain insight into the molecular mechanisms underlying tumor survival, the development of targeted therapy appears promising. Thus far, targeted therapy has been proposed in the context of cellular signaling. Arguably the most critical pathway involved in cellular survival, proliferation, differentiation, and growth is the phosphoinositide-3-kinase (PI3K)/Akt/mTOR pathway [12]. Inhibition of the PI3K pathway in gliomas has been studied well, and the data shows that small molecule inhibitors specific for Akt in glioma may hinder resistant cancer cell survival and invasiveness without affecting the untransformed resident tissue [11]. Cells of the CD133+ are more susceptible to Akt inhibition that CD133- cells, indicating the specificity towards the putative stem cell population in glioma. Such effects have been demonstrated *in vivo* for immunodeficient mice for glioma and may eventually translate to patients [11]. Aside from the use of Akt inhibitors, PI3K and mTOR inhibition has demonstrated anti-proliferative effects [12].

Targeted therapy for cancer stem cells has been studied by a few groups with some *in vitro* success. For instance, stem cells of glioblastoma multiforme express the chloride channel CLIC1, which mediates efflux of nitrosureas commonly used in cancer chemotherapy [52]. Antagonism of this channel has been shown to help induce apoptosis in glioma cancer stem cells while restoring chemosensitivity to nitrosureas [52]. As another example, viral-mediated therapy has been attempted for breast cancer stem cells [53]. Cells of the CD44+/CD24- phenotype were targeted by a lytic virus of the Reovirus family [53]. Nonetheless, specificity was not established, as the reovirus induced apoptosis in both the CD44+/CD24- and the non-stem cancer cells [53]. Lack of specificity leaves behind the possibility that normal resident tissue can destroyed. Attempts at targeted therapy for breast cancer have resulted in successful elimination of CD44+/CD24^{low} cells by cytotoxic T cells primed with the Numb-1 peptide [54]. This suggests that sensitization of lymphocytes by particular antigens may be gear the immune towards attacking particular phenotypes [54]. Findings such as these give field hope to prospects on targeted therapy.

Although targeted therapy geared at cancer stem cells has not successfully reached the clinic thus far, the prospects for targeted therapy may become favorable as the science advances [11]. The outlooks on targeted therapy are encouraging based on accumulating evidence on the cancer stem cell phenotype. Important benefits for such therapy include increased effectiveness at eliminating refractory tumors and decreased risk of cytotoxic side effects [11]. Central to all therapeutic endeavors is that the molecular mechanisms governing the tumor-initiating phenotype must be determined before success is achieved in the clinic.

Challenges to the cancer stem cell hypothesis are well recognized. Two of the foremost challenges include the successful culturing of these cells *in vitro* and the identification of a targetable phenotype [10]. Phenotypes may be tissue-specific, so attempts at universal characterization are unlikely to be successful. Once a phenotype is established, isolation of these cells is critical for characterization of the subpopulations. Downstream applications may include molecular and functional characterization of the subpopulations, which will ultimately allow for development of targeted therapy [6]. As studies continue on the cancer stem cell hypothesis, science may hold promising therapies for the treatment of the chemo-resistant and radio-resistant tumors that are responsible for the high mortality rates in cancer.

References

[1] Tomasson, MH. Cancer stem cells: a guide for skeptics. *J Cell Biochem* 2009; 106:745-9.

[2] Li, L, Borodyansky, L and Yang Y. Genomic instability en route to and from cancer stem cells. *Cell Cycle* 2009; 8:1000-2.

[3] Kakarala, M. and Wicha MS. Implications of the cancer stem-cell hypothesis for breast cancer prevention and therapy. *J Clin Oncol* 2008; 26:2813-20.

[4] Palapattu, GS, Wu, C, Silvers, CR, Martin, HB, Williams, K, Salamone, L, Bushnell, T, Huang, LS, Yang, Q, Huang and J. Selective expression of CD44, a putative prostate cancer stem cell marker, in neuroendocrine tumor cells of human prostate cancer. *Prostate* 2009. [In press]

[5] Suva, ML, Riggi, N, Stehle, JC, Baumer, K, Tercier, S, Joseph, JM, Suvà, D, Clément, V, Provero, P, Cironi, L, Osterheld, MC, Guillou, L and Stamenkovic I. Identification of cancer stem cells in Ewing's sarcoma. *Cancer Res* 2009; 69:1776-81.

[6] Al-Hajj, M, Wicha, MS, Benito-Hernandez, A, Morrison, SJ and Clarke, MF. Prospective identification of tumorigenic breast cancer cells. *Proc Natl Acad Sci U S A* 2003; 100:3983-8.

[7] Santisteban, M, Reiman, JM, Asiedu, MK, Behrens, MD, Nassar, A, Kalli, KR, Haluska, P, Ingle, JN, Hartmann, LC, Manjili, MH, Radisky, DC, Ferrone, S and Knutson, KL. Immune-Induced Epithelial to Mesenchymal Transition In vivo Generates Breast Cancer Stem Cells. *Cancer Res* 2009. [In press]

[8] Oates, JE, Grey, BR, Addla, SK, Samuel, JD, Hart, CA, Ramani, V, Brown, MD and Clarke, NW. Hoechst 33342 side population identification is a conserved and unified mechanism in urological cancers. *Stem Cells Dev* 2009. [In press]

[9] Quintana, E, Shackleton, M, Sabel, MS, Fullen, DR, Johnson, TM and Morrison, SJ. Efficient tumour formation by single human melanoma cells. *Nature* 2008; 456:593-8.

[10] Yu, SC, Ping, YF, Yi, L, Zhou, ZH, Chen, JH, Yao, XH, Gao, L, Wang. JM and Bian, XW. Isolation and characterization of cancer stem cells from a human glioblastoma cell line U87. *Cancer Lett* 2008; 265:124-34.

[11] Eyler, CE, Foo, WC, LaFiura, KM, McLendon, RE, Hjelmeland, AB and Rich, JN. Brain cancer stem cells display preferential sensitivity to Akt inhibition. *Stem Cells* 2008; 26:3027-36.

[12] Endersby, R and Baker, SJ. PTEN signaling in brain: neuropathology and tumorigenesis. *Oncogene* 2008; 27:5416-30.

[13] Hambardzumyan, D, Becher, OJ, Rosenblum, MK, Pandolfi, PP, Manova-Todorova, K and Holland, EC. PI3K pathway regulates survival of cancer stem cells residing in the perivascular niche following radiation in medulloblastoma in vivo. *Genes Dev* 2008; 22:436-48.

[14] Wojiski, S, Guibal, FC, Kindler, T, Lee, BH, Jesneck, JL, Fabian, A, Tenen, DG and Gilliland, DG. PML-RARalpha initiates leukemia by conferring

properties of self-renewal to committed promyelocytic progenitors. *Leukemia* 2009. [In press]

[15] Polyak, K. and Weinberg, RA. Transitions between epithelial and mesenchymal states: acquisition of malignant and stem cell traits. Nat *Rev Cancer* 2009; 9:265-73.

[16] Wang, Z, Li, Y, Kong, D, Banerjee, S, Ahmad, A, Azmi, AS, Ali, S, Abbruzzese, JL, Gallick, GE and Sarkar, FH. Acquisition of epithelial-mesenchymal transition phenotype of gemcitabine-resistant pancreatic cancer cells is linked with activation of the notch signaling pathway. *Cancer Res* 2009; 69:2400-7.

[17] Kabashima, A, Higuchi, H, Takaishi, H, Matsuzaki, Y, Suzuki, S, Izumiya, M, Iizuka, H, Sakai, G, Hozawa, S, Azuma, T and Hibi, T. Side population of pancreatic cancer cells predominates in TGF-beta-mediated epithelial to mesenchymal transition and invasion. *Int J Cancer* 2009 [In press]

[18] Strizzi, L, Postovit, LM, Margaryan, NV, Seftor, EA, Abbott, DE, Seftor, RE, Salomon, DS and Hendrix MJ. Emerging roles of nodal and Cripto-1: from embryogenesis to breast cancer progression. *Breast Dis* 2008; 29:91-103.

[19] Vincan, E and Barker, N. The upstream components of the Wnt signalling pathway in the dynamic EMT and MET associated with colorectal cancer progression. *Clin Exp Metastasis* 2008; 25:657-63.

[20] Christensen, R, Alsner, J, Brandt Sorensen F, Dagnaes-Hansen, F, Kolvraa S and Serakinci N. Transformation of human mesenchymal stem cells in radiation carcinogenesis: long-term effect of ionizing radiation. *Regen Med* 2008; 3:849-61.

[21] Rodriguez. R, Rubio. R, Masip. M, Catalina, P, Nieto, A, de la Cueva T, Arriero, M, San, Martin N, de la Cueva, E, Balomenos, D, Menendez, P and García-Castro, J. Loss of p53 induces tumorigenesis in p21-deficient mesenchymal stem cells. *Neoplasia* 2009; 11:397-407.

[22] Yamate, J, Ogata, K, Yuasa, T, Kuwamura, M, Takenaka, S, Kumagai, D, Itoh K, LaMarre J. Adipogenic, osteogenic and myofibrogenic differentiations of a rat malignant fibrous histiocytoma (MFH)-derived cell line, and a relationship of MFH cells with embryonal mesenchymal, perivascular and bone marrow stem cells. *Eur J Cancer* 2007; 43:2747-56.

[23] Stingl, J. Detection and analysis of mammary gland stem cells. *J Pathol* 2009; 217:229-41.

[24] Dontu, G. Breast cancer stem cell markers - the rocky road to clinical applications. *Breast Cancer Res* 2008; 10:110.

[25] Lee, CW, Simin, K, Liu, Q, Plescia, J, Guha, M, Khan, A, Hsieh, CC and Altieri DC. A functional Notch-survivin gene signature in basal breast cancer. *Breast Cancer Res* 2008; 10:R97.

[26] Civenni, G and Sommer, L. Chemokines in neuroectodermal development and their potential implication in cancer stem cell-driven metastasis. *Semin Cancer Biol* 2009; 19:68-75.

[27] Liang, Z, Wu, T, Lou, H, Yu, X, Taichman, RS, Lau, SK, Nie, S, Umbreit, J. and Shim, H. Inhibition of breast cancer metastasis by selective synthetic polypeptide against CXCR4. *Cancer Res* 2004; 64:4302-8.

[28] Corcoran, KE, Malhotra, A, Molina, CA and Rameshwar, P. Stromal-derived factor-1alpha induces a non-canonical pathway to activate the endocrine-linked Tac1 gene in non-tumorigenic breast cells. *J Mol Endocrinol* 2008; 40:113-23.

[29] Molloy, AP, Martin, FT, Dwyer, RM, Griffin, TP, Murphy, M, Barry FP, O'Brien, T. and Kerin, MJ. Mesenchymal stem cell secretion of chemokines during differentiation into osteoblasts, and their potential role in mediating interactions with breast cancer cells. *Int J Cancer* 2009; 124:326-32.

[30] Liang, X, Huuskonen, J, Hajivandi, M, Manzanedo, R, Predki, P, Amshey, JR and Pope, RM. Identification and quantification of proteins differentially secreted by a pair of normal and malignant breast-cancer cell lines. *Proteomics* 2009; 9:182-93.

[31] Li, Z, Liu, Y, Tuve, S, Xun, Y, Fan, X, Min, L, Feng, Q, Kiviat, N, Kiem, HP, Disis, ML and Lieber, A. Towards a stem cell gene therapy for breast cancer. *Blood* 2009 [In press]

[32] Xiao, Y, Ye, Y, Yearsley, K, Jones, S, Barsky, SH. The lymphovascular embolus of inflammatory breast cancer expresses a stem cell-like phenotype. *Am J Pathol* 2008; 173:561-74.

[33] Simon, RA, di Sant'Agnese, PA, Huang, LS, Xu, H, Yao, JL, Yang, Q, Liang, S, Liu, J, Yu, R, Cheng, L, Oh, WK, Palapattu, GS, Wei, J and Huang, J. CD44 expression is a feature of prostatic small cell carcinoma and distinguishes it from its mimickers. *Hum Pathol* 2009; 40:252-8.

[34] Patrawala, L, Calhoun, T, Schneider-Broussard, R, Li H, Bhatia, B, Tang, S, Reilly, JG, Chandra, D, Zhou, J, Claypool, K, Coghlan, L, Tang, DG. Highly purified CD44+ prostate cancer cells from xenograft human tumors are enriched in tumorigenic and metastatic progenitor cells. *Oncogene* 2006; 25:1696-708.

[35] Huang, CH, Millenson, MM, Sherman, EJ, Borghaei, H, Mintzer, DM, Cohen, RB, Staddon, AP, Seldomridge, J, Treat, OJ, Tuttle, H, Ruth, KJ and Langer CJ. Promising survival in patients with recurrent non-small cell lung

cancer treated with docetaxel and gemcitabine in combination as second-line therapy. *J Thorac Oncol* 2008; 3:1032-8.

[36] Jiang, F, Qiu, Q, Khanna, A, Todd, NW, Deepak, J, Xing, L, Wang, H, Liu, Z, Su, Y, Stass, SA and Katz RL. Aldehyde dehydrogenase 1 is a tumor stem cell-associated marker in lung cancer. *Mol Cancer Res* 2009; 7:330-8.

[37] Balicki, D. Moving forward in human mammary stem cell biology and breast cancer prognostication using ALDH1. *Cell Stem Cell* 2007; 1:485-7.

[38] Yang, Y, Qiu, Y, Ren, W, Gong, J and Chen, F. An identification of stem cell-resembling gene expression profiles in high-grade astrocytomas. *Mol Carcinog* 2008; 47:893-903.

[39] Nern, C, Sommerlad, D, Acker, T and Plate, KH. Brain tumor stem cells. *Recent Results Cancer Res* 2009; 171:241-59.

[40] Wu, A, Oh, S, Wiesner, SM, Ericson, K, Chen, L, Hall, WA, Champoux, PE, Low, WC and Ohlfest, JR. Persistence of CD133+ cells in human and mouse glioma cell lines: detailed characterization of GL261 glioma cells with cancer stem cell-like properties. *Stem Cells Dev* 2008; 17:173-84.

[41] Annabi, B, Lachambre, MP, Plouff,e K, Sartelet, H and Béliveau, R. Modulation of invasive properties of CD133(+) glioblastoma stem cells: A role for MT1-MMP in bioactive lysophospholipid signaling. *Mol Carcinog* 2009. [In press]

[42] Diaz Miqueli, A, Rolff, J, Lemm, M, Fichtner, I, Perez, R, Montero, E. Radiosensitisation of U87MG brain tumours by anti-epidermal growth factor receptor monoclonal antibodies. *Br J Cancer* 2009; 100:950-8.

[43] Bednar, F and Simeone, DM. Pancreatic cancer stem cells and relevance to cancer treatments. *J Cell Biochem* 2009 [In press]

[44] Baba, T, Convery, PA, Matsumura, N, Whitaker, RS, Kondoh, E, Perry T, Huang, Z, Bentley, RC, Mori, S, Fujii, S, Marks, JR, Berchuck, A and Murphy, SK. Epigenetic regulation of CD133 and tumorigenicity of CD133+ ovarian cancer cells. *Oncogene* 2009; 28:209-18.

[45] Cabana, R, Frolova, EG, Kapoor, V, Thomas, RA, Krishan, A and Telford, Wg. The Minimal Instrumentation Requirements for Hoechst Side Population Analysis: Stem Cell Analysis on Low-Cost Flow Cytometry Platforms. *Stem Cells* 2006; 24: 2573-2581.

[46] Bleau, AM, Hambardzumyan, D, Ozawa, T, Fomchenko, EI, Huse, JT, Brennan, CW and Holland, EC. PTEN/PI3K/Akt pathway regulates the side population phenotype and ABCG2 activity in glioma tumor stem-like cells. *Cell Stem Cell* 2009; 4:226-35.

[47] Ho, MM, Ng, AV, Lam, S and Hung, JY. Side population in human lung cancer cell lines and tumors is enriched with stem-like cancer cells. *Cancer Res* 2007; 67:4827-33.

[48] Mathew, G, Timm, EA Jr, Sotomayor, P, Godoy, A, Montecinos, VP, Smith, GJ and Huss, WJ. ABCG2-mediated DyeCycle Violet efflux defined side population in benign and malignant prostate. *Cell Cycle* 2009; 8:1053-61.

[49] Di Fiore, R, Santulli, A, Ferrante, RD, Giuliano, M, De Blasio, A, Messina, C, Pirozzi, G, Tirino, V, Tesoriere, G and Vento, R. Identification and expansion of human osteosarcoma-cancer-stem cells by long-term 3-aminobenzamide treatment. *J Cell Physiol* 2009; 219:301-13.

[50] Vander Borght, S, Komuta, M, Libbrecht, L, Katoonizadeh, A, Aerts, R, Dymarkowski, S, Verslype, C, Nevens, F and Roskams, T. Expression of multidrug resistance-associated protein 1 in hepatocellular carcinoma is associated with a more aggressive tumour phenotype and may reflect a progenitor cell origin. *Liver Int* 2008; 28:1370-80.

[51] Krivtsov, AV, Wang, Y, Feng, Z and Armstrong, SA. Gene Expression Profiling of Leukemia Stem Cells. *Methods Mol Biol* 2009; 538:1-16.

[52] Kang, MK and Kang, SK. Pharmacologic blockade of chloride channel synergistically enhances apoptosis of chemotherapeutic drug-resistant cancer stem cells. *Biochem Biophys Res Commun* 2008; 373:539-44.

[53] Marcato, P, Dean, CA, Giacomantonio, CA and Lee, PW. Oncolytic Reovirus Effectively Targets Breast Cancer Stem Cells. *Mol Ther* 2009. [In press]

[54] Mine, T, Matsueda, S, Li, Y, Tokumitsu, H, Gao, H, Danes, C, Wong, KK, Wang, X, Ferrone, S and Ioannides, CG. Breast cancer cells expressing stem cell markers CD44(+) CD24 (lo) are eliminated by Numb-1 peptide-activated T cells. *Cancer Immunol Immunother* 2008. [In press]

In: Pluripotent Stem Cells
Editors: D.W. Rosales et al, pp. 155-171
ISBN: 978-1-60876-738-0

Chapter 6

OUTSTANDING QUESTIONS REGARDING INDUCED PLURIPOTENT STEM (iPS) CELL RESEARCH

Miguel A. Esteban, Jiekai Chen, Jiayin Yang, Feng Li, Wen Li and Duanqing Pei

Chinese Academy of Sciences Key Laboratory of Regenerative Biology,
South China Institute for Stem Cell Biology and Regenerative Medicine,
Guangzhou Institutes of Biomedicine and Health,
Guangzhou 510663, China

Abstract

Terminal somatic cell differentiation is not irreversible. The same route that transforms embryonic stem cells (ESCs) into specific lineages can be walked backwards, e.g. by means of the "induced pluripotent stem (iPS) cell" technology discovered by Shinya Yamanaka in 2006. The implications of iPS are out of proportion and its ease and reproducibility has made it a favorite option compared to other existing approaches including cell fusion or somatic cell nuclear transfer (SCNT). iPS allows the generation of patient specific embryonic like stem cells that are devoid of ethical concerns and may be used for transplantation. iPS has also proven useful to create *in vitro* models that mimic human diseases and this could be used for high throughput drug screening. Besides, thanks to iPS we are now compelled to think of differentiation processes in a bidirectional way, which may be as well cell type and transcription factor specific. Therefore, knowledge is flourishing that will benefit Stem Cell Biology as much as unrelated disciplines. But the pace of discovery has been so quick that every technical advance has raised new issues, creating confusion. Here we will briefly define and try to answer some key questions that in our opinion will shape iPS research and application in following years.

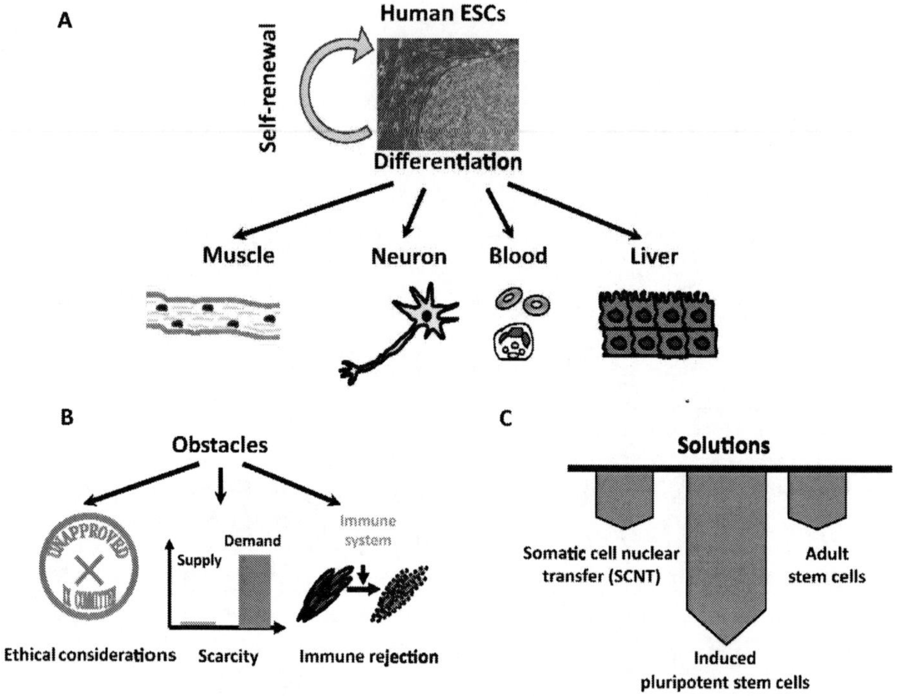

Figure 1. A, Pluripotency and self renewal of ESCs. A capture of human ESCs is shown. B, Some concerns surrounding human ESC research. C, Some solutions to human ESC research and application.

1. Introduction to iPS Technology

ESCs were first isolated (mouse ESCs) in 1981 [1] and are defined by two main characteristics: pluripotency, which means that they have the potential to give rise to all cell types of the adult body, and self renewal, which implies that if cultured under specific conditions they can be maintained undifferentiated indefinitely (Figure 1A). Ever since the discovery of human ESCs (1998) [2], the idea of inducing differentiation "a la carte" to repair damaged tissue has fostered our imagination and stimulated the development of a new branch of Medicine based on tissue regeneration. But on one side the risk of immune rejection, and on the other very important ethical considerations, have hampered human ESC research and application (Figure 1B) [3]. Experiments over the past 50 years have established that, despite the decrease in differentiation potential associated with development, the nuclei of most, if not all, adult cells retain plasticity and can be reset to an ESC-like state. This culminated in 1996 with the birth of Dolly the sheep thanks to SCNT [4]. This technique is founded on the inoculation of somatic cell genomic DNA into an enucleated oocyte that retains the nucleoplasm (nuclear content excluding DNA). The latter may seem irrelevant but indicated that the nucleoplasm contains factors (transcription factors or DNA binding proteins) that drive the nuclear reprogramming. Remarkably, not only whole individuals can be produced this way, the resulting blastocyst may also be broken on feeder layers and cell lines then generated that are similar to ESCs.

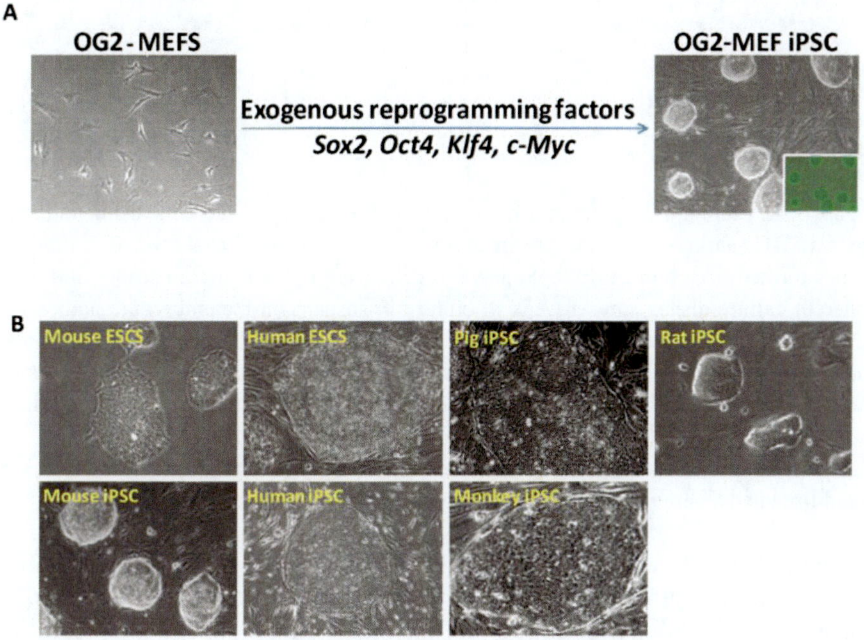

Figure 2. **A**, Schematic representation of iPS cell colony generation from mouse embryonic fibroblasts. Mouse embryonic fibroblasts (MEFs) from mice (OG2 mice) that bear a transgenic Oct4 promoter driving GFP expression were used, the colonies became GFP positive after reactivation of the endogenous ESC program. **B**, Captures of ESCs and iPS cell colonies (iPSC) from different species. All cell lines were generated in our laboratory.

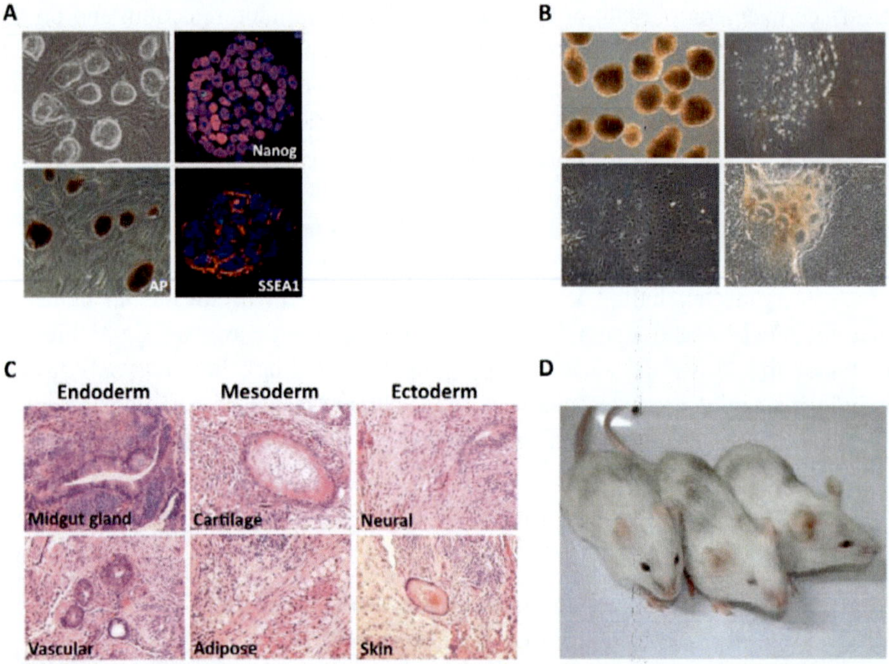

Figure 3. A, Immunofluorescence microscopy captures of mouse iPS cells using antibodies against ESC markers. Alkaline phosphatase (AP) staining is also shown. B, Embryonic bodies formed from human iPS colonies. iPS cells were first cultured in suspension in non adherent culture dishes, after a week of culture in suspension the embryonic bodies were adhered to coverslips and this progressively resulted in differentiation into cells with many shapes and characteristics. Mouse embryonic bodies have similar appearance and behavior (not shown). C, Teratomas derived from mouse iPS cells formed tissues corresponding to the 3 germ layers. D, Captures of chimeric mice produced by injection of iPS cells from black mice into blastocysts from white mice. All experiments in Figure 2 and 3 are unpublished and were performed in our laboratory.

Despite sheep, mice, pigs, and dogs, have been produced this way, the technique is rather inefficient and the reprogramming usually incomplete. Moreover, the procedure is not exempt of ethical considerations either, oocytes are scarce, and SCNT has not yet been achieved in humans [5]. A trendy alternative has been autologous transplantation using cell lineages derived from adult stem cells, for example adipose and bone marrow mesenchymal stem cells (MSCs) [6]. But these cells are not pluripotent, can be obtained in very scarce numbers, and are difficult to expand (self renewal is limited) [7]. With these premises, a major scientific goal of recent years has been to achieve a relatively simple method that can reprogram somatic cells into pluripotent ESC-like cells (Figure 1C). The revolution came in 2006 when Yamanaka and collaborators showed that mouse fibroblasts acquire properties similar to ESCs after retroviral transduction of 4 transcription factors, namely Oct4, Sox2, Klf4, and c-Myc (SKOM), abundant in the nuclei of ESCs [8] (Figure 2A). These cells were called induced pluripotent stem (iPS) cells (Figure 2B). The first generation iPS cells were similar to mouse ESCs in morphology and proliferation, had a normal karyotype, and formed teratomas (Figure 3A-C). However, their global gene expression pattern differed significantly from ESCs and they failed to produce mixed color chimeric mice when injected into blastocysts from a different type of mice. In 2007, chimera competence and germline transmission was achieved [9-11] (Figure 3D), and later on iPS was produced from human fibroblasts [12,13]. Moreover, the technique has been reproduced in multiple laboratories and ever since the pace of discovery has been exponential. Potentially, iPS technology can overcome 2 of the most important problems associated with human ESC application (ethical considerations and immune rejection), but still faces many obstacles, some of which are shared with ESCs (e.g. the bona fide and easy differentiation into given lineages) and others that are unique.

2. Some Essential Questions Surrounding iPS

2.1. Is iPS Originated from Adult Stem Cells Present in the Starting Population? Can iPS be Induced from Cells of Multiple Tissues?

Like it happened with SCNT [14], one of the first tests for iPS was to find out whether any cell is susceptible to this form of reprogramming or only a small minority of cells with inherent stem cell characteristics that are present in skin biopsias. This was particularly important in light of the extremely low efficiency of the initial iPS reports. We know now that besides fibroblasts, also stomach and liver cells, B lymphocytes, pancreatic beta cells, meningeal membrane cells (meningiocytes), keratinocytes, hair follicle cells, and several others, are susceptible to iPS [15-20]. However, this does not imply that stem cells are not easier to reprogram, as this is for example the case of neural stem cells (NSCs) [21]. The exact reason underlying NSC amenability to iPS is unclear but may be related to basal expression of the complementary factors Sox2, Klf4, and c-Myc. It is also interesting to note that like NSCs other cell types derived from the ectoderm, such as meningiocytes and keratinocytes, are more prone to iPS [18,20]. The ectoderm is the first germ layer to appear during development and this may perhaps imply less extended reorganization of the chromatin relative to ESCs and compared to mesoderm and endoderm.

2.2. Can iPS Be Induced with Alternative Combinations of Factors or Using Fewer Factors? Can iPS Be Produced Using Different Delivery Methods Apart from Retroviruses? Can It Be Enhanced Using Chemicals?

The initial approach of Takahashi and Yamanaka included 24 factors expressed by retroviral vectors and then by substitution this narrowed into 4 magic transcription factors [8,22]. Because c-Myc is an oncogene, SKOM iPS resulted in significant risk of tumor formation and decreased life span in the chimeric mice [10]. Several groups then reported mouse and human iPS excluding c-Myc, albeit with a very poor efficiency of colony formation that makes it unpractical [23,24]. In parallel, Thomson *et al.* produced human iPS using an alternative combination (Sox2, Oct4, Nanog, Lin28) [13]. The choice of Nanog seemed logic given its key role in controlling ESC behavior, as for how Lin28 favors iPS it is yet unclear but may be related to its ability to regulate the microRNA let7. By that time chemical enhancers of iPS were discovered, in particular the histone deacetylase inhibitors (HDACi) valproic acid (VPA) and trichostatin (TSA) [25]. Histone modifications, including acetylation and methylation, alter nucleosomes and facilitate or reduce access of transcription factors to their DNA cognate sequences [26]. HDACi not only allowed significant increase of iPS efficiency using fibroblasts and SKOM or SKO, but also iPS using even fewer factors [27]. Whether HDACi also act at least in part through mechanisms independent of their impact on histone acetylation is not known but remains possible. Substitution of Klf4 using chemicals has also been achieved in mouse iPS by means of high throughput screening [28]. Likewise, iPS has been produced using 1 factor (Oct4 in NSCs), and although use of retroviruses still remains the most widespread delivery system other approaches have proliferated recently: excisable piggyBac transposons [29,30], lox-p flanked factors (polycystronic vectors producing factors linked in tandem by means of 2A autocleavable sequences) [31], adenoviruses [32], episomal vectors [33], and recombinant proteins [34,35]. The last three approaches, in particular the proteins, are very appealing but also extremely unproductive and thus may be difficult to reproduce. Moreover, although the general view is that iPS with fewer factors or without transgene integration will result in safer cell lines, things may not be that easy and it is perhaps difficult to achieve complete reprogramming in such conditions, at least in the human model. On the other hand, several groups have increased the number of factors (by combining Yamanaka's and Thomson's combinations and also with other additions) and used lentiviruses to increase human iPS efficiency [36,37]. Likewise, Sox2 can be replaced by Sox1, Klf4 by Klf2 or Klf5 and by estrogen related receptor beta (Esrrb), and c-Myc by n-Myc or l-Myc [38].

2.3. Can iPS Be Produced from Other Mammals in Addition to Mouse and Human?

The demonstration that SKOM can reprogram 2 highly unrelated species transmitted optimism regarding universality of the pluripotency network in mammals and stimulated iPS research on other species. Recently, several groups produced iPS cell lines from Rhesus monkey fibroblasts [39], rat fibroblasts and MSCs [40], and fibroblasts and MSCs from Tibetan [41] and farm pig [42,43]. Rat is a far better model than mouse for physiology and disease-orientated studies, and the generation of rat iPS coincided in time with the discovery of chimera competent and germ line competent ESCs [44,45]. Interest in genetic manipulation of rats has consequently been boosted and many surprises lie ahead. It must be noted however that pluripotency of rat iPS cell lines is reduced compared to ESCs, possibly reflecting partial reprogramming. The same can be said for the pig, but for this animal ESCs haven't been isolated yet despite decades of intense effort [46]. Very likely soon we will see reports on iPS from other non human primates like the marmoset (whose reduced size is an advantage), and domestic animals including dog, cat, rabbit or sheep, as well as subsequent improvements of the respective methodologies. Nevertheless, at some point a standard will need to be set for comparison with humans in the form of preclinical trials. In many countries phylogenetic similarity between monkeys and humans poses a barrier towards research, and in addition monkeys may need to be imported, are expensive, and difficult to breed. Given striking parallelisms with humans, the pig, which is an agricultural commodity in most places, may dominate except for cases such as Parkinson or Huntington disease in which neurological evaluation is easier in primates [47]. In the near future, it is also probable that countries will try to show national pride producing iPS from icon animals such as panda in China or kangaroo in Australia. Besides being a curiosity, one might argue that this could be a way to protect endangered species [48].

2.4.. Are iPS Cells Produced from Different Tissues Identical? What Requisites Must Fulfill an iPS Cell Line to Be Considered Fully Reprogrammed? Are Human iPS Cells Truly Pluripotent?

After the generation of chimera competent mouse iPS, all emphasis was put on the idea that iPS cells and ESCs, either mouse or human, are almost indistinguishable. This was shown using DNA arrays, histone methylation profiling, telomere length, and ultrastructural features, among others [49-51]. However, is the story as simple as this, or iPS is like a make-up, the conversion of a somatic cell to another somatic cell that has the ability to mimic almost all aspects of ESCs? Supporting the idea of some kind of make-up and based on more detailed analysis of data, the paradigm is now emerging that iPS cells differ from ESCs, and iPS from different tissues or generated with different methods are different as well [52-54]. The latter is of particular interest because iPS from a given tissuė may retain some epigenetic memory and that could make it more easily differentiated back into the same tissue than other iPS cell lines or even human ESCs. However, caution is needed when comparing iPS cell lines between themselves and with ESCs, as differences could be only reflection of partial reprogramming in spite of the ability to form teratomas. An extra consideration is that human ESCs from varied sources are not identical and the same applies to mouse ESCs [55]. Numbers, in terms of genes going up or down or other differences, are not vital to answer this question, many genes could be changed and this not mean anything, while differences in one gene could have profound consequences. Besides, it is very important that when iPS cell lines are compared, they have been cultured using the same protocols and have been split for a roughly similar number of times. When profiling iPS cell lines from diverse individuals their ethnic background should also be considered. Whole genome DNA methylation analysis of iPS and ESCs may hold the key to reach a conclusion concerning the identity of iPS cells. But to make it affordable (sequencing each base of the genome at least 5 to 10 times on average) new generation sequencing technologies must be developed further. Moreover, in the near future specific regions will need to be selected and standardized so that the epigenetic characteristics of iPS cell lines can be tested quickly.

2.5. Can iPS Be Used to Model Human Diseases in Vitro? Are There Any Ethical Concerns to Be Considered for iPS Cell Generation and Distribution?

iPS provides an outstanding model to study human genetic diseases in vitro, any hereditary disease in general but in particular those for which animal models don't exist. For example [56], we can generate iPS from a patient with a neurological genetic syndrome, we then characterize those iPS cell lines and make sure that they are truly pluripotent, and finally we differentiate those iPS cells into neurons and compare their functionality with neurons from iPS cell lines derived from unaffected individuals. In the case of monogenic diseases the mutation could be corrected and the neurons from the original or the corrected iPS cell line exhaustively compared. This kind of approach offers the possibility of studying the underlying functional defect at a molecular level, and if properly optimized also high throughput drug screening for compounds that correct the abnormality. For diseases which are not monogenic, like chromosomal abnormalities, the genetic correction is not feasible but the model is no less interesting. In those cases in which the disease has a very complex genetic background the utility is more arguable, and some diseases are not result of one single cell type being affected but very many. For example Alzheimer disease has in cases a familiar history suggestive of genetic predisposition. However, differentiation of iPS cells from these patients into neurons may not yield any conclusion because of the fundamental contribution of the environment and the fact that the disease is consequence of accumulated beta amyloid over many years. One might then argue that challenging those neurons with specific compounds could accelerate the kinetics and this would indeed prove invaluable. Even if this is the case, the analysis of a significant number of patients and comparison with iPS cell lines from unaffected people of the similar social status, age and gender, will be necessary. Likewise, collection of samples from members of one same family, including affected and unaffected is important. Before collecting samples, the individuals should be carefully informed and confidentiality maintained, as these cells may be distributed to other laboratories or even pharmaceutical companies, and they could end up having economic value. The latter would happen if standardized iPS cell lines owned by pharmaceutical companies are commercially distributed for therapeutic purposes in immunologically compatible patients. At this point the Ethics and regulations concerning iPS have not yet been defined [57], but this will likely start soon. In any case, ethical considerations that now apply to human ESCs should not be present in iPS research.

Finally, we would like to state the fact that some still argue that iPS must be banned for the simple reason that it might stimulate scientists to do exhaustive comparisons with human ESCs.

2.6. What Are the Mechanisms of iPS? Is Insertional Mutagenesis a Requisite? Do Barriers Exist That Limit the Reprogramming and Can They be Overcome Through Manipulation?

The mechanisms of iPS remain largely unknown and have been defined as a "black box" [58]. Despite everyone agrees that understanding the molecular machinery will improve the methodology, researchers have so far focused on rather more empirical studies. The quick pace of the field imposed this direction and more laborious mechanistic analysis was set aside with the exception of DNA arrays and ChIP-on-Chip analysis [51,59]. It is known that iPS is a slow process, taking around 15-20 days in the mouse and around 1 month in the human [60]. During this process the first noticeable changes are morphological, cells cluster and start forming aggregates since the first days of reprogramming. Afterwards, alkaline phosphatase staining and suface markers including SSEA1 are progressively acquired. In the last instance, the endogenous ESC program becomes reactivated and the transgenes (at least in the case of retroviruses) become silenced [61]. The latter has been accepted as a criterion for full reprogramming and is based on a self defense reaction of ESCs: methylation of the invading genome [10]. A barrier for exploring iPS has been the low efficiency. Because the population is highly heterogeneous, changes observed in the early phases or reprogramming may not be representative of the internal engine. Low efficiency also raised possibility that the transgenes may need to integrate in specific regions of the genome, and perhaps introduce mutations that activate or silence nearby genes that are in turn critical modulators of iPS. This has not yet been excluded formally but at least it is clear that the integration pattern differs very significantly between different iPS cell lines [62]. Moreover, a single integration of a polycistronic vector can induce iPS [63,64], and iPS can as well be achieved without exogenous insertions [32-35,65]. One might then argue that it is imperative to do single cell analysis using newly developed technologies. But on which basis do we select those cells and how can we be sure they are the "good" ones? If on the top of that we add the fact that time course analysis is needed, then the task is immense, perhaps impossible. DNA arrays produced from time course iPS experiments using secondary fibroblasts generated with doxycicline inducible lentiviruses did not provide clear answers [51]. Addition of the antibiotic produces reactivation of the vectors (lentiviruses are less efficiently silenced than retroviruses) and iPS colonies appear with higher efficiency and quicker kinetics than under standard protocols. Although such approach is powerful, acceleration of the process and biased expression of the integrated factors may alter the whole chain of events that happen in primary cells, and therefore provide wrong conclusions. In the immediate future it is expected that mechanistic investigations will be sorted in three ways: first, use of higher efficiency methods based on previous empirical observations, which may also be coupled to isolation of enriched populations; second, use of high throughput screening assays based on siRNA oligos or vectors; and third, meticulous analysis of pathways relevant to ESCs or to somatic cell functioning in general. Regarding the latter, early stages of reprogramming share similitude with the process of tumorigenesis, as among other things both involve immortalization [66]. Looking at cell cycle check points or tumor suppressor pathways like p21 or p53 will likely shed light into how iPS is accomplished. Manipulating these pathways may as well increase iPS efficiency but since these are guardians of the genome it may also introduce mutations or other abnormalities. This raises the question as to whether the iPS process itself introduces risk of acquiring genomic abnormalities by changing these pathways before the ESC-like identity (and the associated self defense mechanisms) has been achieved. From a different perspective, pre-iPS cell lines, which represent the major part of colonies produced with standard iPS protocols, can be fully reprogrammed by means of chemical additions and this is an outstanding tool to understand iPS mechanisms.

3. Conclusions

Only 3 years ago, what it seemed impossible became real, the fate of somatic cells was changed *in vitro* using a relatively simple methodology. Shinya Yamanaka's approach to induced pluripotency has demolished barriers that politicians could not break with bare talk in over a decade of tense debate surrounding human ESCs. Now everyone talks about iPS, and even if detractors exist, they cannot hide their astonishment. Although many questions remain present, the most difficult step, which is producing the technology, has been accomplished and the rest is only a matter of time. In following years the field is likely to specialize in multiple branches: on one side mechanistic studies coupled to screening of highly susceptible (and easily accessible) cell types and different factor delivery protocols, will converge into a consensus regarding "clinical grade" iPS in humans. On the other, iPS disease models will not rely so much on technical issues or safety, and will look more for ease and robustness. For clinical use of iPS, we will first need to establish adequate large animal models, and the pig will arguably be the reference. Once clinical trials are approved, it is unlikely that autologous transplantation will be a preferred choice, as it is too time consuming and expensive. Creation of an iPS cell bank matching thousands of HLA haplotypes will be instrumental to bring iPS to the general public. Among other things, this would allow use of exhaustively tested iPS cell lines (e.g. teratomas, transcriptome, microRNAs, multilineage differentiation, etc) that with the arrival of new generation sequencing technologies may be studied for existence of insertional or not insertional mutations and their DNA methylation status (other epigenetic marks as well) at a genome wide level. But random banking of iPS cell lines will be unproductive and it is necessary to take advantage of already well established and well characterized cell banks, e.g. of cord blood. iPS from cord blood has not yet been achieved but many laboratories are pursuing this objective and we anticipate a breakthrough soon. Even after this happens, creating an iPS cell bank is an out of dimension enterprise that would benefit from interaction between institutes and countries. An added problem is that pharmaceutical companies will try to purchase large stock of iPS cell lines from laboratories worldwide, and protect the intellectual property; like it happens nowadays with drugs, iPS will at some point move billions. As for the disease models, access to cell banks containing tens or hundreds of well diagnosed patients for every possible disease is equally relevant to achieve effectiveness. So far iPS studies have centered on a very limited number of affected individuals, in occasions 1 or 2, and this is a serious handicap for making serious conclusions. Comparisons between patients of different ethnic groups or countries will be especially valuable to expand credibility. Nevertheless, the study of many genetic diseases will likely be revitalized thanks to iPS. In our opinion, iPS from autosomal recessive diseases is particularly interesting: using homologous recombination techniques the remaining intact allele could be spliced out in a conditional manner that is lineage specific. This could be applied in hereditary cancer syndromes in which the second hit is organ specific (e.g. von Hippel-Lindau syndrome, adenomatous polyposis coli, etc) [67,68]. Apart from all the above considerations, new concepts/approaches may arise from iPS research that could be used to slow down ageing, as this is also in essence a programmed process [69].

References

[1] Evans, M.J. and Kaufman, M.H. (1981). Establishment in culture of pluripotential cells from mouse embryos. *Nature,* **292**, 154-6.

[2] Thomson, J.A., Itskovitz-Eldor, J., Shapiro, S.S., Waknitz, M.A., Swiergiel, J.J., Marshall, V.S. and Jones, J.M. (1998). Embryonic stem cell lines derived from human blastocysts. *Science,* **282**, 1145-7.

[3] Daley, G.Q. et al. (2007). Ethics. The ISSCR guidelines for human embryonic stem cell research. *Science,* **315**, 603-4.

[4] Wilmut, I., Schnieke, A.E., McWhir, J., Kind, A.J. and Campbell, K.H. (1997). Viable offspring derived from fetal and adult. *Science,* **385**, 810-3.

[5] Hwang, W.S. et al. (2004). Evidence of a pluripotent human embryonic stem cell line derived from a cloned blastocyst. *Science,* **303**, 1669-74.

[6] Kern, S., Eichler, H., Stoeve, J., Kluter, H. and Bieback, K. (2006). Comparative analysis of mesenchymal stem cells from bone marrow, umbilical cord blood, or adipose tissue. *Stem Cells,* **24**, 1294-301.

[7] Basem M. Abdallah, Hamid Saeed and Kassem, M. (2009). Human Mesenchymal Stem Cells: Basic Biology and Clinical Applications for Bone Tissue Regeneration. *Trends in Stem Cell Biology and Technology*, pp. 177-190

[8] Takahashi, K. and Yamanaka, S. (2006). Induction of pluripotent stem cells from mouse embryonic and adult fibroblast cultures by defined factors. *Cell,* **126**, 663-76.

[9] Maherali, N. et al. (2007). Directly reprogrammed fibroblasts show global epigenetic remodeling and widespread tissue contribution. *Cell Stem Cell,* **1**, 55-70.

[10] Okita, K., Ichisaka, T. and Yamanaka, S. (2007). Generation of germline-competent induced pluripotent stem cells. *Nature,* **448**, 313-7.

[11] Wernig, M., Meissner, A., Foreman, R., Brambrink, T., Ku, M., Hochedlinger, K., Bernstein, B.E. and Jaenisch, R. (2007). In vitro reprogramming of fibroblasts into a pluripotent ES-cell-like state. *Nature,* **448**, 318-24.

[12] Takahashi, K., Tanabc, K., Ohnuki, M., Narita, M., Ichisaka, T., Tomoda, K. and Yamanaka, S. (2007). Induction of pluripotent stem cells from adult human fibroblasts by defined factors. *Cell,* **131**, 861-72.

[13] Yu, J. et al. (2007). Induced pluripotent stem cell lines derived from human somatic cells. *Science,* **318**, 1917-20.

[14] Hochedlinger, K. and Jaenisch, R. (2002). Monoclonal mice generated by nuclear transfer from mature B and T donor cells. *Nature*, **415**, 1035-8.

[15] Aoi, T., Yae, K., Nakagawa, M., Ichisaka, T., Okita, K., Takahashi, K., Chiba, T. and Yamanaka, S. (2008). Generation of pluripotent stem cells from adult mouse liver and stomach cells. *Science*, **321**, 699-702.

[16] Stadtfeld, M., Brennand, K. and Hochedlinger, K. (2008). Reprogramming of pancreatic beta cells into induced pluripotent stem cells. *Curr Biol,* **18**, 890-4.

[17] Hanna, J. et al. (2008). Direct reprogramming of terminally differentiated mature B lymphocytes to pluripotency. *Cell,* **133**, 250-64.

[18] Qin, D. et al. (2008). Mouse meningiocytes express Sox2 and yield high efficiency of chimeras after nuclear reprogramming with exogenous factors. *J Biol Chem,* **283**, 33730-5.

[19] Eminli, S., Utikal, J., Arnold, K., Jaenisch, R. and Hochedlinger, K. (2008). Reprogramming of neural progenitor cells into induced pluripotent stem cells in the absence of exogenous Sox2 expression. *Stem Cells*, **26**, 2467-74.

[20] Aasen, T. et al. (2008). Efficient and rapid generation of induced pluripotent stem cells from human keratinocytes. *Nat Biotechnol,* **26**, 1276-84.

[21] Silva, J., Barrandon, O., Nichols, J., Kawaguchi, J., Theunissen, T.W. and Smith, A. (2008). Promotion of reprogramming to ground state pluripotency by signal inhibition. *PLoS Biol*, **6**, e253.

[22] Qi, H. and Pei, D. (2007). The magic of four: induction of pluripotent stem cells from somatic cells by Oct4, Sox2, Myc and Klf4. *Cell Res,* **17**, 578-80.

[23] Nakagawa, M. et al. (2008). Generation of induced pluripotent stem cells without Myc from mouse and human fibroblasts. *Nat Biotechnol,* **26**, 101-6.

[24] Wernig, M., Meissner, A., Cassady, J.P. and Jaenisch, R. (2008). c-Myc is dispensable for direct reprogramming of mouse fibroblasts. *Cell Stem Cell,* **2**, 10-2.

[25] Huangfu, D., Maehr, R., Guo, W., Eijkelenboom, A., Snitow, M., Chen, A.E. and Melton, D.A. (2008). Induction of pluripotent stem cells by defined factors is greatly improved by small-molecule compounds. *Nat Biotechnol*, **26**, 795-7.

[26] Bernstein, B.E. et al. (2006). A bivalent chromatin structure marks key developmental genes in embryonic stem cells. *Cell,* **125**, 315-26.

[27] Huangfu, D., Osafune, K., Maehr, R., Guo, W., Eijkelenboom, A., Chen, S., Muhlestein, W. and Melton, D.A. (2008). Induction of pluripotent stem cells from primary human fibroblasts with only Oct4 and Sox2. *Nat Biotechnol,* **26**, 1269-75.

[28] Lyssiotis, C.A. et al. (2009). Reprogramming of murine fibroblasts to induced pluripotent stem cells with chemical complementation of Klf4. *Proc Natl Acad Sci U S A,* **106**, 8912-7.

[29] Kaji, K., Norrby, K., Paca, A., Mileikovsky, M., Mohseni, P. and Woltjen, K. (2009). Virus-free induction of pluripotency and subsequent excision of reprogramming factors. *Nature*, **458**, 771-5.
[30] Woltjen, K. et al. (2009). piggyBac transposition reprograms fibroblasts to induced pluripotent stem cells. *Nature*, **458**, 766-70.
[31] Soldner, F. et al. (2009). Parkinson's disease patient-derived induced pluripotent stem cells free of viral reprogramming factors. *Cell*, **136**, 964-77.
[32] Stadtfeld, M., Nagaya, M., Utikal, J., Weir, G. and Hochedlinger, K. (2008). Induced pluripotent stem cells generated without viral integration. *Science,* **322**, 945-9.
[33] Yu, J., Hu, K., Smuga-Otto, K., Tian, S., Stewart, R., Slukvin, II and Thomson, J.A. (2009). Human induced pluripotent stem cells free of vector and transgene sequences. *Science,* **324**, 797-801.
[34] Zhou, H. et al. (2009). Generation of induced pluripotent stem cells using recombinant proteins. *Cell Stem Cell,* **4**, 381-4.
[35] Kim, D. et al. (2009). Generation of human induced pluripotent stem cells by direct delivery of reprogramming proteins. *Cell Stem Cell,* **4,** 472-6.
[36] Liao, J. et al. (2008). Enhanced efficiency of generating induced pluripotent stem (iPS) cells from human somatic cells by a combination of six transcription factors. *Cell Res,* **18**, 600-3.
[37] Mali, P., Ye, Z., Hommond, H.H., Yu, X., Lin, J., Chen, G., Zou, J. and Cheng, L. (2008). Improved efficiency and pace of generating induced pluripotent stem cells from human adult and fetal fibroblasts. *Stem Cells,* **26**, 1998-2005.
[38] Yamanaka, S. (2009). A fresh look at iPS cells. *Cell*, **137**, 13-7.
[39] Liu, H. et al. (2008). Generation of Induced Pluripotent Stem Cells from Adult Rhesus Monkey Fibroblasts. *Cell Stem Cell*, **3**, 587-590.
[40] Liao, J. et al. (2009). Generation of Induced Pluripotent Stem Cell Lines from Adult Rat Cells. *Cell Stem Cell,* **4**, 11-15.
[41] Esteban, M.A. et al. (2009). Generation of induced pluripotent stem cell lines from tibetan miniature pig. *J Biol Chem,* **284**, 17634.
[42] Wu, Z. et al. (2009). Generation of Pig-Induced Pluripotent Stem Cells with a Drug-Inducible System. *J Mol Cell Biol*, **1**, 46-54.
[43] Ezashi, T., Telugu, B., Alexenko, A.P., Sachdev, S., Sinha, S. and Roberts, R.M. (2009). Derivation of induced pluripotent stem cells from pig somatic cells. *Proc Natl Acad Sci U S A*, **106**, 10993-8.
[44] Li, P. et al. (2008). Germline competent embryonic stem cells derived from rat blastocysts. *Cell,* **135**, 1299-1310.

[45] Buehr, M. et al. (2008). Capture of authentic embryonic stem cells from rat blastocysts. *Cell*, **135**, 1287-1298.

[46] Hall, V. (2008). Porcine embryonic stem cells: a possible source for cell replacement therapy. S*tem Cell Rev***,** **4**, 275-82.

[47] Yang, S.H. et al. (2008). Towards a transgenic model of Huntington's disease in a non-human primate. *Nature*, **453**, 921-4.

[48] Trounson, A. (2009). Rats, cats, and elephants, but still no unicorn: induced pluripotent stem cells from new species. *Cell Stem Cell,* **4**, 3-4.

[49] Zeuschner D., Mildner K. , Zaehres, H. and Scholer H,. (2009). Induced Pluripotent Stem Cells at Nano Scale. Stem cells and development. *Epub ahead of print.*

[50] Marion, R.M., Strati, K., Li, H., Tejera, A., Schoeftner, S., Ortega, S., Serrano, M. and Blasco, M.A. (2009). Telomeres acquire embryonic stem cell characteristics in induced pluripotent stem cells. *Cell Stem Cell*, **4**, 141-54.

[51] Mikkelsen, T.S. et al. (2008). Dissecting direct reprogramming through integrative genomic analysis. *Nature,* **454**, 49-55.

[52] Chin, M.H. et al. (2009). Induced pluripotent stem cells and embryonic stem cells are distinguished by gene expression signatures. *Cell Stem Cell*, **5**, 111-23.

[53] Deng, J. et al. (2009). Targeted bisulfite sequencing reveals changes in DNA methylation associated with nuclear reprogramming. *Nat Biotechnol*, **27**, 353-60.

[54] Miura, K. et al. (2009). Variation in the safety of induced pluripotent stem cell lines. *Nat Biotechnol*, **27**, 743-5.

[55] Sharova, L.V., Sharov, A.A., Piao, Y., Shaik, N., Sullivan, T., Stewart, C.L., Hogan, B.L. and Ko, M.S. (2007). Global gene expression profiling reveals similarities and differences among mouse pluripotent stem cells of different origins and strains. *Dev Biol,* **307**, 446-59.

[56] Ebert, A.D., Yu, J., Rose, F.F., Jr., Mattis, V.B., Lorson, C.L., Thomson, J.A. and Svendsen, C.N. (2009). Induced pluripotent stem cells from a spinal muscular atrophy patient. *Nature*, **457**, 277-80.

[57] Aalto-Setala, K., Conklin, B.R. and Lo, B. (2009). Obtaining consent for future research with induced pluripotent cells: opportunities and challenges. *PLoS Biol*, **7**, e42.

[58] Sridharan, R. and Plath, K. (2008). Illuminating the black box of reprogramming. *Cell Stem Cell*, **2**, 295-7.

[59] Sridharan, R., Tchieu, J., Mason, M.J., Yachechko, R., Kuoy, E., Horvath, S., Zhou, Q. and Plath, K. (2009). Role of the murine reprogramming factors in the induction of pluripotency. *Cell*, **136**, 364-77.

[60] Maherali, N. and Hochedlinger, K. (2008). Guidelines and techniques for the generation of induced pluripotent stem cells. *Cell Stem Cell*, **3**, 595-605.

[61] Hotta, A. and Ellis, J. (2008). Retroviral vector silencing during iPS cell induction: an epigenetic beacon that signals distinct pluripotent states. *J Cell Biochem,* **105**, 940-8.

[62] Hawley, R.G. (2008). Does retroviral insertional mutagenesis play a role in the generation of induced pluripotent stem cells? *Mol Ther*, **16**, 1354-5.

[63] Carey, B.W., Markoulaki, S., Hanna, J., Saha, K., Gao, Q., Mitalipova, M. and Jaenisch, R. (2009). Reprogramming of murine and human somatic cells using a single polycistronic vector. *Proc Natl Acad Sci U S A,* **106**, 157-62.

[64] Sommer, C.A., Stadtfeld, M., Murphy, G.J., Hochedlinger, K., Kotton, D.N. and Mostoslavsky, G. (2009). Induced pluripotent stem cell generation using a single lentiviral stem cell cassette. *Stem Cells*, **27**, 543-9.

[65] Okita, K., Nakagawa, M., Hyenjong, H., Ichisaka, T. and Yamanaka, S. (2008). Generation of mouse induced pluripotent stem cells without viral vectors. *Science*, **322**, 949-53.

[66] Hanahan, D. and Weinberg, R.A. (2000). The hallmarks of cancer. *Cell*, **100**, 57-70.

[67] Kaelin, W.G., Jr. (2002). Molecular basis of the VHL hereditary cancer syndrome. *Nat Rev Cancer*, **2**, 673-82.

[68] Vogelstein, B. and Kinzler, K.W. (2004). Cancer genes and the pathways they control. *Nat Med,* **10**, 789-99.

[69] Kirkwood, T.B. (2005). Understanding the odd science of aging. *Cell,* **120**, 437-47.

In: Pluripotent Stem Cells
Editors: D.W. Rosales et al, pp. 173-184
ISBN: 978-1-60876-738-0

Chapter 7

Lepidopteran Midgut Stem Cells in Culture: A New Tool for Cell Biology and Physiological Studies

Gianluca Tettamanti[1] and Morena Casartelli[2]
[1]Dipartimento di Biotecnologie e Scienze Molecolari, Università degli Studi dell'Insubria, Via Dunant 3, 21100 Varese, Italia
[2]Dipartimento di Biologia, Università degli Studi di Milano, Via Celoria 26, 20133 Milano, Italia

Abstract

Holometabolous insects recruit a wide array of stem cell types to fulfil the growth of larval organs at moulting and their remodelling at metamorphosis, thus achieving the final body organization of the adult.

Over the years a large number of different stem cells, with specific roles in growth and renewal of insect tissues, have been identified in Lepidoptera and Diptera. A particular interest for the stem cells residing within the insect gut is now emerging and the early morphological studies that analyzed the behaviour of these cells are progressively supported by new cellular and molecular data.

After a brief summary of the current knowledge on insect intestinal stem cells, here we will focus on some characteristics of the stem cells in culture of the larval midgut of *Bombyx mori*. These cells can be released from the midgut just before the fourth moult and, once placed in an appropriate medium, they multiply and differentiate in mature cells that are able to perform normal absorptive and digestive functions *in vitro*.

Thereafter we will discuss the use of this reliable *in vitro* system as a tool to study intestinal morphogenesis and differentiation, to investigate the specific roles and reciprocal relationships of autophagy and apoptosis during midgut remodelling, and to analyze physiological functions of midgut cells, such as their ability to internalize different substrates and the mechanisms involved. Studies on midgut stem cells appear of key importance in consideration of the extensive similarities evidenced among mammalian and insect intestinal epithelia in their development, organization and molecular regulatory mechanisms.

Different types of stem cells have been described in several insect organs, where they give rise to a repertoire of tissues during the embryonic, larval and adult stages (for a complete review see [1]). The insect gut makes no exception and an increasing amount of evidence on stem cell behaviour in this organ has been gathered for a long time. More recently, the molecular mechanisms underlying the regulation of these cells have been partially unfolded in species belonging to Diptera and Lepidoptera, the two most widely used *taxa* for the analysis of intestinal stem cell biology. *Drosophila melanogaster* has lately represented a model to analyze stem cells in the adult gut, while in lepidopteran species efforts have been devoted to the larval midgut. The main part of the information reported below will refer to these two systems.

The alimentary canal of insects can be divided into three regions: the foregut, the midgut and the hindgut. The foregut and the hindgut are of ectodermal origin and are covered by a cuticle that is continuous to the epidermal layer one, while the midgut, which has a primary role in nutrient digestion and absorption, is an endodermal derivative devoid of cuticle but lined by a specialized peritrophic membrane. In adult *Drosophila*, the midgut is a pseudostratified epithelium composed mostly of large cells with absorptive function, the enterocytes, and of enteroendocrine cells [2], while the midgut of Lepidopteran larvae consists of a highly folded monolayered epithelium formed by columnar, goblet and endocrine cells [3]. In both cases a further cell type, the stem cells (recently called intestinal stem cells (ISCs) in Diptera and previously indicated as regenerative cells in Lepidoptera and other insects), are located at the base of the midgut epithelium. Following appropriate stimuli, these cells are capable to proliferate and differentiate into the other gut cell types [3].

In adult *Drosophila* ISCs are set in motion to maintain midgut homeostasis: when the midgut epithelial cells become damaged by ingested food, pathogens or toxins, ISCs divide, become enteroblasts, and differentiate into enterocytes or enteroendocrine cells, thus replacing lost cells [2]. While the role of stem cells in midgut homeostasis in the adult fly has been well described *in vivo* [4, 5], the molecular mechanisms by which these cells originate and differentiate into other cell types during development are poorly studied.

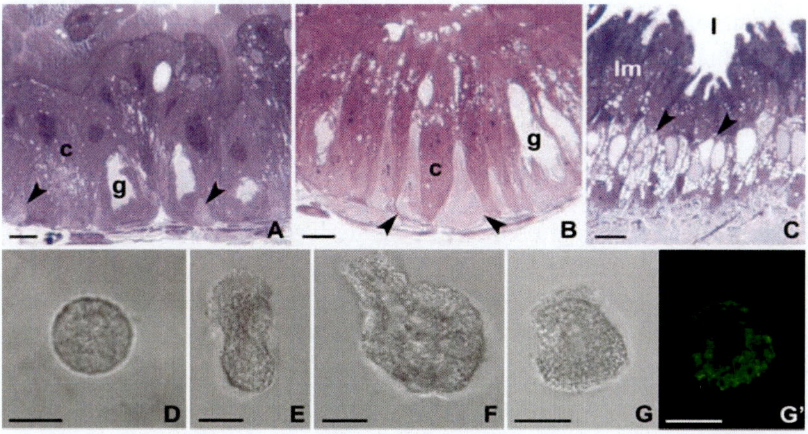

A-C. Cross sections of *B. mori* midgut at different larval stages. **A.** Fourth larval instar. Stem cells (arrowheads) are localized at the base of the midgut epithelium. **B.** Fourth larval moult. Stem cells (arrowheads) proliferate and differentiate into new cells that intercalate among columnar (c) and goblet (g) cells. **C.** Fifth instar. In the prepupal period, stem cells (arrowheads) proliferate underneath the degenerating larval midgut epithelium (lm) and form the new pupal epithelium. l: midgut lumen. Scale bar: 10 μm. **D-G.** Brightfield and confocal laser scanning micrographs of midgut cells in culture. **D.** Typical rounded stem cell. **E.** Mature columnar cell characterized by an apical membrane with well developed microvilli, a centrally placed nucleus and a cylindrical shape. **F.** Mature goblet cell with the typical flask-like shape, the wide cavity, and a basally located nucleus. **G and G'**. Brightfield and confocal laser scanning micrographs (optical sections), respectively, of a columnar cell incubated for 1 h at 25 °C in the presence of 1.4 μM FITC-albumin. The punctuate distribution of FITC-albumin inside the cytoplasm is consistent with a vesicular compartmentalization, which is expected for a protein that is internalized by endocytosis and follows a precise intracellular pathways (Casartelli et al., 2008). Scale bars: 5 μm (D); 10 μm (E-G).

Like in *Drosophila,* in lepidopteran larvae midgut stem cells repair the damaged midgut by replacement [6], maintaining the tissue functional integrity [7]. In addition, it has been long demonstrated that these cells, normally present as single cells during the larval feeding periods (Figure A), proliferate extensively before each moult, forming large nests, or "nidi", and then intercalate between the mature cells of the intestinal monolayer, differentiating into mature columnar and goblet cells during the moult (Figure B) [8, 9]. Besides repair and increase of midgut size along larval growth, stem cells have a key role in the generation of a functional adult midgut. We have recently shown that during the prepupal stage of *Heliothis virescens* larvae, Programmed Cell Death (PCD) events lead to the degradation of the larval midgut monolayer, providing a supply of nutrient molecules that will be readily exploited by the new pupal midgut developing underneath, generated by the massive proliferation and differentiation of stem cells (Figure C) [10].

Although a full comprehension of the mechanisms involved in proliferation and differentiation of midgut stem cells in Lepidoptera is still lacking, in the last fifteen years studies on cultured stem cells derived from the midgut of different lepidopteran species provided several clues on the regulatory factors involved in their proliferation and differentiation, with important outcomes for the setup of primary cultures of midgut cells. Just considering only the most important factors, 20-hydroxyecdysone (20E), that triggers metamorphosis in insects, stimulates the differentiation *in vitro* of stem cells isolated from *Spodoptera littoralis*, while the inactive prohormone ecdysone (E) is very active on their proliferation [11]. 20E also induces the production by the fat body of a Multiplication Factor (MF), a protein that induces the multiplication of stem cells in culture [12]. In Loeb's lab, four different polypeptides that promote differentiation of midgut stem cells have been isolated from midgut cell-conditioned media or pupal hemolymph [13]. These factors, called Midgut Differentiation Factors 1-4 (MDFs 1-4), seem to have partially overlapping functions on midgut stem cells of various Lepidoptera, although the pivotal factor exerting control over stem cell differentiation *in vitro* should be MDF4. The complex interplay of factors regulating proliferation of these stem cells comprehends also α-arylphorin [14], an active mitogen isolated from the fat body, and Bombyxin [15], a member of the insulin family whose source *in vivo* is still unidentified, that acts in concert with α-arylphorin.

Loeb et al. [16] have shown that the administration of these growth factors and insect hormones to stem cells can induce their differentiation towards cell phenotypes identical or similar to those described in larval or pupal midguts *in vivo* and, even more interesting, showed that the cells were sensitive to vertebrate factors like PDGF, EGF and Retinoic Acid, all fundamental for differentiation processes in mammals. These indications are a strong incentive to the identification of insect genes and molecules whose vertebrate counterparts regulate intestinal stem cells.

B. mori can be considered a representative model among Lepidoptera, because of indisputable advantages as a large number of information gathered on its developmental biology, physiology and endocrinology, the availability of numerous genetics and molecular biology tools and a completely sequenced genome.

We have developed a protocol to maintain in culture *B. mori* larval midgut cells, from stem cells to mature cells (Figures D-F). The protocol is described in detail in Cermenati et al. [9], in which all the modifications of the original procedure of Sadrud-Din et al. [17] are specified. Just before the last (fourth) larval-larval moult, stem cells are located in numerous nidi at the base of the epithelium, while during the feeding periods they are few and singly dispersed in the epithelium; therefore, the largest number of stem cells can be isolated in the period just preceding the fourth moult. The stem cells can be easily removed from the surrounding tissue because they are not linked to the other cells by junctions. Following the indications of Sadrud-Din *et al.* [17, 18], with addition of α-arylphorin to the culture medium [14] and the presence of stimulating factors produced by the mature and differentiating cells [13], stable primary cultures of isolated cells in suspension were obtained. A detailed analysis of their evolution with time was performed by counting the different cell types (stem cells, differentiating cells, mature columnar and globlet cells) present since the initial stem cell isolation [9].

Midgut stem cell models *in vivo* are a potent tool to unveil the mechanisms of cell proliferation, differentiation and tissue homeostasis, as recently emphasized by Illa-Bochaca and Montuenga [19]. We believe that the *in vitro* cultured stem cell system from *B. mori* midgut represents a versatile tool to tackle complex issues in different biological contexts that will complement the information acquired by *in vivo* models (*Drosophila, Locusta* and several lepidopterans), exploiting the high degree of conservation of biological processes evidenced to date between these insect species.

Here we will dwell on three topics, that we expect will be of crucial interest in the forthcoming years:

1. *Gut morphogenesis and differentiation.* The presence of ISCs in *Drosophila* has been unambiguously assessed only in recent years, being characterized first in adult fly midgut (mgISCs) [4, 5] and later on in hindgut (hgISCs) [20]. While in the midgut the differentiation of stem cells into enterocytes proceeds from the basal membrane towards the lumen, in the hindgut this renewal process occurs along the antero-posterior axis, with the cells migrating and differentiating from the portion termed hindgut proliferation zone. This latter pattern of proliferation presents large similarities to that occurring within the crypts of mammalian intestine [21]. Subsequent analyses of the signalling

molecules that regulate proliferation and differentiation of stem cells revealed that the similitude of the two systems goes far beyond. In fact, in a fashion similar to the mammalian counterpart, the balance between self-renewal and differentiation of mgISCs is controlled by canonical Wnt and Notch signalling pathways: while Wingless (Wg) is required for the maintenance and proliferation of ISCs, Notch actively controls the determination of the cell fate of ISCs daughter cells. Interestingly, a peculiarity of fly ISCs is that lineage selection and differentiation seem to occur without relying on any identifiable anatomic niche, thus highlighting an active role of stem cells in the cell fate decision of their daughters [22]. These results shed a new light on the importance of this new invertebrate stem cell system. In fact an in depth dissection of the regulatory mechanisms that control crucial phenomena in development will surely benefit from the availability of primary cultures of insect midgut cells, a powerful tool to study biological processes in a simplified experimental context: it will be possible to get further insights into some aspects of Wnt signalling in mammalian crypts [2], to understand the relationships between tissue damage and control of stem cell proliferation [23], and to address some questions about tissue aging and tumour insurgence in the intestine [24].

2. *Dissection of Programmed Cell Death (PCD) processes.* Although the first evidence of the occurrence of PCD processes in midgut cells of insects can be dated back to the '60s, today it is well known that in this tissue two PCD mechanisms are responsible for the disappearance of larval cells at metamorphosis. Besides apoptosis, a second mechanism, namely autophagy, has attracted scientists' attention, making the insect midgut an appealing experimental model to study the regulation of this cell self-eating process. Further, one of the most intriguing and relevant issue that still needs to be addressed is the overlap between apoptosis and autophagy, and more efforts need to be spent to identify the specific regulatory mechanisms and those in common between these two processes. In fact, although some typical apoptotic markers, such as DNA fragmentation and caspase 3 activation, are present in midgut cells at metamorphosis, autophagy represents the most prominent process responsible for the loss of the large majority of cells, as indicated by the increase in lysosomal enzymes, the presence of autophagic compartments [10] and the expression of autophagy specific genes (Cao Y., personal communication). If a co-occurrence of two distinct PCD processes or an

overlap between their signalling pathways occur in this tissue is still an unanswered problem and its solution could serve as a reference for comparative analyses in related biological models. The efficacy of an *in vitro* system to disentangle such an intricate network has been demonstrated in the study of PCD processes in the fat body of Lepidoptera [25]. In the IPLB-LdFB cell line derived from this tissue, it is possible to selectively address cells towards either apoptosis or autophagy, an approach of great help to clarify the dynamics of these two processes. In the literature are reported studies on cultured midgut stem cells from other Lepidoptera, that show perturbations of apoptotic processes induced by 20E [11, 26], a hormone that triggers *in vivo* an increase of the number of lysosomes in midgut stem cells of *B. mori* [26], as well as autophagic processes in *Drosophila* [27]. An appropriate use of activators (e.g. ecdysteroids) and inhibitors of apoptosis and autophagy (e.g. 3-methyladenine and Bafilomycin A1) [28], will allow the manipulation of the two processes also in *B. mori* cultured midgut cells.
Another interesting topic concerns insulin. In fact, members of the insulin family peptides affect the proliferation of lepidopteran cultured stem cells [15] and in *Drosophila* the insulin signalling pathway is critical for ISCs division *in vivo* [23]; moreover, in insects the insulin signalling pathway controlling the nutrition-dependent growth of the cell is strictly coupled to the autophagic process via Target Of Rapamycin (TOR) and Autophagy Gene 1 (ATG1) [29]. We think that these data will be a key starting point for analyzing the links between stem cell proliferation and occurrence of autophagy in midgut cells in culture, derived from stem cell differentiation, under variable nutrient conditions.

3. *Study of midgut cells barrier function.* The movement of orally delivered intact proteins across the digestive system has been shown in numerous insect species (reviewed by Jeffers and Roe [30]). In recent years this field of research has become of particular interest, because a number of proteins with potential insecticide activity has been identified from different biological sources, like viruses, microorganisms, fungi, plants, arthropods (reviewed by Whetstone and Hammock [31]). In most cases, these biopesticides have haemocoelic targets and must pass undegraded the gut barrier to exert their activity when orally administrated. Therefore, an in depth characterization of the mechanisms involved in protein absorption is undoubtedly necessary to develop efficient delivery methods, that would help in reducing the use of broad spectrum chemical

pesticides. As in mammals, the mechanism involved in protein absorption in the midgut of lepidopteran larvae is transcytosis [32, 33], a complex sequence of intracellular events in which the protein is internalized at one pole of the cell membrane and transported by vesicles within the cytoplasm to the plasma membrane at the opposite side. The complete transcellular pathway, i.e. the mechanisms of protein endocytosis, the receptors involved, the cellular compartments implicated in the migration of vesicles along the cytoplasm and the role of cytoskeleton in the entire process, need to be carefully investigated, in order to define possible strategies that would increase the rate of protein permeation across the midgut epithelium. The endocytic mechanism responsible for the internalization of albumin, a protein that crosses the insect midgut by transcytosis [32] has been recently characterized in *B. mori* midgut columnar cells in culture (Figure G-G') [34]. This novel information sheds light on the functional mechanisms of protein absorption in the insect midgut and suggests new opportunities for developing suitable molecular strategies to increase the permeation of proteins through the midgut epithelium. Development of delivery systems to enhance protein movement across the insect digestive system is in its infancy and primary cultures of lepidopteran midgut cells will be a major experimental preparation to improve this field of study.

As highlighted by Whetstone and Hammock [31], viruses have been used for biological control purposes. The arthropods' parvoviruses, named densoviruses, are studied with a renewed interest as potential pest control agents since they are lethal for several insects at larval stages, including agronomical pests and insects vector-borne diseases [35, 36, 37]. However, little is known of the route followed for insect invasion. Since the midgut represents the first barrier that the virus must cross to reach the internal tissues, midgut cells in culture will be an helpful tool to study the infection mechanisms and to optimize the development of viral pesticides.

Finally, isolated midgut cells in culture can also represent a simplified experimental context to study the signalling pathways responsible for mediating and coordinating complex physiological function. It has been recently shown that in the isolated midgut of *Bombyx mori* larvae an increment of cAMP or Ca^{2+} concentration in the cytosol induces the opening of the septate junctions, with a consequent increase of the paracellular permeability [38]. The manipulation of this route may be particularly interesting for the delivery of virulence factors of low molecular weight targeting hemocoelic receptors and therefore the clarification of the signalling cascade and the intracellular effector molecules involved in this process are surely intriguing.

Acknowledgments

The authors are grateful to Prof. Barbara Giordana (Università degli Studi di Milano, Milano, Italia) and Prof. Magda de Eguileor (Università degli Studi dell'Insubria, Varese, Italia) for critically reviewing this manuscript and for their helpful comments. They also thank Prof. Raziel S. Hakim (Howard University, Washington DC, USA) for his support and advise on the preparation of midgut cell cultures and Eleonora Franzetti for image production. G.T.'s work was supported by F.A.R. 2007-2009 grants from the University of Insubria; M.C.'s work was supported by the Italian Ministry of University and Research (PRIN 2006, project n°2006079417).

References

[1] Corley, L.S. and Lavine, M.D. (2006). A review of insect stem cell types. *Semin Cell Dev Biol*, **17**, 510-517

[2] Casali, A. and Batlle, E. (2009). Intestinal stem cells in mammals and Drosophila. *Cell Stem Cell,* **4**, 124-127

[3] Wigglesworth, V.B. (1972). The principles of insect physiology: Digestion and nutrition. *Chapman & Hall.* London, UK; pp 476-552

[4] Micchelli, C.A. and Perrimon, N. (2006). Evidence that stem cells reside in the adult Drosophila midgut epithelium. *Nature*, **439**, 475-479

[5] Ohlstein, B. and Spradling, A. (2006). The adult Drosophila posterior midgut is maintained by pluripotent stem cells. *Nature*, **439**, 470-474

[6] Hakim, R.S.; Baldwin, K.; Smagghe, G. (2010). Regulation of midgut growth, development and metamorphosis. *Annu Rev Entomol*, **55**, 593-608

[7] Spies, A.G.; Spence, K.D. (1985). Effect of sublethal Bacillus thuringiensis crystal endotoxin treatment on the larval midgut of a moth, Manduca: SEM study. *Tissue Cell*, **17**, 379-394

[8] Baldwin, K.M. and Hakim, R.S. (1991). Growth and differentiation of the larval midgut epithelium during molting in the moth Manduca sexta. *Tissue Cell*, **23**, 411-422

[9] Cermenati, G.; Corti, P.; Caccia, S.; Giordana, B. and Casartelli, M. (2007). A morphological and functional characterization of Bombyx mori larval midgut cells in culture. *Invert Survival J* **4**, 119-126

[10] Tettamanti, G.; Grimaldi, A.; Casartelli, M.; Ambrosetti, E.; Ponti, B.; Congiu, T.; Ferrarese, R.; Rivas-Pena, M.L.; Pennacchio, F. and de Eguileor, M. (2007). Programmed cell death and stem cell differentiation are responsible for midgut replacement in Heliothis virescens during prepupal instar. *Cell Tissue Res*, **330**, 345-359

[11] Smagghe, G.; Vanhassel, W.; Moeremans, C.; De Wilde, D.; Goto, S.; Loeb, M.J.; Blackburn, M.B.; Hakim, R.S. (2005). Stimulation of midgut stem cell proliferation and differentiation by insect hormones and peptides. *Ann N Y Acad Sci*, **1040**, 472-475

[12] Smagghe, G.J.; Elsen, K.; Loeb, M.J.; Gelman, DB; Blackburn, M (2003). Effects of a fat body extract on larval midgut cells and growth of lepidoptera. *In Vitro Cell Dev Biol Anim*, **39**, 8-12

[13] Loeb, M.J.; Coronel, ·N.; Natsukawa, D. and Takeda, M. (2004). Implications for the functions of the four known midgut differentiation factors: an immunohistologic study of Heliothis virescens midgut. *Arch Insect Biochem Physiol*, **56**, 7-20

[14] Hakim, R.S.; Blackburn, M.B.; Corti, P.; Gelman, D.B.; Goodman, C.; Elsen, K.; Loeb, M.J.; Lynn, D.; Soin, T. and Smagghe, G. (2007). Growth and mitogenic effects of arylphorin in vivo and in vitro. *Arch Insect Biochem Physiol*, **64**, 63-73

[15] Goto, S.; Loeb, M.J.; Takeda, M. (2005). Bombyxin stimulates proliferation of cultured stem cells derived from Heliothis virescens and Mamestra brassicae larvae. *In Vitro Cell Dev Biol Anim*, **41**, 38-42

[16] Loeb, M.J.; Clark, E.A.; Blackburn, M.; Hakim, R.S.; Elsen, K. and Smagghe, G. (2003). Stem cells from midguts of Lepidopteran larvae: clues to the regulation of stem cell fate. *Arch Insect Biochem Physiol*, **53**, 186-198

[17] Sadrud-Din, S.Y.; Loeb, M.J. and Hakim, R.S. (1996). In vitro differentiation of isolated stem cells from the midgut of Manduca sexta larvae. *J Exp Biol* **199**, 319-325

[18] Sadrud-Din, S.Y.; Hakim, R.S. and Loeb, M.J. (1994). Proliferation and differentiation of midgut cells from Manduca sexta, in vitro. *Invert Reprod Dev* **26**, 197-204

[19] Illa-Bochaca, I. and Montuenga, L.M. (2006). The regenerative nidi of the locust midgut as a model to study epithelial cell differentiation from stem cells. *J Exp Biol*, **209**, 2215-2223

[20] Takashima, S.; Mkrtchyan, M.; Younossi-Hartenstein, A.; Merriam, J.R. and Hartenstein, V. (2008). The behaviour of Drosophila adult hindgut stem cells is controlled by Wnt and Hh signalling. *Nature*, **454**, 651-655

[21] Pitsouli, C and Perrimon, N. (2008). Our fly cousins' gut. *Nature*, **454**, 592-593

[22] Ohlstein, B. and Spradling, A. (2007). Multipotent Drosophila intestinal stem cells specify daughter cell fates by differential notch signaling. *Science*, **315**, 988-992

[23] Amcheslavsky, A.; Jiang, J. and Ip, Y.T. (2009). Tissue damage-induced intestinal stem cell division in Drosophila. *Cell Stem Cell*, **4**, 49-61

[24] Biteau, B.; Hochmuth, C.E. and Jasper, H. (2008). JNK activity in somatic stem cells causes loss of tissue homeostasis in the aging Drosophila gut. *Cell Stem Cell,* 3, 442-455

[25] Tettamanti, G.; Malagoli, D.; Marchesini, E.; Congiu, T.; de Eguileor, M. and Ottavini, E. (2006). Oligomycin A induces autophagy in the IPLB-LdFB insect cell line. *Cell Tissue Res*, **326**, 179-186

[26] Tanaka, Y. and Yukuhiro, F. (1999). Ecdysone has an effect on the regeneration of midgut epithelial cells that is distinct from 20-hydroxyecdysone in the silkworm Bombyx mori. *Gen Comp Endocrinol*, **116**, 382-395

[27] Lee, C.Y.; Cooksey, B.A. and Baehrecke, E.H. (2002). Steroid regulation of midgut cell death during Drosophila development. *Dev Biol*, **250**, 101-111

[28] Rubinsztein, D.C.; Gestwicki, J.E.; Murphy, L.O. and Klionsky, D.J. (2007). Potential therapeutic applications of autophagy. *Nat Rev Drug Discov*, **6**, 304-312

[29] Scott, R.C.; Schuldiner, O.; Neufeld T.P. (2004). Role and regulation of starvation-induced autophagy in the Drosophila fat body. *Dev Cell*, **7**, 167-178

[30] Jeffers, L.A. and Roe, R.M. (2008). The movement of proteins across the insect and tick digestive system. *J Insect Physiol* **54**, 319-332

[31] Whetstone, P.A. and Hammock, B.D. (2007). Delivery methods for peptide and protein toxins in insect control. *Toxicon*, **49**, 576-596

[32] Casartelli, M.; Corti, P.; Leonardi, M.G.; Fiandra, L.; Burlini, N.; Pennacchio, F. and Giordana, B. (2005). Absorption of albumin by the midgut of a lepidopteran larva. *J Insect Physiol*, **51**, 933-940

[33] Casartelli, M.; Corti, P.; Cermenati, G.; Grimaldi, A.; Fiandra, L.; Santo, N.; Pennacchio, F. and Giordana B. (2007). Absorption of horseradish peroxidase in Bombyx mori larval midgut. *J Insect Physiol*, **53**, 517-525

[34] Casartelli, M.; Cermenati, G.; Rodighiero, S.; Pennacchio, F. and Giordana, B. (2008). A megalin-like receptor is involved in protein endocytosis in the midgut of an insect (Bombyx mori, Lepidoptera). *Am J Physiol*, **295**, R1290-R1300

[35] Bergoin, M. and Tijssen, P. (2008) *Encyclopedia of Virology: Parvoviruses of Arthropods.* (B.W.J. Mahy and M.H.V. Van Regenmortel, Editors). Elsevier; Oxford, UK; pp 76-85

[36] Carlson, J.; Suchman, E. and Buchatsky, L. (2006). Densoviruses for control and genetic manipulation of mosquitoes. *Adv Virus Res*, **68**, 361-392

[37] El-Far, M.; Li, Y.; Fediere, G.; Abol-Ela, S. and Tijssen, P. (2004). Lack of infection of vertebrate cells by the densovirus from the maize worm Mythimna loreyi (MlDNV). *Virus Res*, **99**, 17-24

[38] Fiandra, L.; Casartelli, M. and Giordana, B. (2006). The paracellular pathway in the lepidopteran larval midgut: modulation by intracellular mediators. *Comp Biochem Physiol*, **144A**, 464-473

In: Pluripotent Stem Cells
Editors: D.W. Rosales et al, pp. 185-190
ISBN: 978-1-60876-738-0

Chapter 8

ARE EMBRYONIC STEM CELLS REALLY NEEDED FOR REGENERATIVE MEDICINE?

David T. Harris*
Dept. Immunobiology, The University of Arizona, Tucson, AZ 85724

Abstract

It is estimated that as many as 1 in 3 individuals in the United States might benefit from regenerative medicine therapy. Most regenerative medicine therapies have been postulated to require the use of embryonic stem (ES) cells for optimal effect. Unfortunately, ES cell therapies are currently limited by ethical, political, regulatory, and most importantly biological hurdles. These limitations include the inherent allogenicity of this stem cell source and the accompanying threat of immune rejection. Even with use of the rapidly developing iPS technology, the issues of low efficiency of ES/iPS derivation and the threat of teratoma formation limit ES applications directly in patients. The time and cost of deriving and validating mature, differentiated tissues for clinical use further restricts its use to a small number of well-to-do patients with a limited number of afflictions. Thus, for the foreseeable future, the march of regenerative medicine to the clinic for widespread use will depend upon the development of non-ES cell therapies. Current sources of non-ES cells easily available in large numbers can be found in the bone marrow, adipose tissue and umbilical cord blood. Each of these types of stem cells has already begun to be utilized to treat a variety of diseases.

* E-mail address: davidh@email.arizona.edu

For the past decade a political debate has raged regarding the derivation and use of embryonic stem cells for regenerative medicine. The fervour and seriousness of the debate has led the public to believe that their government was deliberately keeping life-saving medical advances from them, thanks to the influence of a small partisan group of conservative advocates. Regardless of one's political persuasion, this long-running debate has at least served to increase awareness of the medical potential of stem cells. Hopefully, this increased awareness will also lead to increased funding, which remains to be seen. Unfortunately, the debate (much of which was led by non-scientists on both sides) has also unreasonably raised expectations of wonder treatments and cures that cannot be readily met.

Embryonic stem (ES) cells (including induced pluripotent stem [or iPS] cells) have been touted as the holy grail of regenerative medicine therapies, while other viable alternatives have been overlooked and disregarded. Now, with many of the political and funding obstacles for ES cell use recently removed from the scientific arena (due to a change in political regime and the development of iPS technology), the question remains as to whether there will be a significant role for non-ES cells in such regenerative therapies? To answer that question, one should be cognizant of the fact that ES and iPS cells have numerous biological roadblocks and limitations that significantly hinder their passage to the clinic and rapid access to patients in need.

The first such limitation is the inherent allogenicity for many versions of this stem cell source and the accompanying threat of immune rejection. To date, most ES cells have been derived by methods that utilize donor oocytes or embryos. Even after nuclear transfer or therapeutic cloning, the derived ES cell is allogeneic to the patient being treated. As life-long immunosuppression is neither desirable nor therapeutically possible in many instances, the need to create patient-specific (i.e., "tissue-matched") ES cells has recently been addressed by the development of induced pluripotentcy methods (i.e., iPS cells) (Byrne et al, 2007; Park et al, 2008). Although the threat of immune rejection can be overcome by derivation of iPS cells directly from patients, the threat of teratoma formation is omnipresent as shown in a recent clinical report (Amariglio et al, 2009). It seems that any type of ES (or iPS) cell that is used directly in patients without prior differentiation of the ES/iPS cells into the desired tissue poses a significant chance of tumor induction. Stem cell tumorigenicity represents the major obstacle to safe regenerative medicine when using either ES or iPS cells. Even with iPS cells, the malignant tumor incidence in chimeric mice constructed with such iPS cells has been observed to be 20% or higher. Recent studies have also shown that construction of iPS cells without the use of Myc still results in tumor formation, implying that the reprogramming process may also activate endogenous oncogenes. It seems that the greater the pluripotency and self-renewal potential of a cell, the greater the potential for tumorigenicity. In fact, the probability of tumor formation is higher for iPS cells than with typical ES cells due to the lack of immune mismatch that might trigger some rejection (reviewed in Knoepfler, 2009). Further, this derivation (and the accompanying validation) process involves large amounts of time and monies, as well as invoking multiple regulatory issues.

It is important to note that for many patients not only will autologous cells and tissues be required, but these tissues must be delivered in a timely fashion for optimal therapeutic benefit. For example, it does little good to wait 2-6 months after a stroke to attempt to replace or rescue damaged nervous tissue and brain function. The requirement for "autologous" stem cells and the inability to derive differentiated cell lines or tissues from newly created patient-specific ES/iPS cells in time to meet the treatment "window" required for successful therapies does not seem to have an answer at this time. At its best, derivation of iPS cell lines requires approximately 1 month of time, differentiation of those iPS cells into a desired tissue requires another month of time, and expansion, validation and purification of those tissues will require an additional 1-3 months of time (Condic and Rao, 2008). Once again, it cannot be overemphasized that when a patient suffers a heart attack or a stroke, these patients require therapy within days if not hours. As most patients will present with a limited time to treat, and as creation of patient-specific ES or iPS cell lines can be expected to require months of effort at best, such an ES/iPS-based therapy should have significant limitations.

There really is a "golden hour" of treatment for most patients, similar to what is seen in stroke patients. Although this "golden hour" may actually be a "golden" day or week or even a year, it is not forever. One must generally treat patients within a confined window of time for the therapy to be effective. That is, once tissue has died and scar tissue has formed, there is very little than can be accomplished. At this time stem cells cannot make their way into the damaged tissue to replace the portion that has been affected or stimulate endogenous repair. Further, reintegration of new tissue at this time would also seem to be problematic. Re-integration of "new" nervous tissue would not necessarily mean re-establishment of memory, personality, etc. as these qualities come from personal experience. Therefore, the most optimal therapeutic approach would seem to be a rescue, or minimal tissue replacement, early on after injury mediated by timely stem cell delivery.

Finally, the overall costs of overcoming each of these limitations must be passed on to either the patient or third-party payers, which ultimately will be the major limiting factor for the progress of ES/iPS cell therapies to the clinic and access to the population in general. It has been conservatively estimated that derivation of each patient-specific ES/iPS cell line/differentiated tissue will cost in the neighborhood of $50,000. A portion of these costs is due to the inherent low efficiency in both ES and iPS derivation. ES cell derivation may require as many as 200 oocytes to derive a single ES cell line (I. Rogers, University of Toronto, personal communication). In general, somatic cell reprogramming by non-viral means occurs at frequencies that are 100-fold lower than with integrating viral vectors. However, recent use of transposons has raised the frequencies to 0.1-1% (similar to viral vectors). The problem remains that one must perform clonal analyses afterwards to identify integration-free, correctly excised clones and insure that no chromosomal rearrangements or point mutations have occurred (Stadtfeld & Hochedlinger, 2009). Directed differentiation is also a very inefficient process and is never 100% successful in driving all the iPS cells to differentiate. It is very difficult to fully and completely differentiate ES/iPS cells to mature cells and tissues, such that the possibility of tumor formation is completely eliminated. Multiple studies in animals have shown tumor formation after implantation of differentiated ES/iPS cells. (Condic & Rao, 2008.). Therefore, even using the transposon approach for iPS generation, all iPS cell lines would need to be cloned and tested for the effects of DNA damage, changes in imprinting and epigenetic changes. (Condic & Rao, 2008.). These stem cells would then require differentiation, followed by some method of additional purification in order to pass FDA and RAC regulatory hurdles; again adding to the time and costs involved. Due to the costs, it is difficult to believe that very many patients would be able to afford to create and bank their own ES or iPS cells, and tissues, in advance of future needs.

It has been postulated that to economize the process it might be possible to create iPS cell banks representing most HLA haplotypes (i.e., tissue types) in the population at large. These banks would then be financed by the nation as a national inventory for anyone's use. However, one must realize, based on the last 30 years of stem cell and organ transplants in a variety of patients, that perfect matching is essential to prevent rejection (and other side-effects). The odds of identifying any two individuals with a 6/6 HLA (i.e., tissue) match ranges from 1 in 40,000 to 1 in 80,000 depending on the ethnicity of the two individuals (Harris, 1998). Therefore, to assure a high probability of locating matches for most patients in need, one would require multi-ethnic iPS banks containing upwards of 1-million total samples (at a cost of $50,000 each, a total of more than 1 trillion dollars). Finally, it is not assured that minor histocompatability antigens that would not typed or considered for matching, would not be capable of eliciting immune reactions as observed for many organ transplant patients (Yamanaka,

2009). The estimate that a million ES lines would be needed to eliminate the need for lifelong immunosuppression would be far in excess of the number of spare embryos approved for use, thus making ES cell derivation impractical (not to mention the fact that ES cells created by SCNT would still express histocompatability genes derived from mitochondrial DNA of the egg donor, and serve as a rejection molecule; Condic & Rao, 2008.). Thus, iPS cells would be the only recourse and the only pluripotent cells that would be truly autologous and might be amenable to such tissue banking, but costs again make this approach impractical. Thus, ES and iPS cell banks are not the answer to making regenerative medicine readily available to the public.

In order for regenerative medicine therapies to be successfully transitioned to the general public, one must identify an autologous source of stem cells that can be obtained from the patient, which is easily and economically harvested or derived, and contains large numbers of stem cells. The stem cells could be either multipotent or pluripotent, depending upon the desired use. Finally, the stem cell based therapy must be as successful as current therapy and must be significantly less expensive. Otherwise, "big pharma" and third-party payers will not agree to fund the development and reimbursement of such therapies, even if such treatments hold greater promise than currently used approaches. Thus, it seems that non-embryonic (and non-iPS) stem cells are the only stem cells that meet these requirements. Stem cells found in umbilical cord blood, bone marrow and adipose tissue seem to be ideal solutions to these problems. Each of these stem cell sources can be harvested directly from patients, in a technically simple and economical fashion, in large stem cell numbers. Bone marrow stem cells have been used in clinical trials for patients with cardiovascular disease and for patients with brain injury. Adipose-derived stem cells have also been used in patients with cardiovascular disease as well as in orthopedic applications. In particular, umbilical cord blood stem cells and umbilical cord blood-based therapies seem to be the most ideal source to meet these requirements as compared to the other two stem cell sources. We believe that cord blood stem cells are the best alternative to ES and iPS cells in that these stem cells appear poised between embryonic and adult stem cells, capable of being utilized in many of the same applications claimed for ES and iPS cells, including cardiac, neurological, orthopedic and ophthalmic applications. Further, cord blood stem cells have already make their way into the clinic, being utilized in regenerative medicine approaches to type 1 diabetes, cerebral palsy and brain injury (Harris & Rogers, 2007; Harris et al, 2008; Harris, 2008; Harris, 2009). For additional information on this topic please see the recent reviews by Harris and colleagues (Harris & Rogers, 2007; Harris et al, 2008; Harris, 2008; Harris, 2009).

References

Amariglio, N., Hirshberg, A., Scheithauer, B.W., Cohen, Y., Loewenthal, R., Trakhtenbrot, L., Paz, N., Koren-Michowitz, M., Waldman, D., Leider-Trejo, L., Toren, A., Constantini, S., and G Rechavil, G. Donor-Derived Brain Tumor Following Neural Stem Cell Transplantation in an Ataxia Telangiectasia Patient. *PLoS Medicine*, **6**(2), 1-11, 2009.

Byrne, J., Pedersen, D., Clepper, L., Nelson, M., Sanger, W., Gokhale, S., Wolf, D., and Mitalipov, S. Producing primate embryonic stem cells by somatic cell nuclear transfer. *Nature*, **450** (7169), 497-502, 2007.

Condic, ML and Rao, M. Regulatory issues for personalized pluripotent cells. *Stem Cells* **26**: 2753-2758, 2008.

Harris, D.T. Cord Blood Banking: The University of Arizona Experience : Successes, Problems and Cautions. *Cancer Research Therapy and Control.* 7:63-67, 1998

Harris, D.T. and Rogers, I. Umbilical cord blood: a unique source of pluripotent stem cells for regenerative medicine. *Current Stem Cell Research and Therapy*, **2:** 301-309, 2007.

Harris, D.T., Badowski, M, Ahmad, N and Gaballa, M. The Potential of Cord Blood Stem Cells for Use in Regenerative Medicine**.** *Expert Opinion on Biological Therapy* **7**(9): 1311-1322, 2008.

Harris, D.T. Cord Blood Stem Cells: A Review of Potential Neurological Applications. *Stem Cell Reviews* **4**(4), 269-274, 2008.

Harris, D.T. Non-Haematological Uses of Cord Blood Stem Cells, *British Journal of Haematology,* In Press, 2009.

Knoepfler, P.S. Deconstructing stem cell tumorigenicity: a roadmap to safe regenerative medicine. *Stem Cell.* **27**: 1050-1056, 2009.

Park, I.H., Lerou, P.H., Zhao, R., Huo, H. and Daley, G.Q. Generation of human-induced pluripotent stem cells. *Nature Protocols*, **3**, 1180–1186, 2008.

Stadtfeld, M and Hochedlinger, K. Without a trace? PiggyBac-ing towards pluripotency. *Nature Methods* **6**(5): 329-330, 2009.

Yamanaka, S. A fresh look at iPS cells. *Cell* **137**: 13-17, 2009.

In: Pluripotent Stem Cells ISBN 978-1-60876-738-0
Editors: D.W. Rosales et al, pp. 191-211

Chapter 9

GENETIC STABILITY OF MURINE PLURIPOTENT AND SOMATIC HYBRID CELLS MAY BE AFFECTED BY CONDITIONS OF THEIR CULTIVATION

Shramova Elena Ivanovna, Larionov Oleg Alekseevich, Khodarovich Yurii Mikhailovich and Zatsepina Olga Vladimirovna*
Shemyakin and Ovchinnikov Institute of Bioorganic Chemistry, Russian Academy of Sciences

Abstract

Using mouse pluripotent teratocarcinoma PCC4aza1 cells and proliferating spleen lymphocytes we obtained a new type of hybrids, in which marker lymphocyte genes were suppressed, but expression the *Oct-4* gene was not effected; the hybrid cells were able to differentiate to cardiomyocytes. In order to specify the environmental factors which may affect the genetic stability and other hybrid properties, we analyzed the total chromosome number and differentiation potencies of hybrids respectively to conditions of their cultivation. Particular attention was paid to the number and transcription activity of chromosomal nucleolus organizing regions (NORs), which harbor the most actively transcribed – ribosomal – genes. The results showed that the hybrids obtained are characterized

*Corresponding Address: ul. Mikluho-Maklaya, 16/10, Moscow 117997, Russia; Tel: +7-495-3306465; Fax: +7-495-3350812

by a relatively stable chromosome number which diminished less than in 5% during 27 passages. However, a long-term cultivation of hybrid cells in non-selective conditions resulted in preferential elimination of some NO-chromosomes, whereas the number of active NORs per cell was increased due to activation of latent NORs. On the contrary, in selective conditions, i.e. in the presence of hypoxantine, aminopterin and thymidine, the total number of NOR-bearing chromosomes was not changed, but a partial inactivation of remaining NORs was observed. The higher number of active NORs directly correlated with the capability of hybrid cells for differentiation to cardiomyocytes.

Keywords: PCC4aza1 cells, mouse splenocytes, tetraploid hybrids, chromosomes, nucleolus organizing regions, FISH, Ag-NOR, reprogramming, differentiation, cardiomyocytes.

1. Introduction

The term 'nuclear reprogramming' is currently understood as the process of modification of the gene expression pattern specific for a cell that leads to a change of the cell properties and phenotype [1]. Reprogramming can be induced by transfer of a somatic cell nucleus to an enucleated oocyte (the nuclear transfer method) [2], by introduction in the differentiated cells of specific factors responsible for the nuclear reprogramming by the use of retroviruses [3, 4], or by *in vitro* hybridization of a pluripotent or a multipotent cell with a differentiated somatic cell [5]. In the last case, embryonic stem (ES) cells and embryonal carcinoma (EC) cells are the most often used as the starting material for fusion with somatic cells. Fusion of the parental cells is achieved in the presence of polyethylene glycol, inactivated Sendai virus or by electric pulses, and is followed by cultivation of the cells in selective medium. The choice of selective conditions is directed by the properties of parental cells and is aimed to eliminate non-fused cells within the first 3–5 days after fusion [6, 7]. During the last years, various types of reconstructed hybrids between ES or EC cells and somatic cells have been obtained [6-13]. In such hybrids the key somatic genes become repressed, whereas the majority of pluripotent or multipotent cell genes, including *Oct-4*, remain expressed.

EC cells belong to the tumor-forming stem cells which possess a significant similarity to cells of early (preimplantation) embryos [14]. They are capable to develop teratocarcinomas in isogenic animals, are included in various tissues of an adult organism [15], and in the presence of inducers can differentiate into embryoid bodies, neuronal cells and cardiomyocytes *in vitro* [16]. Unlike ES cells, EC cells do not demand special culture conditions and thus are more convenient for obtaining intercellular hybrids and analyzing their properties. The study of EC cells hybrids provides many new insights into the mechanisms of differentiation, relationship between pluripotency and tumor genesis, to examine the fundamental mechanisms of the somatic genome reprogramming, and to analyze the impact of environmental conditions on stability and other properties of hybrid cells.

In the present work, we obtained for the first time the stable hybrids between a proliferating mouse spleen lymphocyte and an EC PCC4aza1 cell. We showed that the genetic stability and differentiation potencies of PCC4aza1$\times$ lymphocyte hybrid cells may be affected by conditions of their cultivation. A few parameters, including the total number of chromosomes and the number and activity of chromosomal nucleolus organizing regions (NORs) have been evaluated. NORs are specific chromosomal loci, where ribosomal genes (rDNA) encoding 18S, 5.8S and 28S rRNA are harbored, in interphase NORs give rise to the functional nucleoli. Ribosomal genes belong to the most actively transcribed genes in eukaryotes, and the level of rDNA transcription is strictly dependent on accessibility of cells to growth factors and cell ploidy [17]. One may expect therefore that the genome reprogramming will result in some assignable changes in the status of chromosomal NORs. However, to the best of our knowledge, the activity and number of NORs as a function of conditions and duration of hybrid cells culturing so far have not been studied.

In the genotype of *Mus musculus* several NO-bearing chromosomes, 12, 15, 16, 18 and 19, are present, but generally only three NORs are transcriptionally active [18]. Active NORs differ from inactive ones by their tight association with the RNA polymerase I transcription complex which has a high affinity to Ag^+ ions and can therefore be revealed by chromosome staining with $AgNO_3$ [19]. The number of active Ag-NORs is used as a measure of activity of rRNA synthesis and cellular metabolism in general [20]. In our study we determined the total number of NO-chromosomes by fluorescence hybridization *in situ* (FISH) with mouse rDNA probes, and compared it with the number of Ag-positive (i.e., active) NORs in PCC4aza1$\times$lymphocyte hybrids at various passages and upon different conditions of cell culturing. Our results show that selective conditions (medium with hypoxantine, aminopterin and thymidine (HAT)) promote inactivation of NORs, but do not affect the number of NO-bearing chromosomes. In contrary, in non-selective medium (i.e. medium without HAT) NO-chromosomes are eliminated, but the total number of active NORs is increased. Noteworthy, differentiation potencies of the hybrids were directly correlated with the number of active NORs.

2. Materials and Methods

2.1. Cells Cultures

All cells used in this study were cultured at 37 °C, 5% CO_2 and in humid atmosphere. Murine embryonal teratocarcinoma PCC4aza1 cells (*hprt*$^-$) were purchased from the Institute of Cytology of the Russian Academy of Sciences (the Russian Cell Culture Collection, St. Petersburg, Russia). The cells of this line have normal mouse karyotype (2n=40). Cells were grown in DMEM medium (PanEco, Russia) containing 8% bovine fetal serum (HyClone, USA) and antibiotics at standard concentrations. To prevent spontaneous differentiation the cells were reseeded every 48 hours.

Mouse spleen cells were isolated from CBA×C57BL/6 F_1 one-and-a half year old male following the standard procedure [21]. Lymphocytes were placed in α-MEM medium (Sigma, USA) containing 15% fetal bovine serum (HyClone) at concentration 10^6 cell/ml. To activate proliferation, the medium was supplemented with 3 μg/ml concanavalin A (PanEco) and 5 μM 5-azacytidine (Sigma) for 5 days.

2.2. Obtaining of Hybrid Cells

PCC4aza1 cells and activated lymphocytes were mixed in a ratio of 1:5 in the presence of 45% polyethylene glycol (PEG, MW 1450, Sigma), 10% dimethyl sulfoxide (DMSO, PanEco) and DMEM medium for 1 min. The cells were then transferred to a HAT-containing medium (10^{-4} M hypoxantine, 7×10^{-7} M aminopterin and 10^{-5} M thymidine, Flow Laboratories, UK) for 24 hours, and then transferred to a medium without HAT. Incubation of PCC4aza1 cells in HAT-containing medium resulted in death of all the cells within 24 hours.

2.3. Polymerase Chain Reaction (PCR)

Genome DNA for PCR was isolated using SiO_2-coated magnetic particles by the usage of approximately 10^6 cells per isolation. PCR was carried out in 10 μl of a reaction mix containing 2 mM $MgCl_2$, 1 unit of Taq DNA-polymerase, 200 μM of each dNTP, primers (for microsatellite markers D1Mit155, D2Mit30, D6Mit15, D6Mit102, D7Mit145, D7Mit178, D8Mit4; for RT-PCR Oct4_(F/R), Act_(F/R), CD11_(F/R), CD45_(F/R)) in the final concentration of 1 pmol/μl and 0.2-1 μg DNA or cDNA. The annealing temperature and elongation time were optimized for the each primer pair used. Parameters for denaturation and elongation reactions were adjusted based on the standard parameters for Taq polymerase functioning. The primer sequences used for PCR microsatellite analysis are listed in Table 1.

Table 1. Primers* used for the microsatellite analysis of PCC4aza1×lymphocyte hybrids, PCC4aza1 cells (originated from the mouse strain 129/Ola) and of mouse spleen lymphocytes (obtained from a CBA×C57BL/6 F_1 mice).

Microsatellite marker (chromosome)	Primers sequences (from 5' to 3' ends)	Lengths of the PCR-fragments for the 129/Ola line, CBA line or C57BL/6 line, respectively, bp
D1Mit155 (1)	ATGCATGCATGCACACGT ACCGTGAAATGTTCACCCAT	252 and 216 (CBA), 252 (C57BL/6)
D2Mit30 (2)	CATCCAAGCAGTAACGTAGACG AAATGTTACACCCTCTGCGG	280 and 136 (CBA), 320 (C57BL/6)
D6Mit15 (6)	CACTGACCCTAGCACAGCAG TCCTGGCTTCCACAGGTACT	170 and 195 (CBA)
D6Mit102 (6)	CCATGTGGATATCTTCCCTTG GTATACCCAGTTGTAAATCTTGTGTG	177 and 145 (C57BL/6)
D7Mit145 (7)	CAGGTGACCTTGGTCATGG AGAGCCCAGGGGTTTTAAGA	148 and 200 (C57BL/6)
D7Mit178 (7)	ACCTCTGATTTCAGAACCCTTG TAGAGAGCCACTAGCATATCATAACC	165 and 210 (C57BL/6)
D8Mit4 (8)	CCAACTCATCCCCAAAGGTA GTATGTTCAAGGCTGGGCAT	156 and 195 (CBA), 156 (C57BL/6)

*The primer sequences were selected using the data base provided by Jackson Laboratory, Bar Harbor, Maine, USA (www.informatics.jax.org).

Expression of *Oct4* and *β-actin* genes was analyzed using the following pairs of primers: Oct4_F (5'-GGAGCTAGAACAGTTTGC-3'), Oct4_R (5'-CTTCCTCCACCCACTTC-3') and Act_F (5'-GAAATCGTGCGTGACATC-

AAAG-3'), Act_R (5'-TGTAGTTTCATGGATGCCACAG-3'), respectively. To analyze the expression of *CD11* and *CD45* genes which are markers of T-lymphocytes the following primer pairs were used: CD11_F (5'-ACA-CTGTGGCCTGGATGACCTC-3'), CD11_R (5'-GGTAAGTGAACACTC-GGCCTCC-3') and CD45_F (5'-GCGAAGGAAAGCAGACTTATGGAG-3'), CD45_R (5'-CGAGGATGGATGCATGCTTGTG-3').

Total RNA was isolated from 10^6 cells using the YellowSolve kit (Sileks, Russia). The RT-PCR reaction was carried out using a kit for the first cDNA chain synthesis and a mixture of random hexaprimers (Sileks).

2.4. Isolation of Metaphase Plates

Adhesive cells were synchronized at metaphase by incubation with 50 ng/ml nocodazol (Sigma) for 1–2 hours, treated with 0.56% KCl for 10 min at 37 °C and fixed in a mixture of absolute methanol and glacial acetic acid (3:1) at -20 °C for 3 hours. Spleen lymphocytes were also synchronized at metaphase by means of nocodazol, collected by centrifugation, incubated with 0.56% KCl and fixed by the same way as adhesive cells. The cells were dropped onto wet microscope slides, and the quality of metaphase plates was controlled under an ICM 405 (Opton, Germany) microscope. The preparations were stored at room temperature for up to one month.

2.5. Probes used for Fluorescent *in situ* Hybridization

Two probes for murine rDNA used in the study are depicted in Fig. 1. Probe 1 (the *Eco*RI-*Eco*RI fragment of rDNA, 6.6 kbp, from +5.635 to +12.235) contains a part of the 18S rDNA sequence, the first internal transcribed spacer (ITS1), 5.8S rDNA, the second internal transcribed spacer (ITS2) and about 80% of the 28S rDNA sequence. Probe 2 (an *Eco*RI-*Eco*RI fragment of rDNA, 4.3 kbp, from +12.235 to +16.535) encodes the remaining part of the 28S rDNA and the 3' external transcribed spacer (3'ETS). The rDNA fragments were labeled with digoxigenin by nick translation using the Dig-Nick-Translation Mix (Roche, France) following the manufacturers recommendations.

2.6. Fluorescence *in situ* Hybridization

Fluorescence *in situ* hybridization was performed as described earlier [22]. Chromosome preparations were treated with 100 μg/ml RNase A in a 2× SSC-

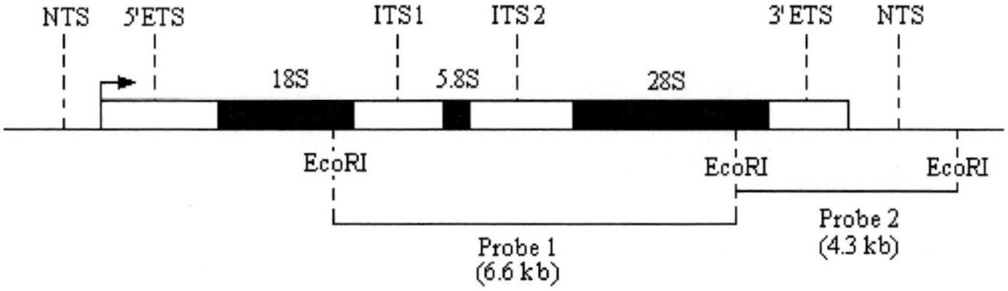

Figure 1. The scheme of the mouse ribosomal repeat and rDNA probes used for fluorescence *in situ* hybridization. NTS – intergenic non-transcribed spacer; 5'ETS – 5'-external transcribed spacer; ITS1 and ITS2 – the first and second internal transcribed spacers correspondingly; 3'ETS – 3'-external transcribed spacer; *Eco*RI – sites of *Eco*RI restriction.

buffer (0.3 M NaCl; 0.03 M sodium citrate, pH 7.3) for 1 h at 37 °C, and then with 0.01% pepsin in 0.05 M sodium citrate, (pH 2.0) for 2–4 min at ambient temperature. Preparations were washed in PBS, dried and incubated with hybridization mixture containing 10–25 ng/μl labeled rDNA, 50% deionized formamide and 10% dextransulfate in 2× SSC. Denaturation of the rDNA probes and specimens was made simultaneously at 85 °C for 10 min. *In situ* hybridization was performed at 37 °C for 16–18 hours. Specimens were washed in 50% formamide in 4× SSC/Tween 20 buffer at 42 °C for 10 min, then in 2× SSC for 10 min at room temperature, incubated with rhodamine-conjugated antibodies to digoxigenin, stained with 1 μg/ml Hoechst 33342 for 10 min at room temperature and mounted in Mowiol (Calbiochem, USA). Samples were examined under an Axiovert 200 microscope (Carl Zeiss, Germany) equipped with a 100× PlanApochromat objective (numerical aperture 1.3). The images were recorded by means of a 12-bit monochrome CCD camera CoolSnap$_{cf}$ (Roper Scientific, USA) and processed using Adobe Photoshop software (version 7.0).

2.7. Ag-NOR Staining of Chromosomes

Revealing active NORs of chromosomes was performed according Howell and Black [19]. Two parts of 50% $AgNO_3$ in bidistilled water and one part of 2% gelatin containing 1% formic acid were placed onto a slide with cells. Specimen incubated at 37 °C for 15 min, thoroughly washed in distilled water, counterstained with 1 μg/ml Hoechst 33342 and mounted in Mowiol. The preparations were then studied as described above.

2.8. Differentiation of Hybrid Cells *in vitro*

For differentiation the hybrid cells were seeded in Petri dishes at about 10^5 cells/ml and cultivated during 5 days with 1% DMSO and then without DMSO. Medium was changed every two days. Endodermal-like cells revealed on 6–7 days after differentiation starting. After 7–8 days after DMSO removal isles of beating cells appeared on substrate. Mitochondria were stained by adding to culture media 6 ng/ml rhodamine 6G for 15 min. The cells were then examined under a light microscope BH2 (Olympus, Japan) using a 60× water-immersion objective U PlanApochromat (Olympus, model UPLAPO60×W/1.2, numerical aperture 1.2).

2.9. Statistical Analysis

Correlations were evaluated by simple linear regression analysis. A P value $<0.05\%$ was considered to be significant.

3. Results

3.1. Hybridization of Cells

The hybrids described in this study have been obtained by fusion of mouse EC teratocarcinoma PCC4aza1 cells with proliferating spleen cells of a (CBA× C57BL/6) F_1 mouse adult male. They maintained the morphology of PCC4aza1 cells but were lager in size (Fig. 2A, B). In nuclei of the hybrid cells up to ten nucleoli were clearly seen; PCC4aza1 cells and activated spleen lymphocytes generally contained one or two nucleoli (Fig. 2A, B). PCR analysis of the marker microsatellite sequences for several chromosomes (numbers 1, 2, 6, 7 and 8) showed that at early passages PCC4aza1×lymphocyte hybrids contain chromosomes of the both parental cell types (Fig. 3).

It is known that conditions of culturing have a profound impact on the properties EC cells and EC cells hybrids [6, 23, 24]. To examine whether this regularity is also true for our hybrids, at the 17th passage (i.e., about three weeks)

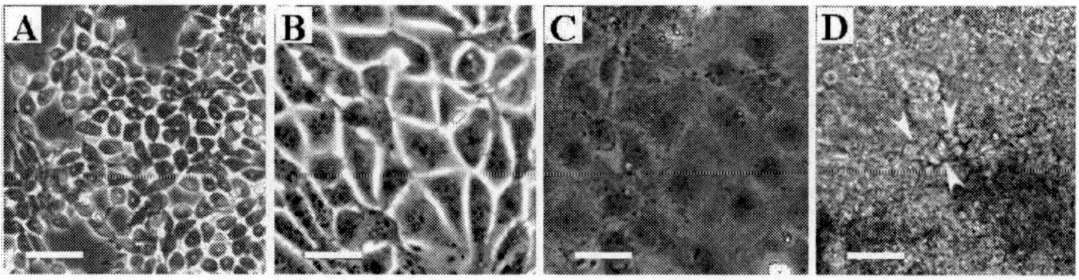

Figure 2. The phenotype of PCC4aza1 cells (A) and PCC4aza1×lymphocyte hybrids in non-selective conditions at the 25th passage of growth (B, C, D). B — non-differentiated hybrid cells; C, D — hybrid cells differentiated to endodermal-like cells (C) or cardiomyocytes (D) in the presence of 1% DMSO. Size bar, 50 μm.

after fusion a portion of hybrid cells were transferred to culture medium supplemented with HAT, and the other cells were continued growing in non-selective medium.

In selective medium the morphology of hybrid cells remained similar to that of hybrids which were cultured without HAT. However, under selective conditions the time period for duplication of the cell number was equal to 24 h, whereas without HAT — to 16 h; the duplication rate of PCC4aza1 cells was about 11 h. The mitotic index of hybrids cultured without HAT was 11.3±1.6%, but with HAT it was diminished to 7.8±2.2%. These observations showed that selective medium inhibits proliferation activity of the obtained hybrid cells.

3.2. Reprogramming of Somatic Genes in Hybrid Cells

Analysis of expression of the lymphocyte marker genes *CD11* and *CD45* in PCC4aza1×lymphocyte hybrids showed that these genes remained not functional in the presence of HAT and without HAT (Fig. 4). These observations evidenced in favor of reprogramming of the lymphocyte nucleus under exposure to factors present in a PCC4aza1 cell. However, similar to teratocarcinoma PCC4aza1 cells, hybrid cells continued to express *Oct4* that is a gene marker of pluripotent cells [11] (Fig. 4).

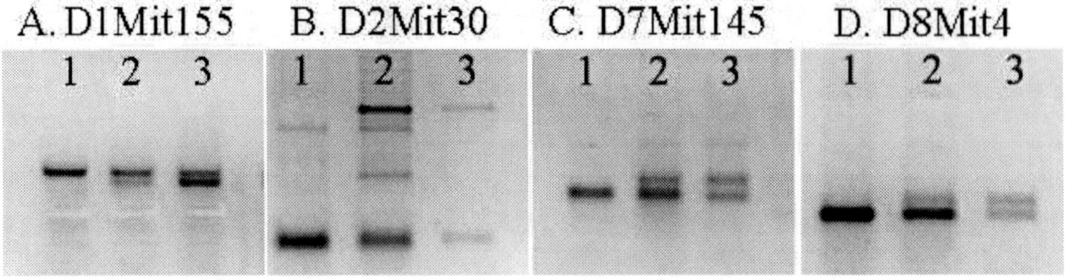

Figure 3. The microsatellite PCR analysis of the chromosomes number 1 (A), 2 (B), 7 (C) and 8 (D) in the mouse strains used to obtain PCC4aza1 cells (129/Ola) and spleen lymphocytes (CBA×C57BL/6). DNA was isolated from PCC4aza1 cells (1), PCC4aza1×lymphocyte hybrids (2), and spleen lymphocytes (3). The length of PCR products for the marker D1Mit155 microsatellite: 252 bp (129/Ola), 216 bp (CBA) and 252 bp (C57BL/6); for the D2Mit30 microsatellite: 280 bp (129/Ola), 136 bp (CBA), and 320 bp (C57BL/6); for the D7Mit145 microsatellite: 148 bp (129/Ola), 148 bp (CBA) and 200 bp (C57BL/6); for the D8Mit4 microsatellite: 156 bp (129/Ola), 195 bp (CBA), and 156 bp (C57BL/6).

3.3. Influence of Selective Medium on the Chromosome Stability in Hybrid Cells

Assessment of the total chromosome number in metaphase plates of PCC4aza1×lymphocyte hybrids grown in non-selective medium showed that at late (25–27th) passages hybrid cells contained an average of 74 (74.4±2.2) chromosomes (Table 2). At the late (26–30th) passages in selective conditions hybrid cells contained an average of 76 (76.1±1.7) chromosomes. As far as these values do not differ statistically significantly, we concluded that conditions of cell culturing have a low impact on the total number of chromosomes in the obtained hybrids. However, the karyotype of the obtained hybrids was not entirely stable: during three months hybrid cells lost four (in selective conditions) or six (in non-selective conditions) chromosomes that is equal to 5–8% of the total chromosome number expected in PCC4aza1×lymphocyte hybrids (Table 2).

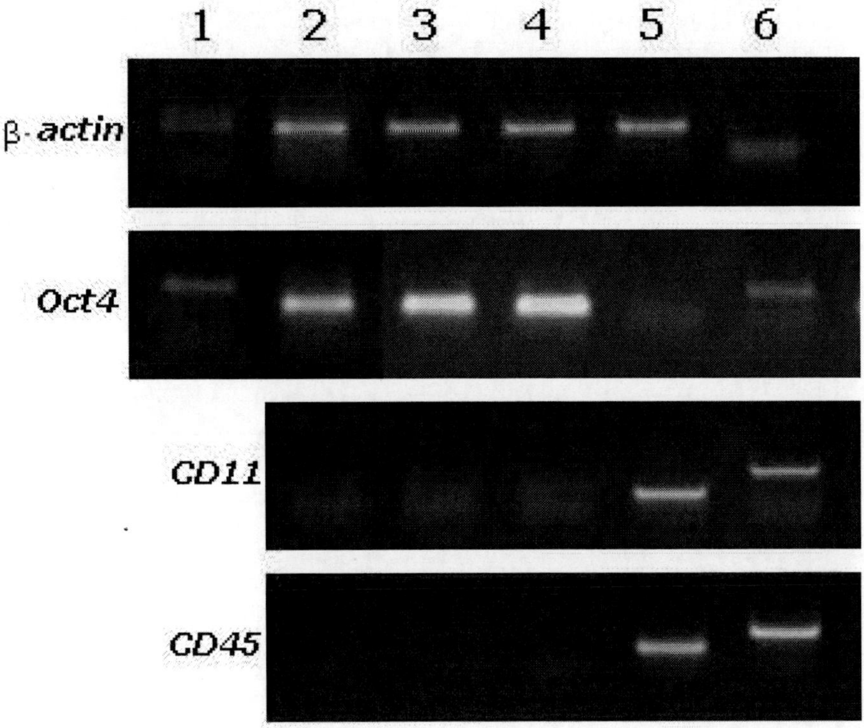

Figure 4. Expression of the *β-actin*, *Oct4*, *CD11* and *CD45* genes in hybrid and parental cells as observed by RT-PCR analysis. The following templates were used: genomic DNA isolated from PCC4aza1 cells (1); cDNA from PCC4aza1 cells (2), cDNA from PCC4aza1 × lymphocyte hybrids at the 27th passage (nonselective conditions) (3) or from hybrids at the 30th passage (selective conditions) (4), cDNA from mouse spleen lymphocytes (5); genomic DNA from spleen lymphocytes (6).

3.4. The Number of NORs Observed by FISH

In laboratory mice *Mus musculus* the number of chromosomal NORs is known to be the strain specific [18, 25], although in all mouse strains, fluorescence *in situ* hybridization (FISH) reveals NORs as singular or double spots located close to the centromeric regions [e.g., 22].

The count of the total number of NORs by FISH was first performed in

Table 2. The average number of chromosomes, FISH-NORs and Ag-NORs in the parental cells and PCC4aza1×lymphocyte hybrid cells. Hybrid cells were cultured for various time periods in non-selective (medium without HAT) or selective (medium with HAT) conditions.

Cell types	Stage	Number of chromosomes	Number of FISH-NORs	Number of Ag-NORs
PCC4aza1	Befor fusion	40	$8(7.9 \pm 0.1)^{\dagger}$	$7(7.0 \pm 0.4)$
Mouse spleen lymphocytes	5th day of activation	40	$7(7.0 \pm 0.1)^{\dagger}$	$6(6.2 \pm 0.5)$
Expected values		80	15	13
Hybrids grown in medium without HAT	6th passage	$78(77.2 \pm 2.4)$	$14(13.9 \pm 0.7)$	$10(10.3 \pm 0.9)$
	17th passage	$76(76.0 \pm 0.8)$	n/d	n/d
	$25–27^{th}$ passage	$74(74.4 \pm 2.2)$	$12(12.0 \pm 0.8)$	$10(10.4 \pm 0.8)^{\ddagger}$
Hybrids grown in medium with HAT	$26–30^{th}$ passage	$76(76.1 \pm 1.7)$	$14(13.9 \pm 0.8)$	$9(8.8 \pm 1.1)^{\ddagger}$

M±m are the mean value and standard deviation from the mean value;
n/d – no data, †, ‡ — data that differ statistically significantly.

metaphase plates obtained from the parental cells — PCC4aza1 and proliferating spleen lymphocytes. PCC4aza1 cells were found to contain eight NORs per cell. In metaphase plates of activated lymphocytes seven FISH-NORs were present. Thus, the expected total number of NORs in the hybrid cells was 15.

Fig. 5 illustrates the typical metaphase chomosomes of PCC4aza1× lymphocyte hybrids obtained in non-selective conditions at an early (6th) (Fig. 5A, D, G) and late ($25 – 27^{th}$) passages (Fig. 5B, E, H). In the majority of metaphase plates from the early passage an average of 14 NO-chromosomes (13.9±0.7) were revealed. At the late passages metaphase plates contained on average of twelve NORs (12.0±0.8). These results showed that cultivation of hybrid cells in non-selective conditions promotes elimination of NO-bearing

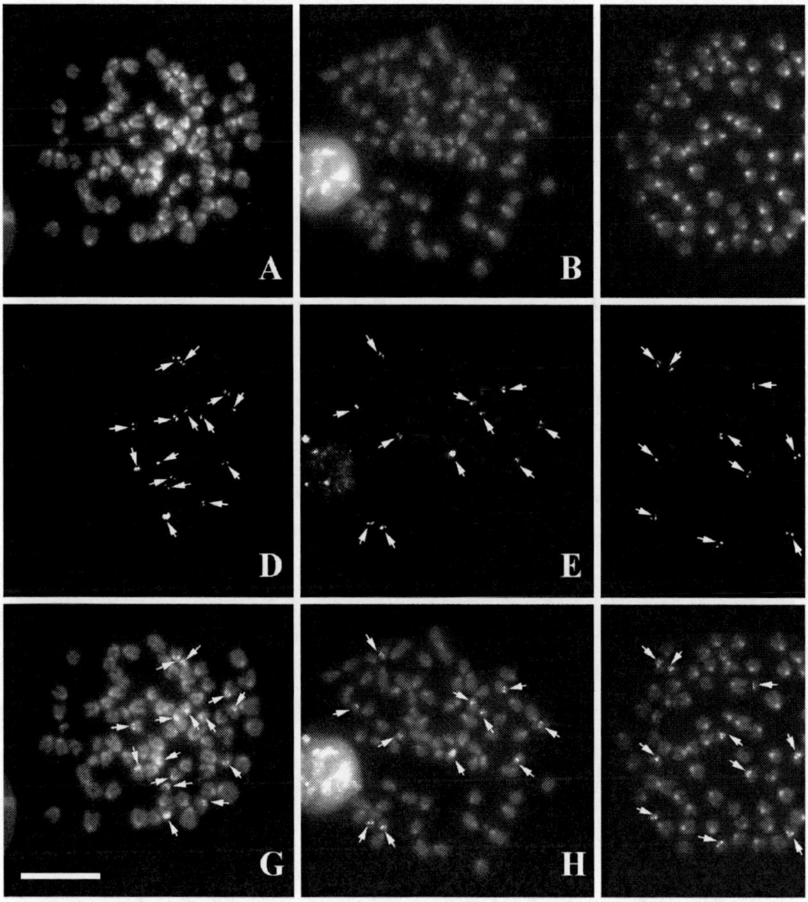

Figure 5. Fluorescence *in situ* hybridization of PCC4aza1×lymphocyte hybrid chromosomes with rDNA probes (D–F) and staining with Hoechst 33342 (A–C) at the 6th (A, D, G) and 27th (B, E, H) passages of cell cultivation in non-selective conditions, and at the 30th passage (C, F, I) of cell cultivation in selective conditions. G–I — overlay of the images. FISH-NORs are indicated by arrows. Size bar, 10 μm.

chromosomes (Table 2).

In contrary, at the late passages 26–30th in selective conditions, PCC4aza1× lymphocyte hybrids contained 13.9±0.8 FISH-NORs (Fig. 5C, F, I; Table 2), and regardless of the total chromosome number about 36% of the metaphase plates analyzed contained 15 NO-chromosomes. These results suggest that cultivation of hybrids under selective pressure favors retaining the NO-bearing chromosomes. The data on the FISH-NOR number at different passages and under various cultivation conditions are summarized in Table 2.

3.5. The Total Number of Ag-NORs

Metaphase plates of the parental PCC4aza1 cells had an average of 7.0±0.4 Ag-NORs per cell and activated lymphocytes — 6.2±0.5 Ag-NORs. Therefore, the expected number of active NORs in hybrid cells was 13. However, in early hybrids (at the 6th passage) only about ten active NORs (10.3±0.9) were present. This value remained almost unchanged in non-selective medium — at the later ($25–27^{th}$) passages an average of 10.4±0.8 Ag-NORs were revealed in hybrid cells. That is, the loss of three NO-bearing chromosomes during hybrid growth under non-selective conditions was not accompanied by any noticeable change in the number of active Ag-NORs (Table 2).

Different results have been obtained in hybrid cells cultivated under selective conditions: at the late ($26–30^{th}$) passages they had 8.8±1.1 Ag-NORs. Processing the data by means of the Student criterion showed that the average numbers of Ag-NORs at the late passages under non-selective (10.4±0.8) and selective (8.8±1.1) conditions differed statistically significantly ($p < 0.05$) (Table 2). It may be concluded that selective media promotes preservation of NO-bearing chromosomes, but favour the inactivation of their NORs.

3.6. Differentiation of PCC4aza1×Lymphocyte Hybrids *in vitro*

The differentiation capability of hybrids was studied by adding 1% DMSO to the culture medium at the early (6th) or late ($25–30^{th}$) passages. Irrespectively to the growth conditions hybrid cells were able to differentiate to endodermal-like cells (Fig. 2C). However, only in non-selective conditions hybrids were able to differentiate to cardiomyocytes as well (Fig. 2D). Differentiation to cardiomyocytes was evidenced by the appearance of clusters of beating cells, in which numerous mitochondria were revealed after staining with rhodamine 6G. It should be noted that PCC4aza1 did not differentiate either along the endodermal path or to cardiomyocytes under the same conditions. Based on these observations we concluded that the ability of hybrid cells for differentiation depends on their cultivation conditions.

4. Conclusion

It is known that some organs (e.g., liver and heart) of mammals and human contain polyploid cells [26, 27]. Therefore, analysis of regularities of the genome reprogramming in tetraploid hybrids that are capable for differentiation has a fundamental and applied significance.

To obtain hybrids between PCC4aza1 and lymphocytes we used mouse spleen cells activated by concanavalin A and treated with 5-azacytidine for 5 days. To our knowledge, hybrids between EC cells and lymphocytes activated for proliferation are described here for the first time. Since cultivation of primary spleen lymphocytes with concanavalin A *in vitro* leads to activation of only T-lymphocytes [28], it is highly likely that the obtained hybrid cells were resulted from fusion of a PCC4aza1 cell and a T-lymphocyte.

5-azacytidine is known to promote demethylation of DNA and to inhibit activity of DNA methyltransferases [29–31]. It has been shown that treatment of cells with 5-azacytidine induces reprogramming of the somatic genome in hybrids between somatic and ES cells [7] and after nuclei transfer to enucleated oocytes [32, 33]. DNA methylation is known to influence regulation of expression of ribosomal genes, and incubation of cells with 5-azacytidine increases the number of active NORs [34]

In hybrids PCC4aza1×lymphocyte expression of the genes specific to T-lymphocytes, *CD11* and *CD45*, ceased whereas expression of *Oct4*, a gene marker of pluripotent cells, was not repressed. Down regulation of *CD11* and *CD45* expression was not due to a loss of the chromosomes bearing these genes (chromosomes 7 and 1 respectively), that was confirmed by microsatellite analysis of DNA isolated from the hybrid cells (Fig. 3).

During the last years a number of works have been published, where was shown that the long-lasting cultivation of ES cells lead to the chromosome aberrations and the genetic instability [35–39]. For maintenance of chromosome stability, hybrid cells are routinely cultivated in selective media, for example, in media containing HAT [23, 24, 40]. Without selective pressure chromosomes are readily lost in intraspecific hybrids between mouse teratocarcinoma and thymus cells [40], EC cells and lymphocytes [24], ES cells and spleenocytes [6] as well as in interspecies hybrids between mouse EC and rat intestinal villus cells [41]. However, in hybrid cells obtained in the present work, the chromosome number was rather stable and diminished only in 5–8% in various conditions of hybrid cultivation (Table 2).

Predominant elimination of NO-chromosomes in PCC4aza1×lymphocyte hybrids grown in non-selective conditions has been described here for the first time. To the best of our knowledge, similar phenomena have so far been described only in hybrids of a plant origin. For example, in hybrids of the somatic potato cells chromosomes with more active NORs were eliminated preferentially [42, 43]. The authors the cited works supposed that elimination of NO-chromosomes was genetically controlled and resulted from their spatial associations [42]. This assumption can explain the predominant elimination of NO-chromosomes observed in our hybrids under non-selective conditions, where metabolic activity of cells appeared to be higher than that in HAT-containing medium.

Fusion of PCC4aza1 cells with lymphocytes resulted in partial inactivation of NORs. Indeed, if all NORs of the parental cells used in the study would remain active, the total number of Ag-NORs in PCC4aza1×lymphocyte hybrids should be 13. However, the maximal number of Ag-NORs observed in hybrid cells was always less (Table 2). This observation is a good line with literature data on the hybrids between mouse and human somatic cells, which show that respectively to the line of somatic cells used, activity of either human or mouse NORs was suppressed so that in hybrids the total number of active Ag-NORs was less than the sum of the Ag-NORs present in the parental cells [44, 45].

Suppression of NOR activity in PCC4aza1×lymphocyte hybrids occurred by one of the two ways — either by elimination of NO-bearing chromosomes (in non-selective conditions) or by inactivation of some NORs (in selective conditions). We concluded that elimination of NO-chromosomes is the most radical mechanism controlling the overall activity of ribosomal genes and synthesis of ribosomes in hybrid cells.

By now the question of relationship between activity of ribosomal genes and differentiation remains to be elucidated. Results of the present work show that hybrid cells possessing a higher number of active NORs (in non-selective conditions; Table 2) also have a higher potencies for differentiation *in vitro* as compared with the parental PCC4aza1 cells or hybrid cells grown in the presence of HAT. Since the amount of Ag-binding material associated with NORs in mitosis directly correlates with transcriptional activity of ribosomal genes in interphase [46, 47], one may assume that lower differentiation potencies of hybrid cells observed in HAT-containing medium are resulted from down-regulation of rDNA transcription and ribosome production and finally lead to depletion of protein factors responsible for differentiation.

Acknowledgments

The study was supported by the Russian Academy of Sciences (the program Molecular and Cell Biology) and in part by the Russian Foundation for Basic Researches (grant 08-04-00854).

References

[1] Sullivan, S., Pells, S., Hooper, M., Gallagher, E. & McWhir, J. (2006). Nuclear reprogramming of somatic cells by embryonic stem cells is affected by cell cycle stage. *Cloning Stem Cells*, **8**, 174-188.

[2] Gurdon, J. B. (2006). From nuclear transfer to nuclear reprogramming: the reversal of cell differentiation. *Annu Rev Cell Dev Biol*, **22**, 1-22.

[3] Takahashi, K. & Yamanaka, S. (2006). Induction of pluripotent stem cells from mouse embryonic and adult fibroblast cultures by defined factors. *Cell*, **126**, 663-676.

[4] Yu, J., Vodyanik M. A., Smuga-Otto, K., Antosiewicz-Bourget, J., Frane, J. L., Tian, S., Nie, J., Jonsdottir, G. A., Ruotti, V., Stewart, R., Slukvin, I. I. & Thomson, J A. (2007). Induced pluripotent stem cell lines derived from human somatic cells. *Sceince*, **318**, 1917-1920.

[5] Serov, O., Matveeva, N., Kuznetsov, S., Kaftanovskaya E. & Mittmann, J. (2001). Embryonic hybrid cells: a powerful tool for studying pluripotency and reprogramming of the differentiated cell chromosomes. *An Acad Bras Cienc*, **73**, 561-568.

[6] Matveeva, N. M., Shilov, A. G., Kaftanovskaya, E. M., Maximovsky, L. P., Zhelezova, A. I., Golubitsa, A. N., Bayborodin, S. I., Fokina, M. M. & Serov, O. L. (1998). In vitro and in vivo study of pluripotency in intraspecific hybrid cells obtained by fusion of murine embryonic stem cells with splenocytes. *Mol Reprod Dev*, **50**, 128-138.

[7] Do, J. T. & Schler, H. R. (2004). Nuclei of embryonic stem cells reprogram somatic cells. *Stem Cells*, **22**, 941-949.

[8] Mittmann, J., Kerkis, I., Kawashima, C., Sukoyan, M., Santos, E. & Kerkis, A. (2002). Differentiation of mouse embryonic stem cells and their hybrids during embryoid body formation. *Genet Mol Biol*, **25**, 103-111.

[9] Pells, S., Di Domenico, A. I., Gallagher, E. J. & McWhir, J. (2002). Multipotentiality of neuronal cells after spontaneous fusion with embryonic stem cells and nuclear reprogramming in vitro. *Cloning Stem Cells*, **4**, 331-338.

[10] Terada, N., Hamazaki, T., Oka, M., Hoki, M., Mastalerz, D. M., Nakano, Y., Meyer, E. M., Morel, L., Petersen, B. E. & Scott, E. W. (2002). Bone marrow cells adopt the phenotype of other cells by spontaneous cell fusion. *Nature*, **416**, 542-545.

[11] Flasza, M., Shering, A. F., Smith, K., Andrews, P. W., Talley, P. & Johnson, P. A. (2003). Reprogramming in inter-species embryonal carcinoma-somatic cell hybrids induces expression of pluripotency and differentiation markers. *Cloning Stem Cells*, **5**, 339-354.

[12] Tada, M., Takahama, Y., Abe, K., Nakatsuji, N. & Tada, T. (2001). Nuclear reprogramming of somatic cells by in vitro hybridization with ES cells. *Curr Biol*, **11**, 1553-1558.

[13] Cowan, C. A., Atienza, J., Melton, D. A. & Eggan, K. (2005). Nuclear reprogramming of somatic cells after fusion with human embryonic stem cells. *Science*, **309**, 1369-1373.

[14] Martin, G. R. (1975). Teratocarcinomas as a model system for the study of embryogenesis and neoplasia. *Cell*, **5**, 229-243.

[15] Mintz, B. & Illmensee, K. (1975). Normal genetically mosaic mice produced from malignant teratocarcinoma cells. *Proc Natl Acad Sci USA*, **72**, 3585-3589.

[16] Martin, G. R., Wiley, L. M. & Damjanov, I. (1977). The development of cystic embryoid bodies in vitro from clonal teratocarcinoma stem cells. *Dev Biol*, **61**, 230-244.

[17] Mayer, C. & Grummt, I. (2005). Cellular stress and nucleolar function. *Cell Cycle*, **4**, 1036-1038.

[18] Long, E. O. & Dawid, I. B. (1980). Repeated genes in eukaryotes. *Annu Rev Biochem*, **49**, 727-764.

[19] Howell, W. M. & Black, D. A. (1980). Controlled silver-staining of nucleolus organizer regions with a protective colloidal developer: a 1-step method. *Experientia*, **36**, 1014-1015.

[20] Hadjiolov, A. A. (1985). *The nucleolus and ribosome biogenesis. In: Cell Biology Monographs*, Vol. 12, New York: Springer-Verlag, 1-263.

[21] StGroth, S. F., de & Scheidegger, D. (1980). Production of monoclonal antibodies: strategy and tactics. *J Immunol Methods*, **35**, 1-21.

[22] Romanova, L. G., Anger, M., Zatsepina, O. V. & Schultz, R. M. (2006). Implication of nucleolar protein SURF6 in ribosome biogenesis and preimplantation mouse development. *Biol Reprod*, **75**, 690-696.

[23] Mise, N., Sado, T., Tada, M., Takada, S. & Takagi, N. (1996). Activation of the inactive X chromosome induced by cell fusion between a murine EC and female somatic cell accompanies reproducible changes in the methylation pattern of the Xist gene. *Exp Cell Res*, **223**, 193-202.

[24] Forejt, J., Saam, J. R., Gregorova, S. & Tilghman, S. M. (1999). Monoallelic expression of reactivated imprinted genes in embryonal carcinoma cell hybrids. *Exp Cell Res*, **252**, 416-422.

[25] Savino, T. M., Gebrane-Younes, J., De Mey, J., Sibaritac, J. B. & Hernandez-Verduna, D. (2001). Nucleolar assembly of the rRNA processing machinery in living cells. *J Cell Biol*, **153**, 1097-1110.

[26] Adler, C. P., Friedburg, H., Herget, G. W., Neuburger, M. & Schwalb, H. (1996). Variability of cardiomyocyte DNA content, ploidy level and nuclear number in mammalian hearts. *Virchows Arch*, **429**, 159-164.

[27] Gupta, S. (2000). Hepatic polyploidy and liver growth control. *Semin Cancer Biol*, **10**, 161-171.

[28] Stobo, J. D. (1972). Phytohemagglutin and concanavalin A: probes for murine 'T' cell activivation and differentiation. *Transplant Rev*, **11**, 60-86.

[29] Taylor, S. M. & Jones, P. A. (1979). Multiple new phenotypes induced in 10T1/2 and 3T3 cells treated with 5-azacytidine. *Cell*, **17**, 771-779.

[30] Cheng, X. (1995). DNA modification by methyltransferases. *Curr Opin Struct Biol*, **5**, 4-10.

[31] Fukuda, K. (2001). Development of regenerative cardiomyocytes from mesenchymal stem cells for cardiovascular tissue engineering. *Artif Organs*, **25**, 187-193.

[32] Jones, K. L., Hill, J., Shin, T. Y., Lui, L. & Westhusin, M. (2001). DNA hypomethylation of karyoplasts for bovine nuclear transplantation. *Mol Reprod Dev*, **60**, 208-213.

[33] Enright, B. P., Kubota, C., Yang, X. & Tian, X. C. (2003). Epigenetic characteristics and development of embryos cloned from donor cells treated by trichostatin A or 5-aza-2'-deoxycytidine. *Biol Reprod*, **69**, 896-901.

[34] Ferraro, M. & Lavia, P. (1983). Activation of human ribosomal genes by 5-azacytidine. *Exp Cell Res*, **145**, 452-457.

[35] Brimble, S. N., Zeng, X., Weiler, D. A., Luo, Y., Liu, Y., Lyons, I. G., Freed, W. J., Robins, A. J., Rao, M. S. & Schulz, T. C. (2004). Karyotypic stability, genotyping, differentiation, feeder-free maintenance, and gene expression sampling in three human embryonic stem cell lines derived prior to August 9, 2001. *Stem Cells Dev*, **13**, 585-597.

[36] Draper, J. S., Smith, K., Gokhale, P., Moore, H. D., Maltby, E., Johnson, J., Meisner, L., Zwaka, T. P., Thomson, J. A. & Andrews, P. W. (2004). Recurrent gain of chromosomes 17q and 12 in cultured human embryonic stem cells. *Nat Biotechnol*, **22**, 53-54.

[37] Inzunza, J., Sahln, S., Holmberg, K., Strmberg, A. M., Teerijoki, H., Blennow, E., Hovatta., O. & Malmgren, H. (2004). Comparative genomic hybridization and karyotyping of human embryonic stem cells reveals the occurrence of an isodicentric X chromosome after long-term cultivation. *Mol Hum Reprod*, **10**, 461-466.

[38] Hanson, C. & Caisander, G. (2005). Human embryonic stem cells and chromosome stability. *APMIS*, **113**, 751-755.

[39] Maitra, A., Arking, D. E., Shivapurkar, N., Ikeda, M., Stastny, V., Kassauei, K., Sui, G., Cutler, D. J., Liu, Y., Brimble, S. N., Noaksson, K.,

Hyllner, J., Schulz, T. C., Zeng, X., Freed, W. J., Crook, J., Abraham, S., Colman, A., Sartipy, P., Matsui, S., Carpenter, M., Gazdar, A. F., Rao, M. & Chakravarti, A. (2005). Genomic alterations in cultured human embryonic stem cells. *Nat Genet*, **37**, 1099-1103.

[40] Rousset, J. P., Bucchini, D. & Jami, J. (1983). Hybrids between F9 nullipotent teratocarcinoma and thymus cells produce multidifferentiated tumors in mice. *Dev Biol*, **96**, 331-336.

[41] Kamp, van der, A. W., Roza-de Jongh, E. J., Houwen, R. H., Magrane, G. G., van Dongen, J. M. & Evans, M. J. (1984) Developmental characteristics of somatic cell hybrids between totipotent mouse teratocarcinoma and rat intestinal villus cells. *Exp Cell Res*, **154**, 53-64.

[42] Pijnacker, L. P., Ferwerda, M. A., Puite, K. J. & Roest, S. (1987). Elimination of Solanum phureja nucleolar chromosomes in S. tuberosum + S. phureja somatic hybrids. *Theor Appl Genet*, **73**, 878- 882.

[43] Pijnacker, L. P., Ferwerda, M. A., Puite, K. J. & Schaart, J. G. (1989). Chromosome elimination and mutation in tetraploid somatic hybrids of Solanum tuberosum and Solanum phureja. *Plant Cell Reports*, **8**, 82-85.

[44] Miller, D. A., Dev, V. G., Tantravahi, R. & Miller, O. J. (1976a). Suppression of human nucleolus organizer activity in mouse-human somatic hybrid cells. *Exp Cell Res*, **101**, 235-243.

[45] Miller, O. J., Miller, D. A., Dev, V. G., Tantravahi, R. & Croce, C. M. (1976b). Expression of human and suppression of mouse nucleolus organizer activity in mouse-human somatic cell hybrids. *Proc Natl Acad Sci USA*, **73**, 4531-4535.

[46] Derenzini, M., Sirri, V., Pession, A., Trer, D., Roussel, P., Ochs, R. L. & Hernandez-Verdun, D. (1995). Quantitative changes of the two major Ag-NOR proteins, nucleolin and protein B23, related to stimulation of rDNA transcription. *Exp Cell Res*, **219**, 276-282.

[47] Sirri, V., Roussel, P. & Hernandez-Verdun, D. (2000). The AgNOR proteins: qualitative and quantitative changes during the cell cycle. *Micron*, **31**, 121-126.

In: Pluripotent Stem Cells
Editors: D.W. Rosales et al, pp. 213-226
ISBN: 978-1-60876-738-0

Chapter 10

RECENT ADVANCEMENTS TOWARDS THE DERIVATION OF IMMUNE-COMPATIBLE PATIENT-SPECIFIC HUMAN PLURIPOTENT STEM CELL LINES

Micha Drukker *
Institute for Stem Cell Biology and Regenerative Medicine, Beckman Center B261, 279 Campus Drive, Stanford, CA 94305-5323, USA

Abstract

The derivation of human embryonic stem cell lines from blastocyst stage embryos, first achieved almost a decade ago, demonstrated the potential to prepare virtually unlimited numbers of therapeutically beneficial cells *in vitro*. Assuming that large-scale production of differentiated cells is attainable, it is imperative to develop strategies to prevent immune responses towards the grafted cells following transplantation. This paper presents recent advances in the production of pluripotent cell lines using three emerging techniques: somatic cell nuclear transfer into enucleated oocytes and zygotes, parthenogenetic activation of unfertilized oocytes and induction of pluripotency in somatic cells. These techniques have a remarkable potential for generation of patient-specific pluripotent cells that would be tolerated by the immune system.

* E-mail address: dmicha@stanford.edu

Keywords: Human embryonic stem cells (hESCs); Immunogenicity; Parthenogenesis; Somatic cell nuclear transfer (SCNT); Induction of pluripotent stem (iPS) cells.

Introduction

Human embryonic stem cells (hESCs) have the capacity perpetuate themselves indefinitely in culture conditions while maintaining the potential to differentiate to all cell types of the body upon induction [1, 2]. These cells offer a considerable therapeutic advantage over the lineage-committed adult stem cell types such as hematopoietic stem cells (HSCs) and neuronal stem cells, since they may serve as virtually an infinite source for all cell lineages. Therefore, the isolation of hESCs has lead to numerous studies that aim to isolate beneficial cells for therapeutics [1]. The goal now remains to develop methodologies for harnessing the potential of hESCs in tissue replacement, repair, maintenance, and/or enhancement of function.

As a first step towards this goal, multiple laboratories have developed an array of differentiation protocols to derive specialized cell types, such as neuronal cells, cardiomyocytes, endothelial cells, hematopoietic precursors and hepatocytes (reviewed in [3]). Yet, other aspects of cellular therapeutics should be addressed before successful therapeutic application of hESC-derived cells is possible. For example, differentiation protocols need to improve to the point that homogenous preparations of particular cell types can be produced without any remaining undifferentiated (and potentially teratogenic) cells. In addition, derivation, propagation and differentiation of hESCs should be carried out in animal product-free culture conditions to prevent cross-specie contaminations. Finally, implanted cells must successfully integrate into the patient's tissue without prompting immune responses towards the graft. This review summarizes the current knowledge about the immune properties of hESCs and their differentiated derivatives (for detailed review see [4]) followed by an discussion of novel strategies that could potentially generate histocompatible patient-specific hESC lines.

Immunogenicity of Human Embryonic Stem Cells and Differentiated Cells

The two arms of the immune system, innate and adaptive, can interact with transplanted allogeneic cells (from genetically non-identical individual) leading to their rejection. Clearly, the major assaults on allogeneic tissues are mediated either directly through the action of cytotoxic T cells or by alloantibodies that are produced by alloreactive B cells against graft-derived antigens (reviewed in [5]). Class I and II MHC proteins (MHC-I and MHC-II, respectively), which are encoded by a highly variable set of human leukocyte antigens (HLA), lie at the heart of these acute allogeneic responses (reviewed in [6]). Following transplantation, foreign MHC molecules, which are expressed on grafted cells, can interact with the recipient's T cells leading to their sensitization and maturation into cytotoxic T cells that attack the transplant (direct recognition) [7]. In addition, host professional antigen presenting cells can processes foreign MHC molecules and present them to host T and B cells leading to alloantibodies secretion by B cells (indirect recognition) [6]. When alloantibodies enter circulation, they bind to transplanted cells and target them for destruction by phagocytosis and the complement system.

To evaluate whether hESCs and their derivatives could potentially induce allogeneic responses, the expression of MHC molecules on these cells was tested in a number of studies [8, 9]. It was found that undifferentiated hESCs express low levels of MHC-I proteins and that differentiation and application of interferons (IFNs) induces 100-fold increase to somatic levels. In contrast, MHC-II proteins seem to be absent under all tested conditions probably due to minimal differentiation towards hematopoietic fate (MHC-II expression is largely restricted to this lineage). Furthermore, together with colleagues, we tested the immunogenicity of hESCs *in vitro* by incubating the cells with pre-stimulated human T cells. We found that following MHC-I induction by IFNs kT cells specifically recognize and lyse hESCs. In contrast, human T-cell response against differentiated hESCs in mice was very weak most probably due to low expression of co-stimulatory signals (CD80 and CD86) that are necessary for T activation [10]. These data indicate that hESCs express sufficient levels of MHC-I molecules to elicit rejection by primed cytotoxic T cells, but have a reduced potential to stimulate T cells.

Another line of immune defense that can potentially reject foreign grafts is natural killer (NK) cells. Theses are cytotoxic lymphocytes that lyse cells based on the balance between stimulating and inhibiting signals that are provided by target cells. It is possible that low expression of MHC-I in hESCs and their derivatives could result in their targeting by NK cells since these molecules serve as ligands for NK-cell inhibitory receptors [11]. When we examined the NK-cell response towards hESCs *in vitro*, we found that irrespective of MHC expression NK cells do not readily lyse hESCs [9]. Additional studies are required to determine whether hESCs are sensitive to NK-mediated rejection *in vivo*, and whether NK cells might pose a significant obstacle to hESC therapeutics. At least in one case, it has been shown that hematopoietic progenies of mouse ES are rejected by NK cells *in vivo* [12].

Based on the existing data regarding antigenicity and immunogenicity of hESCs, a complex picture of their immunological status can be drawn. Differentiation to specialized somatic cell types is likely to induce moderate levels of MHC-I expression and in the case of hematopoietic differentiation MHC-II and co-stimulatory molecules will also be expressed [13-15]. Thus, T-cell mediated immune responses are likely to be directed at differentiated hESCs, and in the case of hematopoietic transplantation this reaction may be even more severe. Also, alloantibodies and NK cells may play a role in graft rejection. Therefore, these immune factors must be considered when designing strategies for preventing rejection of hESC-derived transplants.

Strategies for Immune Protection of Differentiated Human Embryonic Stem Cells

Excluding immunosuppression, currently five major approaches may be used to diminish or abolish the immune response against transplanted hESCs (i-iv were reviewed in [4, 16]). These options include: *i*) transplantation of differentiated therapeutic cells to natural environments that restrict immune responses (immune-privileged sites), such as the brain and testis. *ii*) Generation of large hESC line banks will allow matching MHC haplotypes between patients and cell lines. *iii*) Genetic manipulation of the genes that encode for MHC antigens and other immune modulators in hESC. *iv*) Induction of hematopoietic chimerism – a state that allows acceptance of allografts from the donor cell line that is used for hematopoietic stem cell transplantation. *v*) Generation of genetically identical hESC lines specifically for each patient. The latter approach would alleviate most immunological considerations, but until very recently seemed improbable due to technical and ethical issues. This view is changing now as several seminal advancements made within the last two years have indicated that tailored derivations of patient specific syngeneic (genetically close or identical) hESC lines could be done in the near future. I will discuss these developments hereafter (summarized in table 1).

Table 1. Proposed pathways for derivation of patient specific hESC lines

Method	Cell sources		Gender specificity	Immunological considerations for transplantation	Demonstrated in:	
					Mouse	Human
Parthenogenesis	Metaphase II oocytes [19]		Yes, female	Preferentially, MHC heterozygous cells should be used	+	+
Somatic cell nuclear transfer	Oocytes [28]	+ Somatic nucleus	No	Mitochondrial mHAgs might induce immune responses	+	-
	Zygotes [30]					
Fusion with hESCs	Fibroblasts [34]		No	Should be used only as diploid cells	+	+
			No			
Induced pluripotency	Embryonic and adult fibroblasts [36-41]		No	Unknown	+	+

Parthenogenetically Activated Oocytes Give Rise to Syngeneic ES Cell Lines

Parthenogenesis is the process of embryonic development without male fertilization. Mammals do not reproduce by parthenogenesis, but for many species activation of arrested metaphase oocytes by chemical regents can lead to development into diploid blastocyst stage embryos. Protocols for ESC-derivation from pseudo-zygotes were developed for mouse [17], macaque monkey [18] and recently human embryos by Revazova et al., [19]. Quite strikingly, this study showed that about half of the human oocytes that were chemically activated (23 of 46 embryos) progressed to the blastocyst stage, and of these, six parthenogenetic ESC (pESCs) lines were successfully produced. In mice and presumably also in humans, parthenogenetic embryos do not develop past the early limb bud stage as embryonic development require expression from the two parental genomes [20]. Still, the differentiation capacity of mouse, macaque monkey and human pESCs is striking; for example, mouse pESCs differentiate *in vitro* and contribute to multiple tissues in chimeric mice. When transplantation compatibility of these cells was tested, it was found that differentiated pESC lines engrafted only in MHC matched animals, meaning that they are histocompatible with the nucleus donor [21]. Similarly, human pESCs (phESCs) form embryoid bodies (EBs) in culture and teratomas that include cell types of the three embryonic germ layers, however, their immunological properties are yet to be determined [19].

The extent of homozygosity in parthenogenetic cells depends on oocyte activation stage, metaphase-I or metaphase-II and on recombination events. Activation of metaphase-I arrested oocytes (before first polar body extrusion) gives rise to pESC lines that are identical to the donor as they contain the two maternal chromosome homologs. However, it is unlikely that these cells would be used for therapeutics since experiments in mice showed that they were tetraploid or aneuploid. Metaphase-II arrested mouse and human oocytes (before second polar body extrusion) give rise to pESC lines containing duplicated hemizygote genome and have normal karyotype [17]. Therefore, the latter may be clinically applicable.

Although phESC lines are histocompatible with the oocyte donor, NK cells may actually respond against the cells if they lack one set of MHC genes. This phenomenon is thought to be relevant mainly to rejection of bone marrow by NK cells following transplantation (reviewed in [22]) and therefore should be examined carefully prior clinical application. It seems that all metaphase-II derived phESC lines that were reported by Revazova et al., contained full heterozygosity in the MHC region [19]. This means that during oocyte development, recombination occurred between the centromere and the MHC region on chromosome 6 homologs, and the resulting recombinant sister chromatids contain the whole MHC milieu. Therefore, NK-cell response against differentiated phESCs that retain heterozygosity seems unlikely.

It should be noted that phESCs were probably also derived in experiments carried out by Hwang's group in South Korea. Although the team reported the derivation of "cloned" embryo-derived hESCs they could not provide definitive proof to show that the cell lines were not result of parthenogenesis. Recently, Kim et al., found that the most of the genes in pESCs are heterozygous, but close to the centromere the gene copies show predominant homozygosity [23]. In contrast, nuclear transfer-derived ESCs (ntESCs) contain heterozygosity throughout the genome. Analysis of a hESC line that was claimed to be derived from a cloned embryo [24] showed that the cells contain extensive homozygosity in the MHC loci indicating that this cell line is actually parthenote [23].

PhESC lines that carry only one set of MHC genes (when recombination does not occur) could potentially prove beneficial not only for the oocyte donor but also for genetically related individuals. For example, there is a 50% chance that a cell line that is derived for a patient will be histocompatible to any of her children. Moreover, if a sizable depository of MHC homozygous phESC lines that carry MHC alleles that are common in the population were to be generated, it may serve as a hESC MHC matching bank [25]. In summary, if it would be possible to produce phESC lines as effectively as reported, such cells may become a major source of therapeutic histocompatible cell lines for fertile women, genetically related individuals and the general public. It is important to note that the extent of the NK-cell response against such transplants remains unclear and must be further examined. Immune responses against minor histocompatibility antigens and mitochondrial antigens may jeopardize grafted cells from genetically non-identical hESC lines (discussed below). It is likely that additional factors such as the tissue in question, the transplantation site and the extent of donor-derived vasculature would also influence transplantation outcomes.

Derivation of Embryonic Stem Cells from Somatic Cell Nuclear Transferred Oocytes and Zygotes

The seminal experiment of producing live sheep from oocytes that had their nucleus replaced by somatic nucleus (somatic cell nuclear transfer - SCNT) proved for the first time that the genetic information in the somatic mammalian nucleus could be reprogrammed to the embryonic state [26]. Since then, this technique has been successfully translated to other species, including mouse, rabbit, cat, pig, cow and goat (reviewed in [27]). Cloned mouse embryos can give rise to ESC lines with a relatively high success rate [28]. Since the nucleus donor and the ESC line are genetically identical, except for mitochondrial antigens (discussed below), it has been suggested that differentiated tissues derived from human reprogrammed cell lines would not be rejected by the immune system of the donor.

Currently, there is still no proof for isolation of ntESCs from cloned humans oocytes and previous publications that described the derivation of such lines have been retracted [29, 24]. Nevertheless, these studies were probably the first to report derivation of hESCs from parthenogenetic embryos. If SCNT into human oocytes and the generation of histocompatible ESC lines could be achieved, a significant obstacle lies in acquiring the large numbers of oocytes that would be necessary for the clinical application of this technique. A novel approach that may alleviate this issue utilizes mitotically arrested zygotes to reprogram injected mitotic somatic nuclei, following chromosome removal [30]. After release from mitotic arrest, ~20% of the mouse cloned embryos developed to the blastocyst stage, and of these, ~5% developed to full term following transfer to pseudopregnant recipients (no live births were recorded). Cloned blastocysts could give rise to ESC lines that were shown to contribute extensively to chimeric embryos following injection into recipient blastocysts. The authors went on to prove that murine aneuploid zygotes (containing more than 2 polar bodies) could also serve as recipients to chromosome transfer following zygotic chromosome removal. This means that abnormal human embryos containing more than two nuclei and are therefore discarded following in vitro fertilization (about 5% of the embryos), could potentially be used to generate patient specific hESC lines. Still, it is important to note that SCNT into human oocytes or zygotes was not demonstrated to date.

One final immunological issue not addressed by derivation of hESC lines through SCNT is the potential immune response directed towards mitochondrial histocompatibility antigens. It is known that in mouse and rats certain amino acid substitutions in mitochondrial proteins can lead to generation of specific alloreactive cytotoxic T cells [31]. Therefore, it is possible that certain mitochondrial protein polymorphisms might become antigenic and initiate immune responses following transplantation of differentiated hESCs that were generated following SCNT. But, the small number of encoded proteins in mitochondria and the relatively small number of mitochondrial single nucleotide polymorphisms (~170), suggests that the risk of immune response towards donor-derived mitochondrial antigens would be considerably smaller than mismatched genomes. In accordance, it has been shown in cows that transplantation of organs derived from cloned embryos to the adult nuclear donor did not lead to immune response even though they express different mitochondrial haplotypes [32].

Reprogramming of Somatic Cells by Fusion with Embryonic Stem Cells

Similarly to the reprogramming effects of oocytes and zygotes, ESCs also have the capacity to reprogram somatic nucleus to the ESC-state. Since ESCs are small and have a high nucleus-to-cytoplasm ratio, reprogramming by SCNT into these cells is technically challenging and has not been reported to date. Still, fusion of somatic cells with ESC partners has a similar reprogramming effect on the somatic nucleus leading to reactivation of embryonic genes [33]. This concept has been proven recently for human somatic cells fused with hESCs in two studies that used foreskin fibroblasts and hESC-derived myeloid progenitors as fusion partners [34, 35]. In both cases, the resulting hybrid cell lines could gave rise to EBs in vitro and teratomas in vivo. Therefore, fusion of patient's somatic cells with hESCs could potentially circumvent the need for oocytes or embryos as vehicles to reprogram somatic cells to the ESC-stage.

Still, it seems unlikely that tetraploid hybrid cells would be considered suitable as therapeutic reagents due to their genomic instability. Moreover, such cell lines contain 4 copies of the MHC region and therefore, MHC matching is improbable. It is possible that in the future technical advancements will allow elimination of the ESC chromosomes before or after cell fusion. Alternatively, enucleated hESCs may preserve the capacity to reprogram the somatic genome. If these techniques will be developed, issues such as the extent of somatic reprogramming and full differentiation capacity of hESC/somatic cell fusions will have to be investigated further.

Reprogramming Somatic Cells by Defined Factors

Successful experiments showing nuclear reprogramming by SCNT and by fusion of somatic cells with ESCs have led to the realization that oocytes, early zygotes and ESCs contain reprogramming factors. Successful reprogramming by fusion is of particular importance in trying to isolate these factors since measurements of gene expression can be carried out reliably in ESCs but not in oocytes and zygotes. Using this rationale, Shinya Yamanaka and colleagues have recently examined the ability of 24 genes that are preferentially expressed in mouse ESCs to reprogram somatic cells [36]. Introduction of the genes was carried out by retroviral transduction and then selection of cells that obtained the pluripotent state was carried out by a knock-in of drug resistance cassette into a gene that is specifically expressed in ES cells. They found that co-transfecting all the 24 factors into murine fetal fibroblasts could induce pluripotent state and colonies that had ESC morphology and expressed pluripotency markers were formed. They went on to determine which of 24 factors are necessary for the process and found that the four transcription factors that are critical for induction of pluripotent stem (iPS) cells are Oct3/4, Klf4, Sox2 and c-Myc. The authors also showed that iPS cells can differentiate into EBs, teratomas and contribute to all cell lineages including germline by generating adult chimeras [37].

During the past year, additional two independent laboratories have confirmed these results [38, 39] and very recently Yamanaka [40] and Thomson [41] groups showed that induction of pluripotency is also applicable to human cells. Yamanaka's group used the same four factors to induce pluripotency in human cells whereas Thomson group used Nanog and Lin28 instead of Klf4 and c-Myc. Furthermore, Yamanaka's group showed that iPS colonies could be isolated just by morphological criteria without the use of gene selection [40]. This elegant investigation showed for the first time that pluripotency can be induced using a relatively simple method of over-expressing transcription factors in somatic cells. From the immunological perspective, iPS cells would be fully compatible with the donor since there is no addition of genetic information to the cells.

Since induction of pluripotency by transcription factors is a very recent development it is still undetermined whether introduction of transgenes expressing Oct3/4, c-Myc and Klf4 is safe for clinical use. For example, as a result of c-Myc reactivation, tumors were found in about a fourth of the F1 offspring that were born to iPS cell injected chimeras [37]. Therefore, strategies to induce pluripotency without stable integration of oncogenes and retroviruses must be developed. If these issues can be met, iPS cells will be generated per patient needs and it is very likely that they will become the primary source of differentiated cells.

Conclusion

The extent to which hESC-derived tissues will be used for therapeutics depends first and foremost on the capacity to develop differentiation protocols and methods for isolation of therapeutically relevant cells free from hazardous undifferentiated cells. Once that is successfully achieved, the immunological response represents the next obstacle that will strongly influence transplantation outcomes and hence the feasibility of such treatments. Our current knowledge indicates that following differentiation, hESCs express MHC-I and possibly MHC-II molecules and therefore might be rejected by adaptive immune responses. Circumventing this hurdle depends on the capacity to either actively prevent the immune response, for example by genetic manipulation of the MHC genes, or by the generation and use of patient specific hESC lines. Until very recently, it seemed that generating patient specific hESC lines would be possible only by SCNT into donated oocytes but the scarcity of donated oocytes, as well ethical issues regarding their obtainment and use, represent considerable obstacles for implementation of this technique.

Outlined in the review, several new key developments may now enable derivation of patient specific "tailor made" hESC lines. Parthenogenetic hESC lines that have the full donor MHC repertoire may be derived, but still their derivation and use is likely to be practical only for fertile women. In contrast, SCNT into genetically abnormal zygotes may be used to produce genetically identical hESC lines for virtually any nucleus donor (although mitochondrial antigens may still vary). It seems that the ethical and religious considerations using these two options would be minimal since parthenogenetic embryos cannot fully develop and abnormal zygotes are routinely discarded. Perhaps the most significant breakthrough, however, is the demonstration that human pluripotent stem cells can be induced in somatic cells by the introduction of four pluripotency-inducing genes. Adaptation of this technique for derivation of transplantation-safe patient-specific human pluripotent cell lines would bypass significant technical, as well as ethical issues that are associated with oocyte and zygote usage [42]. Relevant to all these derivation pathways, is the fact that *in vitro* differentiated hESCs might have somewhat modified expression signature of immunological antigens and other molecules that participate in immune responses. Hence, analysis of their immune properties will need to be further pursued prior to clinical use.

Acknowledgments

I would like to thank Mr. C. Tang and Drs. T. Serwold, R. Ardehali and Y. Mayshar for critical reading of the manuscript. M.D. is supported by a Human Frontier Science Program postdoctoral fellowship.

References

[1] Thomson, J. A. Itskovitz-Eldor, J. Shapiro, S. S. Waknitz, M. A. Swiergiel, J. J. Marshall, V. S. and Jones, J. M. (1998). Embryonic stem cell lines derived from human blastocysts. *Science,* **282**, 1145-1147.

[2] Reubinoff, B. E. Pera, M. F. Fong, C. Y. Trounson, A. and Bongso, A. (2000). Embryonic stem cell lines from human blastocysts: somatic differentiation in vitro. *Nat. Biotechnol.*, **18**, 399-404.

[3] Hyslop, L. A. Armstrong, L. Stojkovic, M. and Lako, M. (2005). Human embryonic stem cells: biology and clinical implications. *Expert Rev. Mol. Med*, **7**, 1-21.

[4] Drukker, M. and Benvenisty, N. (2004). The immunogenicity of human embryonic stem-derived cells. *Trends. Biotechnol.*, **22**, 136-141.

[5] Rogers, N. J. and Lechler, R. I. (2001). Allorecognition. *Am. J. Transplant.*, **1**, 97-102.

[6] Lechler, R. I. Sykes, M. Thomson, A. W. and Turka, L. A. (2005). Organ transplantation--how much of the promise has been realized? *Nat. Med*, **11**, 605-613.

[7] Suchin, E. J. Langmuir, P. B. Palmer, E. Sayegh, M. H. Wells, A. D. and Turka, L. A. (2001). Quantifying the frequency of alloreactive T cells in vivo: new answers to an old question. *J. Immunol,* **166**, 973-981.

[8] Draper, J. S. Pigott, C. Thomson, J. A. and Andrews, P. W. (2002). Surface antigens of human embryonic stem cells: changes upon differentiation in culture. *J. Anat.,* **200**, 249-258.

[9] Drukker, M. Katz, G. Urbach, A. Schuldiner, M. Markel, G. Itskovitz-Eldor, J. Reubinoff, B. Mandelboim, O. and Benvenisty, N. (2002). Characterization of the expression of MHC proteins in human embryonic stem cells. *Proc. Natl. Acad. Sci. U. S. A.,* **99**, 9864-9869.

[10] Drukker, M. Katchman, H. Katz, G. Even-Tov Friedman, S. Shezen, E. Hornstein, E. Mandelboim, O. Reisner, Y. and Benvenisty, N. (2006). Human embryonic stem cells and their differentiated derivatives are less susceptible to immune rejection than adult cells. *Stem Cells*, **24**, 221-229.

[11] Raulet, D. H. (2006). Missing self recognition and self tolerance of natural killer (NK) cells. *Semin. Immunol*, **18**, 145-150.

[12] Rideout, W. M., 3rd Hochedlinger, K. Kyba, M. Daley, G. Q. and Jaenisch, R. (2002). Correction of a genetic defect by nuclear transplantation and combined cell and gene therapy. *Cell*, **109**, 17-27.

[13] Anderson, J. S. Bandi, S. Kaufman, D. S. and Akkina, R. (2006). Derivation of normal macrophages from human embryonic stem (hES) cells for applications in HIV gene therapy. *Retrovirology*, **3**, 24.

[14] Kaufman, D. S. Hanson, E. T. Lewis, R. L. Auerbach, R. and Thomson, J. A. (2001). Hematopoietic colony-forming cells derived from human embryonic stem cells. *Proc. Natl. Acad. Sci. U. S. A.,* **98**, 10716-10721.

[15] Slukvin, II Vodyanik, M. A. Thomson, J. A. Gumenyuk, M. E. and Choi, K. D. (2006). Directed differentiation of human embryonic stem cells into functional dendritic cells through the myeloid pathway. *J. Immunol,* **176**, 2924-2932.

[16] Bradley, J. A. Bolton, E. M. and Pedersen, R. A. (2002). Stem cell medicine encounters the immune system. *Nat. Rev. Immunol*, **2**, 859-871.

[17] Allen, N. D. Barton, S. C. Hilton, K. Norris, M. L. and Surani, M. A. (1994). A functional analysis of imprinting in parthenogenetic embryonic stem cells. *Development*, **120**, 1473-1482.

[18] Cibelli, J. B. Grant, K. A. Chapman, K. B. Cunniff, K. Worst, T. Green, H. L. Walker, S. J. Gutin, P. H. Vilner, L. Tabar, V. Dominko, T. Kane, J. Wettstein, P. J. Lanza, R. P. Studer, L. Vrana, K. E. and West, M. D. (2002). Parthenogenetic stem cells in nonhuman primates. *Science,* **295**, 819.

[19] Revazova, E. S. Turovets, N. A. Kochetkova, O. D. Kindarova, L. B. Kuzmichev, L. N. Janus, J. D. and Pryzhkova, M. V. (2007). Patient-Specific Stem Cell Lines Derived from Human Parthenogenetic Blastocysts. *Cloning Stem Cells*.

[20] Kaufman, M. H. Barton, S. C. and Surani, M. A. (1977). Normal postimplantation development of mouse parthenogenetic embryos to the forelimb bud stage. *Nature*, **265**, 53-55.
[21] Kim, K. Lerou, P. Yabuuchi, A. Lengerke, C. Ng, K. West, J. Kirby, A. Daly, M. J. and Daley, G. Q. (2007). Histocompatible embryonic stem cells by parthenogenesis. *Science*, **315**, 482-486.
[22] Hoglund, P. Sundback, J. Olsson-Alheim, M. Y. Johansson, M. Salcedo, M. Ohlen, C. Ljunggren, H. G. Sentman, C. L. and Karre, K. (1997). Host MHC class I gene control of NK-cell specificity in the mouse. *Immunol. Rev*, **155**, 11-28.
[23] Kim, K. Ng, K. Rugg-Gunn, P., G. Shieh, J. Kirak, O. Jaenisch, R. Wakayama, T. Moore, M., A. Pedersen, R., A. and Daley, G., Q. (2007). Recombination Signatures Distinguish Embryonic Stem Cells Derived by Parthenogenesis and Somatic Cell Nuclear Transfer. *Cell Stem Cell*, **1**, 1-7.
[24] Hwang, W. S. Ryu, Y. J. Park, J. H. Park, E. S. Lee, E. G. Koo, J. M. Chun, H. Y. Lee, B. C. Kang, S. K. Kim, S. J. Ahn, C. Hwang, J. H. Park, K. Y. Cibelli, J. B. and Moon, S. Y. (2004). Evidence of a Pluripotent Human Embryonic Stem Cell Line Derived from a Cloned Blastocyst. *Science.*
[25] Taylor, C. J. Bolton, E. M. Pocock, S. Sharples, L. D. Pedersen, R. A. and Bradley, J. A. (2005). Banking on human embryonic stem cells: estimating the number of donor cell lines needed for HLA matching. *Lancet,* **366**, 2019-2025.
[26] Campbell, K. H. McWhir, J. Ritchie, W. A. and Wilmut, I. (1996). Sheep cloned by nuclear transfer from a cultured cell line. *Nature,* **380**, 64-66.
[27] Gurdon, J. B. and Byrne, J. A. (2003). The first half-century of nuclear transplantation. *Proc. Natl. Acad. Sci. U. S. A*, **100**, 8048-8052.
[28] Hochedlinger, K. and Jaenisch, R. (2003). Nuclear transplantation, embryonic stem cells, and the potential for cell therapy. *N. Engl. J. Med,* **349**, 275-286.
[29] Hwang, W. S. Roh, S. I. Lee, B. C. Kang, S. K. Kwon, D. K. Kim, S. Kim, S. J. Park, S. W. Kwon, H. S. Lee, C. K. Lee, J. B. Kim, J. M. Ahn, C. Paek, S. H. Chang, S. S. Koo, J. J. Yoon, H. S. Hwang, J. H. Hwang, Y. Y. Park, Y. S. Oh, S. K. Kim, H. S. Park, J. H. Moon, S. Y. and Schatten, G. (2005). Patient-specific embryonic stem cells derived from human SCNT blastocysts. *Science*, **308**, 1777-1783.
[30] Egli, D. Rosains, J. Birkhoff, G. and Eggan, K. (2007). Developmental reprogramming after chromosome transfer into mitotic mouse zygotes. *Nature*, **447**, 679-685.

[31] Loveland, B. Wang, C. R. Yonekawa, H. Hermel, E. and Lindahl, K. F. (1990). Maternally transmitted histocompatibility antigen of mice: a hydrophobic peptide of a mitochondrially encoded protein. *Cell*, **60**, 971-980.

[32] Lanza, R. P. Chung, H. Y. Yoo, J. J. Wettstein, P. J. Blackwell, C. Borson, N. Hofmeister, E. Schuch, G. Soker, S. Moraes, C. T. West, M. D. and Atala, A. (2002). Generation of histocompatible tissues using nuclear transplantation. *Nat. Biotechnol*, **20**, 689-696.

[33] Tada, M. Takahama, Y. Abe, K. Nakatsuji, N. and Tada, T. (2001). Nuclear reprogramming of somatic cells by in vitro hybridization with ES cells. *Curr. Biol*, **11**, 1553-1558.

[34] Cowan, C. A. Atienza, J. Melton, D. A. and Eggan, K. (2005). Nuclear reprogramming of somatic cells after fusion with human embryonic stem cells. *Science*, **309**, 1369-1373.

[35] Yu, J. Vodyanik, M. A. He, P. Slukvin, II and Thomson, J. A. (2006). Human embryonic stem cells reprogram myeloid precursors following cell-cell fusion. *Stem Cells*, **24**, 168-176.

[36] Takahashi, K. and Yamanaka, S. (2006). Induction of pluripotent stem cells from mouse embryonic and adult fibroblast cultures by defined factors. *Cell*, **126**, 663-676.

[37] Okita, K. Ichisaka, T. and Yamanaka, S. (2007). Generation of germline-competent induced pluripotent stem cells. *Nature*, **448**, 313-317.

[38] Maherali, N. Sridharan, R. Xie, W. Utikal, J. Eminli, S. Arnold, K. Stadtfeld, M. Yachechko, R. Tchieu, J. Jaenisch, R. Plath, K. and Hochedlinger, K. (2007). Directly Reprogrammed Fibroblasts Show Global Epigenetic Remodeling and Widespread Tissue Contribution. *Cell Stem Cell,* **1**, 55-70.

[39] Wernig, M. Meissner, A. Foreman, R. Brambrink, T. Ku, M. Hochedlinger, K. Bernstein, B. E. and Jaenisch, R. (2007). In vitro reprogramming of fibroblasts into a pluripotent ES-cell-like state. *Nature*, **448**, 318-324.

[40] Takahashi, K. Tanabe, K. Ohnuki, M. Narita, M. Ichisaka, T. Tomoda, K. and Yamanaka, S. (2007). Induction of pluripotent stem cells from adult human fibroblasts by defined factors. *Cell*, **131**, 861-872.

[41] Yu, J. Vodyanik, M. A. Smuga-Otto, K. Antosiewicz-Bourget, J. Frane, J. L. Tian, S. Nie, J. Jonsdottir, G. A. Ruotti, V. Stewart, R. Slukvin, II and Thomson, J. A. (2007). Induced Pluripotent Stem Cell Lines Derived from Human Somatic Cells. *Science*.

[42] Green, R. M. (2007). Can we develop ethically universal embryonic stem-cell lines? *Nat. Rev. Genet*, **8**, 480-485.

In: Pluripotent Stem Cells
Editors: D.W. Rosales et al, pp. 227-246
ISBN: 978-1-60876-738-0

Chapter 11

PLURIPOTENT CELLS IN EMBRYOGENESIS AND IN TERATOMA FORMATION

O.F. Gordeeva
Institute of Developmental Biology Russian Academy of Sciences, Moscow, 119991, Russia

Abstract

Pluripotent cells of the early preimplantation embryo originate all types of somatic cell and germ cells of the adult organism. Permanent pluripotent cell lines (ES and EG cells) that were derived from an inner cell mass of blastocysts and primordial germ cells have a high proliferative potential and ability to differentiate in vitro into a wide variety of somatic and extraembryonic tissues as well as germ cells and to contribute to different organs of chimeric animals. In some cases pluripotent cells and primordial germ cells can generate teratomas, teratocarsinomas and some kinds of seminomas as the results of damages of differentiation programme of these cells. Experimental teratomas which formed after transplantation of undifferentiated ES and EG cells into immunocompromiced mice may provide a unique opportunity to study pluripotent cell specification and to develop novel approaches in carcinogenesis investigations. Research of signaling and metabolic pathways regulating the pluripotent cell maintenance and their multilineage differentiation are essential to search molecular targets to eliminate undifferentiated cells in tumors. Analysis of interactions between pluripotent cells and differentiated cells of the recipient animals, identification of the factors that may drive differentiation ES and EG cells in vivo contribute in understanding the mechanisms involved in the determination of cell fate during normal development and tumorigenesis. These data are important for development of effective and safe stem cell based technologies for prospective clinical treatment.

Introduction

Stem cells of adult animals have remarkable features: the ability to self-renew throughout all life generating new stem cells and to produce cells which can differentiate into various cell types. Strict control of the balance between proliferation and differentiation processes provides the maintenance of morphological stability and homeostasis in tissues with high cell turnover. The capacity of stem cells to reproduce themselves gives them the potential for unlimited life span and proliferation. When mechanisms underlying control proliferation rate in stem cells is injured they transit to abnormal tumor growth without terminal differentiation into appropriate somatic cells. Cancer stem cells arise from normal stem cells as a result of a direct genetic insult in themselves and disrupting cross talk between stem cells and their environmental niche. It was shown that abnormal stem cells are "the real culprits in cancer" in different tissues [1-5].

Pluripotent cells in early embryo as rapidly dividing and undifferentiated cells, similar with adult stem cells, potentially, can become cancer initiating cells in defined conditions and results in failure of the animal developmental program. Pluripotent cells can originates special kind of tumor called teratoma and teratocarcinoma. Teratoma tumor resembles disintegrated embryogenesis with a set of different immature histological structures that develop anisochronously whereas teratocarcinoma represented by undifferentiated cell mass displays the inability of pluripotent cells to start the differentiation [6]. Mechanisms that prevent tumor progression in the developing organism exist and lead to different malformations and then loss of vitality of embryos, but sometimes embryonic cancer cells survive and expand. Pluripotent cell lines of ES and EG cells represent a novel and interesting experimental system for fundamental research of the regulatory mechanisms that control stem cell pluripotency to understand and appreciate how stem cells orchestrate generation and maintenance different tissues and how to prevent and suppress abnormal growth and differentiation.

Embryo-Derived Pluripotent Stem Cell Lines

Pluripotent cells in a developing embryo appear in the late morula stage (at E3.0 for mouse) and are present until pre-gastrulating stages as early epiblast cells

(E5.5). According to their spatial position the outer cell layer of morula becomes the trophoblast and the internal layer becomes the inner cell mass – a tiny little cell cluster that gives rise toall cell types of the adult organism and certain extraembryonic tissues. Pluripotent cells of inner cell mass generate parietal and visceral extraembryonic endoderm as well as a primitive ectoderm also called epiblast. At the start of gastrulation (egg cylinder, E6.5) pluripotent state terminates after segregation of the founders of primordial germ cells from other epiblast cells that originate ectodelmal, mesodermal and endodermal lineage. During this short period pluripotent cells fall within a diverse cell environment and are affected by different extracellular signals that promote subsequent developmental events (Figure 1). Interestingly, pluripotent cells have similar molecular profiles with primordial germ cells (PGC) exceptionally, despite the fact that PGCs are the committed cell population [7-10]. In particular, it was shown, that octamer-binding transcription factor Oct4 is crucial for the regulation of the pluripotent state and viability of germ cells [11].

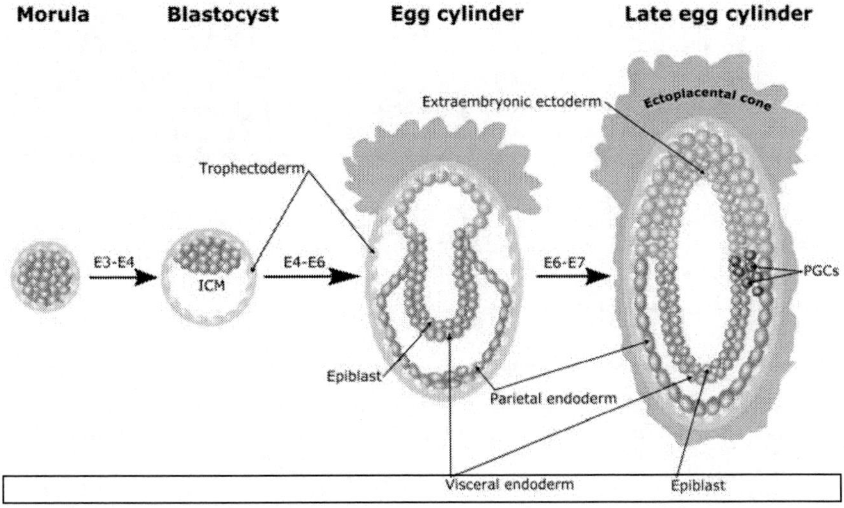

Figure 1. Pluripotent cells in early mammalian development. Pluripotent cells in developing embryo appear in late morula stage and are present until pre-gastrulating stages as early epiblast cells. Founders of primordial germ cells are recognized in distal epiblast prior to gastrulation.

To improve the research of early mammalian development were established permanent embryo-derived cell lines – **embryonic stem cells (ES cells)**, trophoblast stem (TS cells) cells and extraembryonic endoderm cells(XEN) [12-

14] were established. Pluripotent ES cell lines were derived from the inner cell mass of the blastocyst and early epiblast cells (Figure 2). At first, inner cell mass of mouse blastocyst was placed onto mitotically inactivated mouse primary embryonic fibroblasts and was grown in media conditioned by teratocarcinoma cell supplemented by fetal bovine serum. [13] At present, these conditions with mouse fibroblast feeder cells are most effective for derivation of ES cell lines of different species including human ES cells and most suitable for the propagation and expansion ES cells in vitro and preservation their stability [15].

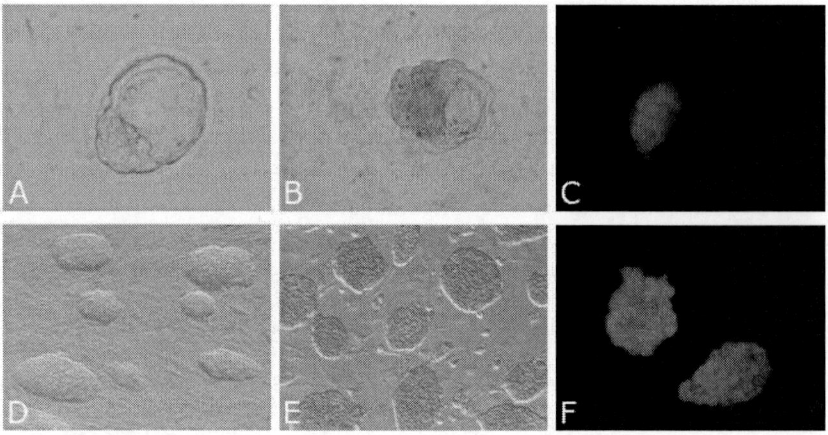

Figure 2. Pluripotent cells in mouse blastocyst (A-C) and in colonies of ES cells (D-F). Pluripotent ES cell lines were derived from the inner cell mass of blastocyst and retained similar features and expression of specific markers: alkaline phosphatase (B,E) and transcriptional factors Oct4 (C, F). Magnification 300x.

Later, cell lines ehich possessed similar properties were derived from the primordial germ cells of post-implantation stage embryos and called **embryonic germ cells (EG cells)**. ES and EG cells retain pluripotency during prolonged cultivation in vitro and can incorporate into embryoblasts and participate in development of all somatic tissues as well as germ line cells after transplantation into donor blastosysts [14,16-18]. EG cells distinguish from ES cells in their origin but after propagation in artificial culture conditions they take on similar characteristics and become capable to differentiate into somatic cells too (Figure 3). Recently, **spermatogonial stem cells (GS cells)** were derived from neonatal and adult mouse testis [19,20]. They display ES-like morphology, express a pluripotent cell marker, form teratomas after transplantation into immunocompromised mice and give rise chimerical animals with germ line transmission. Thus, primordial germ cells and spermatogonial cells can be reprogrammed in vitro in a cell population which has identical features with ES cells. No convincing and reproducible evidence about the derivation from the pluripotent cell line from the fetal or adult somatic cells without reprogramming procedure were presented yet (Figure 2).

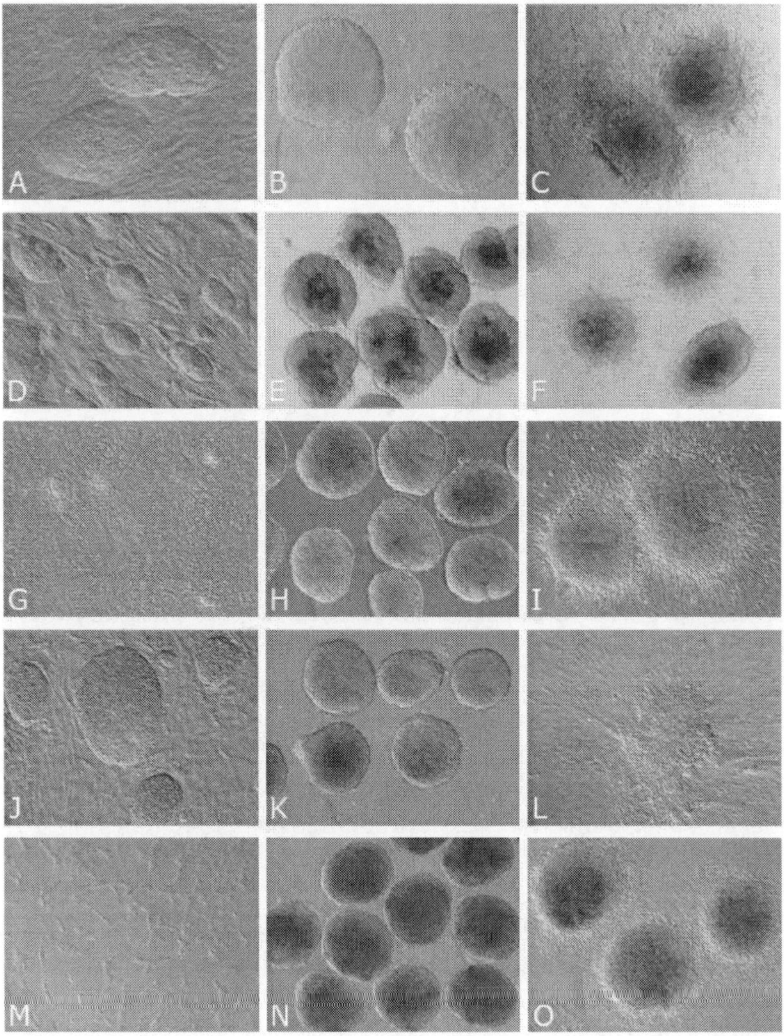

Figure 3. The initial stages of in vitro differentiation of ES, EG and EC cells. Dispite different origins all cell lines can form embryoid bodies of similar morphology. Mouse ES R1 cells (A-C), mouse EGC-10 cells (D-F), mouse EC F9 (G-I), human ES M1 (J-L), human EC PA-1 (M-O). Magnification: A, B 300x, rest 200x.

Embryonal teratocarcinoma cell (EC) lines are malignant counterparts of ES and EG cells that were derived from different genital tumors. However, EC cell lines unlike ES and EG cells vary in their differentiation potential, pluripotent cell lines have the ability to differentiate into derivatives of three germ layers and nullipotent cell lines have restricted capacity for self-renewal only [21,22]. This distinction is tightly connected with the features and lineage of tumor initiating cells which were the founders of the EC cell line. Mintz and Illmensee injected METT1 teratocarcinomal cells into mouse blastocysts and produced viable chimerical mice, that contained cells with donor genotype in somatic tissues and germ cells. Tumorigenesis rate in the adult mosaic animals was insignificantly higher than in the reference group. This experiment demonstrated the opportunity of the EC cells to contribute in embryogenesis and the transmission of teratocarcinomal genotype to germ line and then to the next generation [23-25] but it indicated that the successful result can be achieved only in the case of using euploid teratocarcinomal cell lines. Authors hypothesized that the changes in gene expression due to tissue disorganization and may apply to some malignancies of stem cells of certain tissues. Unfortunately, these data were not reproduced in other laboratories and question about normalization of malignant teratocarcinomal cells in embryogenesis is still open [26]

At present, ES, EG, and EC cell pluripotency is evaluated by producing chimeric animal with germ line transmission and generation of experimental teratomas in adult immunocompromised mice. It is well known that mammalian ES, EG and EC cells form teratomas and teratocarcinomas when they engraft into an immuno-deficient host (Nude and SCID/Beige mouse strain). Furthermore, it is the only way to test the pluripotency of human and primate ES cells because there are ethical limitations. Teratomas formed by pluripotent cells consist of the variety of differentiated tissues representative of three germ layers. Undoubtedly, histological analysis of teratomas is more reliable for estimation of developmental potential than immunofluorescent assays of differentiating cells in vitro [27].

Reconstructed ES cells or NTES cells generated by somatic nuclear transfer and by fusion ES cells with differentiated cells have the similar developmental potentials with wild type ES cells. These results prove the postulate that nuclei from terminal differentiated cells didn't restrict their potential to support the animal development. In case of multiple genetic and epigenetic changes in the donor nucleus or resulted from nuclear injuries during manipulation procedures cloned mice are dying during early development and the surviving clones have different defects whereas ES cell lines can be derived successfully. Efficiency of cloned mice generation is significantly lower than rate of reconstructed ES establishment (2% vs. 20%) [28].

The crucial question about capacity of cancer cell nucleus to support normal development was investigated recently [29,30]. Nuclear transplantation of tumor cells into oocytes resulted in generation cloned fetus and adult animals only in the case of medulloblastoma, melanoma and three pluripotent teratocarcinoma cell lines. Interestingly, F9 NT ES cells showed neither differentiation into teratomas nor contribution to mosaic embryos while several P19 NT ES chimeras developed into term but pups were afflicted with head and neck teratocarcinomas and were unviable, furthermore differentiation this line in teratomas was limited. METT-1 NT ES chimeric adult animals were morphologically normal [29]. Strikingly, teratoma analysis of corresponding EC and EC NT ES cell lines displayed an identical potential of parental and NT ES cell lines. R. Jaenisch and colleagues show that nuclei of leukemia, lymphoma and breast cancer cells can support the development to the blastocyst stage but they failed to produce NT ES cell lines. However, NTES cells and chimerical animals can be generated from RAS-inducible melanoma cell clone blastocysts. Note, that all chimeras produced from melanoma NT ES cells developed multiple primary melanoma lesions [30].

Study of reprogramming of somatic cells by fusion between ES or EG cells and differentiated cells demonstrated the dominance of pluripotent partner phenotype over a differentiated cell one. In most stable tetraploid hybrids somatic cell chromosomes undergo reprogramming via demethylation, reactivation of pluripotency-associated gene expression and activation of the silent somatic X-chromosome [31-35].

Together, these results suggest the following conclusions:

(1) Pluripotency as a capacity of cells to differentiate into various cell type including germ cells with equal probability, can be realized only in genetically and epigenetically stable ES, EG and some EC cell lines maintaining the characteristic gene expression profile of pluripotent cells
(2) Chimerical animals producing and experimental teratoma generation may be used for measuring of pluripotency tests
(3) In the most cases NT ES cell developmental potential depends on the corrected genetic and epigenetic state of the donor nucleus and the absence of genome abnormalities that hinder their differentiation into various cell types.

Molecular Mechanisms Underlying Pluripotency of ES, EG and EC Cells

The pluripotency is maintained by a complex of extracellular and intracellular factors that set up a specific pattern of the gene expression. Molecular signaling network that working in pluripotent cells controls self-renewal and maintenance of the pluripotent cell identity. When the external signals from the environment niche (culture media for pluripotent cell lines) do change and the balance of proliferation and differentiation promoting factors alters then the pluripotent cells are involved in the lineages' determination.

Octamer-binding homeobox transcriptional factor POU family Oct4 was the first identified factor that sustained the pluripotent phenotype in ES and EC cells as well as in pluripotent cells of pre-implantation embryo and in germ cells [11,36]. Two other transcriptional factors Sox2 and FoxD3 can interact with Oct4, in particular, Sox2 and Oct4 bind to adjacent cites within the enhancer of several target genes and act cooperatively to stimulate the transcription [37]. Recently, the second homeodomain transcription factor Nanog that regulate the plutipotent state was identified in the mouse and human. Nanog expression is detected firstly in late morulae stage and then it decreases in epiblast cells. Nanog is detectable in migrating primordial germ cells and residing in early gonocytes but it is not expressed in adult gonads [38-41].

Obviously, Oct4, Nanog and Sox2 function as suppressors of differentiation of inner cell mass into extraembryonic lineages – trophoblast and extraembryonic endoderm but they act cooperatively with many other genes that are elements of developmental programme of pluripotent cells. Another component of the regulation of gene expression pattern in mouse and human ES cells is the polycomb group (PcG) proteins that directly repress a large cohort of differentiation regulators. Using genome-wide location analysis in murine ES cells, there was found that the Polycomb repressive complexes PRC1 and PRC2 co-occupied 512 genes, many of which encode transcription factors with important roles in development [42, 43].

The investigation of signaling pathways that underlay pluripotent state maintenance in ES cells demonstrated that several differences exist between mouse and human ES cells. It was shown that leukemia inhibitory factor (LIF, and differentiation inhibitory factor Dia) is essential for self-renewal mouse ES and EG cells but it is not necessary for pre-gastrulating mouse development [44-47]. LIF is bound to the LIF receptor and activates the signal transducer and activator of transcription STAT-3. Phosphorilated STAT-3 translocates into the nucleus and regulates target genes transcription. Mouse ES cells growing without feeder cells begin to differentiate after several days of LIF withdrawal. On the other hand, human ES cells are not sensitive to LIF absence and the supplement to this factor to culture media does not prevent differentiation [48]. With the presence of LIF, bone morphogenetic protein BMP4 enhance the self-renewal of ES cells and activate Id (inhibitor of differentiation) genes. On the contrary, without LIF, BMP4 activates other signaling cascades that promote the differentiation of mouse ES cells. BMP4 also stimulates human ES cells to differentiate into trophoblast cell or mesodermal precursors [41, 49-51].

The activation of the WNT pathway leads to inhibition of glycogen-synthase kinase (GSK3) in undifferentiated mouse and human ES cells and blocks their differentiation [52-54]. Several groups demonstrated that the preserving of an undifferentiated state of human ES cells requires Activin and Nodal signaling interaction with FGF2 cascade [55, 56]. Our experiments for study expression of TGFβ superfamily factors and their receptors at the early stage of differentiation of human and mouse ES and EC do not reveal significant differences in expression profiles despite the diverse origin and species differences of studied cell lines [57]. We suppose that expression of Nodal, Activin, BMP and TGFβ factors in ES and EC cells reflects the situation in pre-gastrulating epiblast where spatial-temporal distribution of this factor drives the development of different areas of an embryo. However, the position information characteristic for the developing embryo is disturbed in ES and EC cells growing in vitro and spatial-temporal gradients of these signal factors are absent and therefore, every cell secrets whole set of ligands. The strict control of transcription and protein activity balance of TGFβ superfamily factors prevents differentiation more probably, than promote the self-renewal ES and EC cells. The unique combinatorial complex of signal pathways existing in ES cells provides the equal expectancies to initiate the differentiation of ectodermal, endodermal and mesodermal precursors. It is still unclear why nullipotent EC F9 cells that have similar to ES cells signaling pathways cannot initiate the spontaneous differentiation in vitro and in vivo. It is necessary to ascertain the disrupted components of regulation pathways that can direct EC cell differentiation and prevent their overgrowth.

Spontaneous and Experimental Teratomas and Teratocarcinomas

Germ cell tumors of the testis and the ovary have been studied extensively in humans and experimental animals. These spontaneous and experimentally induced tumors provide numerous data about the differentiation of tumor stem cells and the regulation of their growth. Teratomas and teratocarcinomas proved to be one of the best experimental models for elucidating the histogenesis of these tumors and the nature of their undifferentiated stem cells. The malignancy of teratocarcinoma stem cells is determined genetically but can be regulated epigenetically. Development of teratocarcinoma stem cells parallels the events in the normal embryo, suggesting that events in the tumor have their normal regulatory counterparts in the embryogenesis. Cumulative data indicate that neoplastic development of murine embryonic cells is just one of the possible ontogenic pathways these cells can take while proliferating in various developmental fields.

Spontaneous testicular and ovarian teratomas and teratocarcinamas were described in human, mouse and horses as rare tumors [6,58-60]. Stevens and Little demonstrated that teratomas arised in the testes of about 1% male of 129 strain mice [6]. Ovarian teratomas or benign ovarian cysts arisen from parthenogeneticaly activated oocytes begun development and then became disorganized embryonic cell structures [58]. Testicular germ cell tumors that were detected in young post-pubertal man, probably, arose from abnormal gonocytes in seminal tubules and progressed after birth. These cancers can either be benign or malignant. All of the well-known germinal tumors are divided into seminomas that consist of the cells resembling primordial germ cells and non-seminomas that contain a heterogeneous somatic cell population with undifferentiated teratocarcinoma cells. Recently, it was shown in the diagnostic study of different types of germ cell tumor that specific cancer-testicular antigen MAGE-4 is expressed only in classical seminoma cells while non-seminoma cells are negative for this antigen [61]. Hypothesis about the origin of germinal tumor from primordial germ cells was confirmed in the numerous experimental studies of teratomas that were induced by transplantation of genital ridge cells of mouse fetuses, between 11-13,5 days of development, into ectopic sites [22, 62,63]. Some of these experimental tumors were evidently highly malignant and reproduced the parental tumor phenotype in serial transplantation experiments. Later, the tumorigenic cell populations were expanded in vitro and permanent embryonal teratocarcinoma (EC) cell lines were established. Kleinsmith and Pierce demonstrated the stem-cell feature of EC cells in experiment with EC cell transplantation into the secondary host [64]. Inner cell mass and epiblast cells as well as ES and EG cells can initiate experimental teratomas after transplantation of them into different tissue sites of adult animals [65,66]. After human ES and EG cell lines were derived they were tested on the capacity to form experimental teratomas for the confirmation of their pluripotent state.

Teratomas test may also be helpful and informative to understand the developmental and tumorigenic potential of different precursor cells that originate from embryonic or adult stem cells differentiating in vitro. For example, developmental potential of undifferentiated mouse ES cells and embryoid bodies that have differentiated before in vitro during 4-5 days was compared in dynamic of the teratoma formation [67,68]. Approximately 3x105 cells in ES colonies or embryoid bodies growing on an acetate-cellulose membrane were implanted into peritoneal cavities of irradiated mice and then observed grafting cell differentiation within 2,3,4 and 6 week. Two weeks after the onset of each experimental series, cell aggregations resulting from proliferation and migration of the grafted cells appeared on the implanted membranes. By that time, the colonies of undifferentiated ESC had merged and acquired an asymmetric shape, while outgrowths of the embryoid bodies had increased in size. The cell aggregations contained no morphologically differentiated cell types. In addition to ESC, numerous fibroblasts-like cells of the recipient encapsulating the foreign body were found on the filters. These fibroblasts-like cells were also present on the membranes isolated from the abdominal cavity of the control animals. Note that small teratomas have been revealed in three out of five animals that received the implants of membranes with the embryoid bodies.

After three and six weeks, all experimental animals developed tumors in the region of contact between the membrane and loops of the small intestine, which were much larger than the tumors found after two weeks. No tumor growth was detected in other tissues.

Histological analysis revealed various types of differentiated cells in the tumors, including ectodermal (keratinized epithelium and neural ganglion cells, neural rosettes), mesodermal (hyaline cartilage and bone, striated and smooth muscles, adipocytes and connective tissue), and endodermal (secreted and ciliated epithelium of intestinal and respiratory types) lineages (Figure 4). Lacunar blood vessels (most likely originating from the recipient) and large hemorrhagic zones were found in the tumors.

Our experiments have revealed no significant differences in the types of differentiation of pluripotent cells in the ESC colonies and inner cells of the embryoid bodies, although the embryoid bodies attached to the substrate are a heterogeneous population including pluripotent, differentiated, and committed cells. On the other hand, the embryoid body cells have produced tumors much more rapidly, which agrees with the concept that they are an activated cell population.

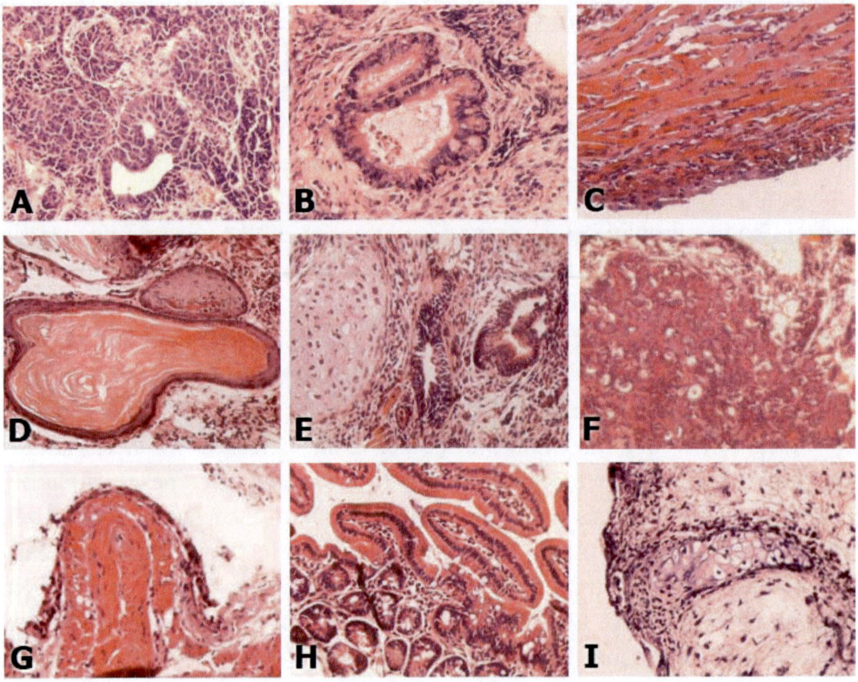

Figure 4. Differentiation of ES, EG and EC cells in experimental teratomas formed after transplantation into peritoneal cavities of immunocompromised hosts. Histological analysis revealed various types of differentiated cells in the tumors, including ectodermal, mesodermal and endodermal lineages: neural rosettes in mouse ES cell teratoma (A), ciliated epithelium of intestinal type in mouse ES cell teratoma (B), striated muscles in mouse (C) and human ES teratotoma (G), keratinized epithelium in mouse EG cell teratoma (D), hyaline cartilage in mouse EG cell teratoma (E) and human ES cell teratoma (I), intestinal crypts in human ES cell teratoma (H) and undifferentiated teratocarcinoma cell of mouse EC F9 line (F).

To understand whether pluripotent cells remain in experimental teratomas we evaluated expression of pluripotent and germ line specific genes in ES cells and embryoid bodies prior to transplantation and in all types of experimental teratomas. Expression analysis showed that in all studied tumors cell populations exist, they expressed Oct4, Nanog, Stella, Fragilis, Dazl and Vasa/Mvh genes which are expressed by the initial transplanted cells [68, and unpublished data]. The same pattern of expression was revealed for mouse EG and EC cells and in teratomas formed by these cells into peritoneal cavities of Nude strain immunodeficient mice (Figure 5).

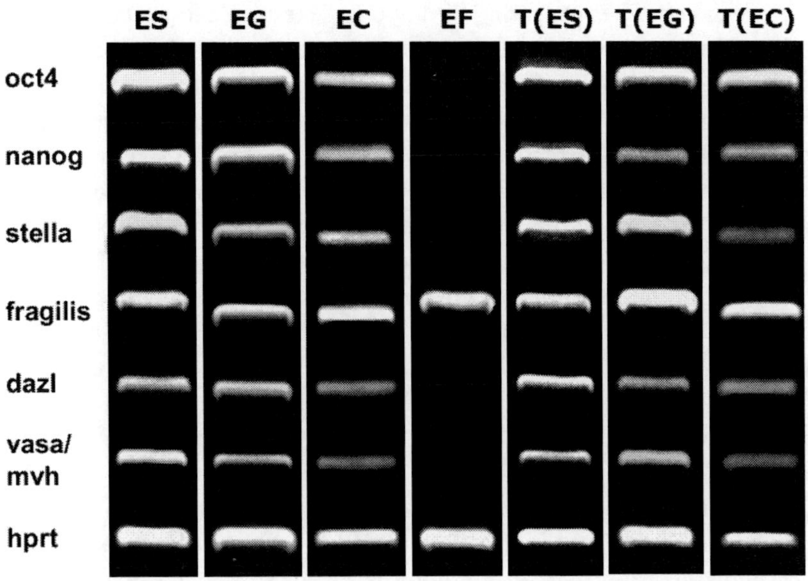

Figure 5. Expression of genes specific for pluripotent and germ line cells in mouse ES, EG and EC cells and in teratomas formed by these lines.

Our results and that of other laboratories demonstrated that undifferentiated ES and EG cells and differentiating embryoid bodies have similar developmental potencies to differentiate into derivatives of three germ layers in teratomas that dramatically diverse from teratocarcinomas generating by EC F9 cell which contain only undifferentiated cells. It remains unclear whether these Oct4, Nanog, Stella, Dazl, Vasa positive cells in different types of experimental ES and EG teratomas have normal or cancer nature and why residual undifferentiated cells remained there so long together with well-differentiated structures. The first assumption, that undifferentiated cells in ES and EG teratomas are teratocarcinoma cells that resulted after transformation events during their differentiation in vivo. It was shown that human ES cells accumulate different mutations and epigenetic modifications during propagation in vitro and the number of aneuploid cells increases at the late passages especially when trypsin and collagenase are used for splitting cells [69-71]. Most likely, different genetic rearrangements may take place during experimental teratoma formation too.

Another hypothesis, which explains the existence of residual undifferentiated cells in experimental teratomas, based on fundamental features of ES and EG cells. Comparative transcriptional profiling studies of ES, EG, EC cells and different embryonic and adult cells display the dissimilarity of ES cells from well-characterized cell types appearing during ontogenesis of this species. ES and EG cells have intermediate status between epiblast cells and primordial germ cells. This steady state provides them the same possibilities to proliferate actively (symmetric divisions) and to start differentiation of all the lineages with equal expectancy. During differentiation in teratomas ES and EG cells realize their developmental potentials and they give rise to the representative of all somatic lineages and early primordial germ cells. Precursors of germ cells stay immature like the most other histological structures presented in teratomas. This statement may be true for nullipotent teratocarcinomal cells that have only one cell destined to be abnormal intermediate progenitors of primordial germ cells. It will be interesting to model the experimental situations when teratomas would not contain the undifferentiated cell or these cells completely differentiate into different types of somatic cells. It is necessary to determine the critical cell number of grafted pluripotent and teratocarcinoma cells for growth and differentiation of experimental teratomas. What genetic mechanisms are involved in transformation of ES cells to EC cells? What are the ways to exterminate the cancer initiating cells? These questions need answers to understand the basic mechanisms underlying the early events of embryogenesis and for development of ES cell technologies for future therapeutic applications. Resent advances in stem cells research provide new insight in mechanisms of tissues development and function in embryo and adult individual and open new perspectives in understanding the cause of many pathologies including different cancers.

Conclusion

One of the most important lessons that came from the recent studies of stem cells biology postulates that the deregulation of signaling pathways that involved control of self-renewal and differentiation of stem cells and progenitors leads to tumorigenesis in tissues with high cell turnover [1,5]. Pluripotent cells that originate all cell types of organisms and some extraembryonic tissues theoretically can be transformed into wide variety of embryonic tumors. ES and EG cells are artificial counterparts of pluripotent cells of embryos and they retain their features. Obviously, genetic failures and epigenetic modifications in stem cells resulting in uncontrolled growth are true cases of tumorigenesis. Embryonic stem cells and different rapidly dividing multipotent cells deriving from pluripotent cells can became cancer initiating cells after long-term propagation in vitro and may be dangerous for therapeutic stem cells application.

On the other hand, embryonic stem cell lines may be used as a powerful experimental model and tool to develop new approaches in cancer research that directed towards the understanding of lineages of different embryonic and neonatal tumors. The combination of different genetic engineering technologies with transplantation assays provides new opportunities for cancer research focused on searching target genes involved in development of teratomas, teratocarcinomas or other embryonic malignancies. Utilizing of mutant ES cell lines may help us to discover many connections between normal stem cells and tumor initiating cells and to develop effective drugs target in cancer stem cells.

References

[1] Reya, T., Morrison, S.J., Clarke, M.F. and Weissman, I.L. (2001). Stem cells, cancer, and cancer stem cells. *Nature,* **414**, 105-111.

[2] Appelbaum, F.R., Rowe, J.M., Radich, J. and Dick, J.E. (2001*).* Acute myeloid leukemia. *Hematology Am Soc Hematol Educ Program.*, 62-86.

[3] Dick, J.E. (2003). Breast cancer stem cells revealed. *PNAS,* **100**, 3547-3549.

[4] Clarke, M.F. and Becker, M.W. (2006). *Stem cells: The Real Culprits in Cancer?* Scientific American, July, 53-59.

[5] Morrison, S.J. and Kimble, J. (2006). Asymmetric and symmetric stem-cell divisions in development and cancer. *Nature*, **441**, 1068-1074.

[6] Stevens, L.C. and Little, C.C. (1954). Spontaneous testicular teratomas in an inbred strain of mice. *Proc Natl Acad Sci U S A*, **40**, 1080-1087.

[7] D'Amour K.A. and Gage F.H. (2003). Genetic and functional differences between multipotent neural and pluripotent embryonic stem cells. *Proc. Natl. Acad. Sci.* USA., **100** (suppl 1), 11866-11872.

[8] Ramalho-Santos, M., Yoon S., Matsuzaki Y., Mulligan R.C. and Melton D.A. (2002). «Stemness»: transcriptional profiling of embrionic and adult stem cells. *Science*, **298**, 597-600

[9] Tanaka, T.S., Kunath, T., Kimber, W.L., Jaradat, S.A., Stagg, C.A., Usuda, M., Yokota, T., Niwa, H., Rossant. J. and Ko, M.S. (2002). Gene expression profiling of embryo-derived stem cells reveals candidate genes associated with pluripotency and lineage specificity. *Genome Res*, **12**, 1921-1928

[10] Tanaka, T.S., Jaradat, S.A., Lim, M.K., Kargul, G.J., Wang, X., Grahovac, M.J., Pantano, S., Sano, Y., Piao, Y., Nagaraja, R., Doi, H., Wood, W.H. 3rd, Becker, K.G. and Ko. M.S (2000). Genome-wide expression profiling of mid-gestation placenta and embryo using a 15,000 mouse developmental cDNA microarray. *Proc. Natl. Acad. Sci.* U S A., **97**(16), 9127-9132.

[11] Palmieri, S.L., Peter, W., Hess, H. and Scholer, H.R. (1994). Oct-4 transcription factor is differentially expressed in the mouse embryo during establishment of the first two extraembryonic cell lineages involved in implantation. *Dev Biol.*, **166**, 259-267.

[12] Evans, M.J.and Kaufman, M.H. (1981). Establishment in culture of pluripotential cells from mouse embryos. *Nature*, **292**, 154-156.

[13] Martin, G.R. (1981). Isolation of pluripotent cell line from early mouse embryo cultured in medium conditioned by teratocarcinoma stem cells. *Proc. Natl. Acad. Sci. USA.*, **78**, 7634-7638.

[14] Rossant, J. (2001). Stem cells from mammalian blastocyst. *Stem Cells*, **19**, 477-482.

[15] Thomson, J.A., Itskovitz-Eldor, J., Shapiro, S.S., Waknitz, M.A., Swiergiel, J.J, Marshall, V.S. and Jones J.M. (1998). Embryonic stem cell lines derived from human blastocysts. *Science*, **282**(5391), 1145-1147.

[16] Matsui, Y., Zsebo, K., Hogan, B.L. (1992). Derivation of pluripotential embryonic stem cells from murine primordial germ cells in culture. *Cell*, **70**, 841-847

[17] Resnick, J.L., Bixler, L.S., Cheng, L and Donovan, P.J. (1992). Long-term proliferation of mouse primordial germ cells in culture. *Nature*, **359**, 550-551

[18] Bradley, A., Evans, M., Kaufman, M.H. and Robertson, E. (1984). Formation of germ-line chimaeras from embryo-derived teratocarcinoma cell lines. *Nature,* **309**,255-256.

[19] Kanatsu-Shinohara, M., Inoue, K., Lee, J., Yoshimoto, M., Ogonuki, N., Miki, H., Baba, S., Kato, T., Kazuki, Y., Toyokuni, S., Toyoshima, M., Niwa, O., Oshimura, M., Heike, T., Nakahata, T., Ishino, F., Ogura, A. and Shinohara, T.(2004). Generation of pluripotent stem cells from neonatal mouse testis. *Cell*, **119**, 1001-1012.

[20] Guan, K., Nayernia, K., Maier, L.S., Wagner, S., Dressel, R., Lee, J.H., Nolte, J., Wolf, F., Li, M., Engel, W. and Hasenfuss, G. (2006). Pluripotency of spermatogonial stem cells from adult mouse testis. *Nature*, **440**, 1199-1203.

[21] Martin, G.R. and Evans, M.J. (1975). Differentiation of clonal lines of teratocarcinoma cells: formation of embryoid bodies in vitro. *Proc Natl Acad Sci U S A*, **72**, 1441-1445.

[22] Andrews, P.W. (2002*).* From teratocarcinomas to embryonic stem cells. *Philos Trans R Soc Lond B Biol Sci.*, **357**, 405-417.

[23] Mintz, B. and Illmensee, K. (1975). Normal genetically mosaic mice produced from malignant teratocarcinoma cells. *Proc Natl Acad Sci U S A.*, **72**, 3585-3589.

[24] Illmensee, K. and Mintz, B. (1976). Totipotency and normal differentiation of single teratocarcinoma cells cloned by injection into blastocysts. *Proc Natl Acad Sci U S A*, **73**, 549-553.
[25] Stewart, T.A. and Mintz, B. (1981). Successive generations of mice produced from an established culture line of euploid teratocarcinoma cells. *Proc Natl Acad Sci U S A*, **78**, 6314-6318.
[26] Rossant, J. and McBurney, M.W (1982). The developmental potential of a euploid male teratocarcinoma cell line after blastocyst injection. *J Embryol Exp Morphol*, **70**, 99-112.
[27] Przyborski, S.A. (2005). Differentiation of Human Embryonic Stem Cells After Transplantation in Immune-Deficient Mice. *Stem Cells*, 23, 1242-1250.
[28] Hochedlinger, K. and Jaenisch, R. (2006). Nuclear reprogramming and pluripotency. *Nature*, 441, 1061-1067
[29] Blelloch, R.H., Hochedlinger, K., Yamada, Y., Brennan, C., Kim, M., Mintz, B., Chin, L. and Jaenisch, R. (2004). Nuclear cloning of embryonal carcinoma cells. *Proc Natl Acad Sci U S A*, **101**, 13985-13990.
[30] Hochedlinger, K., Blelloch, R., Brennan, C., Yamada, Y., Kim, M., Chin, L. and Jaenisch, R. (2004). Reprogramming of a melanoma genome by nuclear transplantation. *Genes Dev.*, **18**, 1875-1885.
[31] Tada, M., Tada, T., Lefebvre, L., Barton, S.C. and Surani, M.A. (1997). Embryonic germ cells induce epigenetic reprogramming of somatic nucleus in hybrid cells. *EMBO J.*, **16**, 6510-6520.
[32] Tada, M., Takahama, Y., Abe, K., Nakatsuji, N. and Tada, T. (2001). Nuclear reprogramming of somatic cells by in vitro hybridization with ES cells. *Curr Biol.*, **11**, 1553-1558.
[33] Tada, M., Morizane, A., Kimura, H., Kawasaki, H., Ainscough, J.F., Sasai, Y., Nakatsuji, N. and Tada, T. (2003). Pluripotency of reprogrammed somatic genomes in embryonic stem hybrid cells. *Dev Dyn.*, **227**, 504-510.
[34] Bortvin, A., Eggan, K., Skaletsky, H., Akutsu, H., Berry, D.L., Yanagimachi, R., Page, D.C. and Jaenisch, R. (2003). Incomplete reactivation of Oct4-related genes in mouse embryos cloned from somatic nuclei. *Development,* **130**, 1673-1680.
[35] Cowan, C.A, Atienza, J., Melton, D.A. and Eggan, K. Nuclear reprogramming of somatic cells after fusion with human embryonic stem cells. *Science*, **309**, 1369-1373.
[36] Niwa, H., Miyazaki. J. and Smith, A.G. (2000). Quantitative expression of Oct-3/4 defines differentiation, dedifferentiation or self-renewal of ES cells. *Nat Genet.*, **24**, 372-376.

[37] Boiani, M. and Schöler, H.R. (2005). Regulatory networks in embryo-derived pluripotent stem cells. *Nat. Rev. Mol. Cell Biol.*, **6,** 872-884.

[38] Chambers, I., Colby, D., Robertson, M., Nichols, J., Lee, S., Tweedie, S. and Smith, A. (2003). Functional expression cloning of Nanog, a pluripotency sustaining factor in embryonic stem cells. *Cell*, **113**, 643-655.

[39] Mitsui, K., Tokuzawa, Y., Itoh, H., Segawa, K., Murakami, M., Takahashi, K., Maruyama, M., Maeda, M. and Yamanaka, S. (2003). The homeoprotein Nanog is required for maintenance of pluripotency in mouse epiblast and ES cells. *Cell*, **113**, 631-642.

[40] Hart, A.H., Hartley, L., Ibrahim, M. and Robb, L. (2004). Identification, cloning and expression analysis of the pluripotency promoting Nanog genes in mouse and human. *Dev Dyn.*, **230**, 187-198.

[41] Chambers, I. and Smith, A. (2004). Self-renewal of teratocarcinoma and embryonic stem cells. *Oncogene*, **23**, 7150-7160.

[42] Boyer, L.A., Plath, K., Zeitlinger, J., Brambrink, T., Medeiros, L.A., Lee, T.I., Levine, S.S., Wernig, M., Tajonar, A., Ray, M.K., Bell, G.W., Otte, A.P., Vidal, M., Gifford, D.K., Young, R.A. and Jaenisch, R. (2006). Polycomb complexes repress developmental regulators in murine embryonic stem cells. *Nature*, **441**, 349-353.

[43] Lee, T.I., Jenner, R.G., Boyer, L.A., Guenthe, M.G., Levine, S.S., Kumar, R.M., Chevalier, B., Johnstone, S.E., Cole, M.F., Isono, K., Koseki, H., Fuchikami, T., Abe, K., Murray, H.L., Zucker, J.P., Yuan, B., Bell, G.W., Herbolsheimer, E., Hannett, N.M., Sun, K., Odom, D.T., Otte, A.P., Volkert, T.L., Bartel, D.P., Melton, D.A., Gifford, D.K., Jaenisch, R. and Young, R.A. (2006). Control of developmental regulators by Polycomb in human embryonic stem cells. *Cell*, **125**, 301-313.

[44] Smith, A.G., Heath, J.K., Donaldson, D.D., Wong, G.G., Moreau, J., Stahl, M. and Rogers, D. (1988). Myeloid leukaemia inhibitory factor maintains the developmental potential of embryonic stem cells. *Nature,* **336**, 684-687.

[45] Boeuf, H., Hauss, C., Graeve, F.D., Baran, N. and Kedinger, C. (1997). Leukemia inhibitory factor-dependent transcriptional activation in embryonic stem cells. *J Cell Biol.,* **138**, 1207-1217.

[46] Niwa, H., Burdon, T., Chambers, I. and Smith, A. (1998). Self-renewal of pluripotent embryonic stem cells is mediated via activation of STAT3. *Genes Dev.,* **12**, 2048-2060.

[47] Nichols, J., Davidson, D., Taga, T., Yoshida, K., Chambers, I. and Smith, A. (1996). Complementary tissue-specific expression of LIF and LIF-receptor mRNAs in early mouse embryogenesis. *Mech Dev.,* **57**, 123-131.

[48] Daheron, L., Opitz, S.L., Zaehres, H., Lensch, W.M., Andrews, P.W., Itskovitz-Eldor, J. and Daley, G.Q. (2004). LIF/STAT3 signaling fails to maintain self-renewal of human embryonic stem cells. *Stem Cells,* **22**, 770-778.

[49] Ying, Q.L., Nichols, J., Chambers, I. and Smith, A. (2003). BMP induction of Id proteins suppresses differentiation and sustains embryonic stem cell self-renewal in collaboration with STAT3. *Cell,* **115**, 281-292.

[50] Gerami-Naini, B., Dovzhenko, O.V., Durning, M., Wegner, F.H., Thomson, J.A. and Golos, T.G. (2004). Trophoblast differentiation in embryoid bodies derived from human embryonic stem cells. *Endocrinology*, **145**, 1517-1524.

[51] Schuldiner, M., Yanuka, O., Itskovitz-Eldor, J., Melton, D.A. and Benvenisty, N. (2000). Effects of eight growth factors on the differentiation of cells derived from human embryonic stem cells. *Proc Natl Acad Sci U S A,* **97**, 11307-11312.

[52] Sato, N., Meijer, L., Skaltsounis, L., Greengard, P., Brivanlou, A.H. (2004). Maintenance of pluripotency in human and mouse embryonic stem cells through activation of Wnt signaling by a pharmacological GSK-3-specific inhibitor. *Nat Med.*, **10**, 55-63.

[53] Paling, N.R., Wheadon, H., Bone, H.K. and Welham, M.J. (2004). Regulation of embryonic stem cell self-renewal by phosphoinositide 3-kinase-dependent signaling. *J Biol Chem.*, **279**, 48063-48070.

[54] Hao, J., Li, T.G., Qi, X., Zhao, D.F. and Zhao, G.Q. (2006). WNT/beta-catenin pathway up-regulates Stat3 and converges on LIF to prevent differentiation of mouse embryonic stem cells. *Dev Biol.*, **290**, 81-91.

[55] Beattie, G.M., Lopez, A.D., Bucay, N., Hinton, A., Firpo, M.T., King, C.C. and Hayek, A. (2005). Activin A maintains pluripotency of human embryonic stem cells in the absence of feeder layers. *Stem Cells*, **23**, 489-495,

[56] Vallier, L., Alexander, M. and Pedersen, R.A. (2005). Activin/Nodal and FGF pathways cooperate to maintain pluripotency of human embryonic stem cells. *J Cell Sci.*, **118**, 4495-4509.

[57] Krasnikova, N.Y. and Gordeeva, O.F. (2006). Nodal signaling in the regulation of pluripotent state ofhuman and mouse ES and EC cells. *FEBS*, **273** (suppl 1), 126.

[58] Stevens, L.C. and Varnum, D.S. (1974). The development of teratomas from parthenogenetically activated ovarian mouse eggs. *Dev Biol.*, **37**, 369-380.

[59] Lefebvre, R., Theoret, C., Dore, M., Girard, C., Laverty, S. and Vaillancourt, D. (2005). Ovarian teratoma and endometritis in a mare. *Can Vet J.,* **46**, 1029-1033.

[60] Carver, B.S., Bianco, F.J. Jr., Shayegan, B., Vickers, A., Motzer, R.J., Bos, G.J. and Sheinfeld, J. (2006). Predicting teratoma in the retroperitoneum in men undergoing post-chemotherapy retroperitoneal lymph node dissection. *J Urol.,* **176**, 100-103;

[61] Aubry, F., Satie, A.P., Rioux-Leclercq, N., Rajpert-DeMeyts, E,, Spagnoli, G.C., Chomez, P., De Backer, O., Jegou, B. and Samson, M. (2001). MAGE-A4, a germ cell specific marker, is expressed differentially in testicular tumors. *Cancer*, **92**, 2778-2785.

[62] Stevens, L.C. (1964). Experimental production of testicular teratomas in mice. *Proc Natl Acad Sci U S A*, **52**,654-561

[63] Bendel-Stenzel, M., Anderson, R., Heasman, J. and Wylie, C. (1998). The origin and migration of primordial germ cells in the mouse. *Semin Cell Dev Biol.*, 9, 393-400.

[64] Kleinsmith, L.J. and Pierce, G.B. Jr. (1964). Multipotentiality of single embryonal carcinoma cells. *Cancer Res.*, 24, 1544-1551

[65] Solter, D., Skreb, N. and Damjanov, I. (1970). Extrauterine growth of mouse egg-cylinders results in malignant teratoma. *Nature*, 227,503-504.

[66] Stevens, L.C. (1970). The development of transplantable teratocarcinomas from intratesticular grafts of pre- and postimplantation mouse embryos. *Dev Biol.*, 21, 364-382.

[67] Gordeeva, O.F., Manuilova, E.S., Paiushina, O.V., Nikonova, T.M., Grivennikov, I.A. and Khrushchev, N.G. (2003*).* Differentiation of pluripotent embryonic stem cells in peritoneal cavity of irradiated mice. *Izv Akad Nauk Ser Biol.*, 3, 371-374.

[68] Gordeeva, O., Zinovieva, R., Smirnova, Y., Payushina, O., Nikonova, T. and Khrushchov, N. (2005). Differentiation of embryonic stem cells after transplantation into peritoneal cavity of irradiated mice and expression of specific germ cell genes in pluripotent cells. *Transplant Proc.*, 37, 295-298.

[69] Rugg-Gunn, P.J., Ferguson-Smith, A.C. and Pedersen, R.A. (2005). Epigenetic status of human embryonic stem cells. *Nat Genet.*, 37, 585-587.

[70] Mitalipova, M.M., Rao, R.R., Hoye,r D.M., Johnson, J.A., Meisner, L.F., Jones, K.L., Dalton, S., Stice, S.L. (2005). Preserving the genetic integrity of human embryonic stem cells. *Nat Biotechnol.*, 23, 19-20.

[71] Maitra, A., Arking, D.E., Shivapurkar, N., Ikeda, M., Stastny, V., Kassauei, K., Sui, G., Cutler, J., Liu, Y., Brimble, S.N., Noaksson, K., Hyllner, J., Schulz, T.C, Zeng, X., Freed, W.J., Crook, J., Abraham, S., Colman, A., Sartipy, P., Matsu,i S., Carpenter, M., Gazdar, A.F., Rao, M., Chakravarti, A. (2005). Genomic alterations in cultured human embryonic stem cells. *Nat Genet.*, 37, 1099-1103.

INDEX

A

B

C

D

E

F

G

H

I

K

L

M

N

O

P

R

S

T

U

V

W

X

Y

Z